Planning, Implementing, and Evaluating Health Promotion Programs

A Primer

FIFTH EDITION

James F. McKenzie, Ph.D., M.P.H., C.H.E.S.
Ball State University

Brad L. Neiger, Ph.D.
Brigham Young University

Rosemary Thackeray, Ph.D., M.P.H.
Brigham Young University

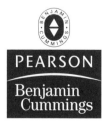

PEARSON

Benjamin Cummings

San Fransicso   Boston   New York
Cape Town   Hong Kong   London   Madrid   Mexico City
Montreal   Munich   Paris   Singapore   Sydney   Tokyo   Toronto

Acquisitions Editor: *Sandy Lindelof*
Project Editor: *Nicole George-O'Brien and Tamara Keller*
Developmental Manager: *Claire Alexander*
Editorial Assistant: *Jacob Evans*
Managing Editor: *Deborah Cogan*
Production Supervisor: *Mary O'Connell*
Manufacturing Buyer: *Dorothy Cox*
Marketing Manager: *Neena Bali*
Cover Designer: *John Rokusek Design*
Production and Composition: *Pre-Press PMG*
Interior Design: *Hespenheide Design*
Copy Editor: *Susan Gilbert*
Cover Printer: *Phoenix Color*
Text Printer: *RR Donnelley*
Cover Design: *Rokusek Design, Inc.*

ISBN-10: 0-3214-9511-X
ISBN-13: 978-0-321-49511-2

Library of Congress Cataloging-in-Publication Data

McKenzie, James F., 1948–
  Planning, implementing, and evaluating health promotion programs: a primer / James F. McKenzie, Brad L. Neiger, Rosemary Thackeray. 5th ed.
    p. ; cm.
  Includes bibliographical references and index.
  ISBN 0-3214-9511-X (pbk.)
1. Health promotion—Planning. 2. Health promotion—Evaluation. 3. Health planning—Methodology. I. Neiger, Brad L. II. Thackeray, Rosemary III. Title.
  [DNLM: 1. Health Promotion. 2. Health Education. 3. Health Planning.
4. Program Evaluation. WA 525 M4785p 2005
  RA427.8.M39 2005
  613'.068—dc22

                                                                2004004984

5 6 7 8 9 10—RRD—11 10
www.aw-bc.com

This book is dedicated to thirteen special people—

Bonnie, Anne, Greg, Mitchell, Julia, Sherry, Lindsay, McKay, Peyton, Jack, Chelsea, Ralph, and NaTel

and to our teachers and mentors—

Marshall H. Becker (deceased), Mary K. Beyer, Noreen Clark, Enrico A. Leopardi, Brad L. Neiger, Lynne Nilson, Terry W. Parsons, Glenn E. Richardson, Irwin M. Rosenstock (deceased), Yuzuru Takeshita, and Doug Vilnius

Contents

Preface

This book is written for students who are enrolled in their first professional course in health promotion program planning. It is designed to help them understand and develop the skills necessary to carry out program planning regardless of the setting. The book is unique among the health promotion planning textbooks on the market in that it provides readers with both theoretical and practical information. A straightforward, step-by-step format is used to make concepts clear and the full process of health promotion planning understandable. This book provides, under a single cover, material on all three areas of program development: planning, implementing, and evaluating.

New Study Card

This edition features a new Study Card providing students with a quick reference to the core concepts of the book.

Learning Aids

Each chapter includes chapter objectives, a list of key terms, presentation of content, chapter summary, review questions, activities, and weblinks. In addition, many of the key concepts are further explained with information presented in boxes, applications, figures, tables, and the appendixes.

Chapter Objectives

The chapter objectives identify the content and skills that should be mastered after reading the chapter, answering the review questions, completing the activities, and using the weblinks. Most of the objectives are written using the cognitive and psychomotor (behavior) educational domains. For most effective use of the objectives, we suggest that they be reviewed before reading the chapter. This will help readers focus on the major points in each chapter and facilitate answering the questions and completing the activities at the end.

Key Terms

Key terms are introduced in each chapter and are important to the understanding of the chapter. The terms are presented in a list at the beginning of each chapter and then are printed in boldface at the appropriate points within the chapter. In addition, all the key terms are presented in the Glossary. Again, as with the chapter objectives, we suggest that readers skim the list before reading the chapter. Then as the chapter is read, particular attention should be paid to the definition of each term.

Presentation of Content

Although each chapter could be expanded—in some cases, entire books have been written on topics we have covered in a chapter or less—we believe that each chapter contains the necessary information to help students understand and develop many of the skills required to be a successful health promotion planner, implementor, and evaluator.

New Applications and Responsibilities and Competencies Boxes

Applications boxes feature real-world examples of the concepts covered in the chapters. Responsibilities and Competencies boxes present chapter-relevant standards from NCHEC, SOPHE, and AAHE (2006).

Chapter Summary

At the end of each chapter, readers will find a one- or two-paragraph review of the major concepts contained in the chapter.

Review Questions

The questions at the end of each chapter provide readers with some feedback regarding their mastery of the content. These questions reinforce the objectives and key terms presented in each chapter.

Activities

Each chapter also includes several activities that allow students to use their new knowledge and skills. The activities are presented in several different formats for the sake of variety and to appeal to the different learning styles of students. It should be noted that, depending on the ones selected for completion, the activities in one chapter can build on those in a previous chapter and lead to the final product of a completely developed health promotion program.

Weblinks

The final portion of each chapter consists of a list of updated links on the World Wide Web. These links allow students to explore a number of different websites that are available to support planning, implementing, and evaluating efforts.

New to This Edition

In revising this textbook, we incorporated as many suggestions from reviewers, colleagues, and former students as possible. In addition to updating material throughout the text, the following points reflect the major changes in this new edition:

- Chapter 1 has been updated and expanded and includes information about the revised Areas of Responsibility and Competencies. In addition, new boxes at the beginning of this and all other chapters identify which Areas of Responsibility and Competencies relate to the material presented in the chapter.

- Chapter 2 still includes essential and updated information on key models used in program planning and evaluation such as PRECEDE-PROCEED, MATCH, CDCyergy, and SMART. In addition, information on the Generalized Model for Program Planning has been expanded to emphasize its importance and value in understanding introductory planning concepts that can then be applied to all planning models as well as parallel processes such as grant writing. Intervention mapping is presented as an alternative planning model, and the relevance of population-based approaches and the ecological framework are more clearly defined in relation to planning and evaluation.

- Chapter 3 has been expanded and now breaks the process of writing a program rationale into manageable steps. The chapter also emphasizes the importance of evidence-based practice in creating both a rationale and a plan.

- Chapter 4 has been updated and expanded and includes some new data collection processes such as windshield tours, or walk-throughs, and photovoice. In addition, the chapter includes more information on community mapping and now combines all the information on data collection that was spread over Chapters 4 and 5 in previous editions.

- Chapter 5 now focuses on the various aspects of measurement and sampling. As noted above, some of the content from the previous edition was moved to Chapter 4 and new information was added on measurement instruments.

- Chapter 6 was also updated and includes new information dealing with the *Healthy People 2010* midcourse review.

- Chapter 7 has been expanded and several new theories and models have been added including the Health Action Process Approach (HAPA) and Community Readiness Model (CRM).

- Chapter 8 has also been expanded and includes information on best practices and intervention development as well as more information on the creation of health education interventions.

- Chapter 9 has been expanded and now includes more information on mapping community capacity.

- Chapter 10 now includes more information on seeking grant dollars to support program planning and on preparing a budget for a program.

- Chapter 11 has been thoroughly reworked and includes more real-life examples of marketing principles and processes; in-depth information on segmentation, including how to evaluate/choose between segments; and on the 4 Ps of marketing.

- Chapter 12's content has been re-ordered and more emphasis placed on safety and ethical issues as they relate to implementation.

- Chapter 13 has been reorganized to help the reader better conceptualize and understand the purposes, sequence, and process of program evaluation. The two basic purposes for evaluation—assessing quality and measuring effectiveness—are more clearly labeled and defined, and the CDC framework for program evaluation provides a clear foundation for all evaluation efforts.

- Chapter 14 has been completely updated with elements of a comprehensive process evaluation and the procedures commonly used in process evaluation. The chapter includes a new classification system for evaluation approaches and designs and better distinguishes process (or formative) evaluation from summative evaluation. Additional informational on pretesting and pilot testing also helps to better inform the reader of the comprehensive nature and value of process evaluation.

- Chapter 15 has been reworked so that the elements of the evaluation report are clarified and more appropriately sequenced, and provides guidelines for how to more effectively present data.

- All chapters include more real-life-planning examples, and new Application boxes have been added in select chapters.

- A revised testbank has been created for this edition.

- Again, as with the previous edition, PowerPoint® presentations are available online.

- Two new features to this edition that should enhance the teaching-learning process are: a Glossary that includes all the key terms, and a companion website <www.aw-bc.com/mckenzie> that includes example student plans created by former students and quizzes that students can access to help them study.

- And finally, we would like to welcome Rosemary Thackeray, Ph.D., M.P.H., as a new co-author to this edition. Her expertise and experience in the field bring many new ideas to the writing team.

Students will find this book easy to understand and use. We are confident that if the chapters are carefully read and an honest effort is put into completing the activities and visiting the weblinks, students will gain the essential knowledge and skills for program planning, implementation, and evaluation.

Acknowledgments

A project of this nature could not have been completed without the assistance and understanding of many individuals. First, we thank all our past and present students, who have had to put up with our "working drafts" of the manuscript.

Second, we are grateful to those professionals who took the time and effort to review and comment on various editions of this book. For the first edition, they included Vicki Keanz, Eastern Kentucky University; Susan Cross Lipnickey, Miami University; Fred Pearson, Ricks College; Kerry Redican, Virginia Tech; John Sciacca, Northern Arizona University; and William K. Spath, Montana Tech. For the second edition, reviewers included Gordon James, Weber State; John Sciacca, Northern Arizona University; and Mark Wilson, University of Georgia. For the third edition, reviewers included Joanna Hayden, William Paterson University; Raffy Luquis, Southern Connecticut State University; Teresa Shattuck, University of Maryland; Thomas Syre, James Madison University; and Esther Weekes, Texas Women's University. For the fourth edition, reviewers included

xvi PREFACE

Robert G. LaChausse, California State University, San Bernardino; Julie Shepard, Director of Health Promotion, Adams County Health Department; Sherm Sowby, California State University, Fresno; and William Kane, University of New Mexico. For this edition, the reviewers include Sally Black, St. Joseph's University; Denise Colaianni, Western Connecticut State University; Sue Forster-Cox, New Mexico State University; Julie Gast, Utah State University; Ray Manes, York College CUNY; and Lois Ritter, California State University East Bay.

Third, we thank our friends for providing valuable feedback on various editions of this book: Robert J. Yonker, Ph.D., Professor Emeritus in the Department of Educational Foundations and Inquiry, Bowling Green State University; Lawrence W. Green, Dr.P.H., Adjunct Professor, Department of Epidemiology and Biostatistics, University of California, San Francisco (UCSF), and UCSF Comprehensive Cancer Center, Bruce Simons-Morton, Ed.D., M.P.H., Senior Investigator, Prevention Research Branch, National Institute of Child Health and Human Development, National Institutes of Health; and Jerome E. Kotecki, H.S.D., Professor, Department of Physiology and Health Science, Ball State University.

Fourth, we appreciate the work of the Benjamin Cummings employees Sandra Lindelof, acquisitions editor for health and kinesiology, who has always been very supportive of our work, and Nicole George-O'Brien, developmental editor, who's keen eye and attention for detail kept all of us on task. We also appreciate the careful work of Lindsay Mateiro at Prepress PMG.

And fifth, we would like to acknowledge the contributions of Jan L. Smeltzer, Ph.D., a co-author on the four previous editions of this book. Her work in the early years was in large part why this book got off the ground in the first place. We appreciate and thank her for that work. We wish her well as her career heads in a new direction.

Finally, we express our deepest appreciation to our families for their support, encouragement, and understanding of the time that writing takes away from our family activities.

J. F. M.
B. L. N.
R. T.

Health Education, Health Promotion, Health Educators, and Program Planning

CHAPTER OBJECTIVES

After reading this chapter and answering the questions at the end, you should be able to:

- Explain the relationship among good health behavior, health education, and health promotion.
- Explain the difference between health education and health promotion.
- Write your own definition of health education.
- Explain the role of the health educator as defined by the Role Delineation Project.
- Explain how a person becomes a Certified Health Education Specialist.
- Explain how the Competency-Based Framework for Health Educators is used by colleges and universities, the National Commission for Health Education Credentialing, Inc. (NCHEC), the National Council for the Accreditation of Teacher Education (NCATE), and the SOPHE/AAHE Baccalaureate Program Approval Committee (SABPAC).
- Identify the assumptions upon which health education is based.
- Define and explain a logic model.

KEY TERMS

advanced-level 1 health educator
advanced-level 2 health educator
entry-level health educator
Framework

health behavior
health education
health educator
health promotion
Healthy People

logic model
primary prevention
Role Delineation Project
secondary prevention
tertiary prevention

Looking back over the twentieth century, we see that much progress was made in the health and life expectancy of Americans: "People are living longer than previously and with greater freedom from the threat of disease" (Breslow, 1999, p. 1031). Since 1900, we have seen a sharp drop in infant mortality (Miniño, Heron, Smith, & Kochanek, 2006); the eradication of smallpox; the elimination of poliomyelitis in the Americas; the control of measles, rubella, tetanus, diphtheria, Haemophilus influenzae type b, and other infectious diseases; better family planning (CDC, 1999d), and an increase of 29.7 years in the average life span of a person in the United States (NCHS, 2006). Over this same time, we have witnessed disease prevention change "from focusing on reducing environmental exposures over which the individual had little control, such as providing potable water, to emphasizing behaviors such as avoiding use of tobacco, fatty foods, and a sedentary lifestyle" (Breslow, 1999, p. 1030). Yet, even with this change in focus "most Americans have not changed their lifestyles sufficiently to reduce their risk of death or illness" (CDC, 2003a, p. 1). "Three modifiable health-damaging behaviors—tobacco use, lack of physical activity, and poor eating habits—are responsible for much of the inordinate suffering and early deaths of millions of Americans. In fact, these three behaviors are responsible for approximately 33% of all U.S. deaths (CDC, 2003a). Many of these deaths are coming in the form of chronic diseases such as heart disease, cancer, and diabetes. Chronic diseases account for 7 of every 10 deaths and affect the quality of life of 90 million Americans. Although chronic diseases are among the most common and costly health problems, they are also among the most preventable" (CDC, 2007) (see **Table 1.1**). Now in the early years of the twenty-first century, behavior patterns continue to "represent the single most prominent domain of influence over health prospects in the United States" (McGinnis, Williams-Russo, & Knickman, 2002, p. 82).

Though the focus on good health, wellness, and **health behavior** (those behaviors that impact a person's health) seem commonplace in our lives today, it was not until the last fourth of the twentieth century that health promotion was recognized for its potential to help control injury and disease and to promote health.

> Most scholars, policymakers, and practitioners in health promotion would pick 1974 as the turning point that marks the beginning of health promotion as a significant component of national health policy in the twentieth century. That year Canada published its landmark policy statement, *A New Perspective on the Health of Canadians* (Lalonde, 1974). In the United States, Congress passed PL 94-317, the Health Information and Health Promotion Act, which created the Office of Health Information and Health Promotion, later renamed the Office of Disease Prevention and Health Promotion. (Green 1999, p. 69).

This led the way for the U.S. government's publication *Healthy People: The Surgeon General's Report on Health Promotion and Disease Prevention* (*Healthy People,* 1979). This document brought together much of what was known about the relationship of personal behavior and health status. The document also presented a "personal responsibility" model that provided Americans with a prescription for reducing their health risks and increasing their chances for good health.

It may not have been the content of **Healthy People** that made the publication so significant, because several publications written before it provided a similar message.

Table 1.1   Comparison of most common causes of death and actual causes of death

Most common causes of death, United States, 2004*	Actual causes of death, United States, 2000**
1. Diseases of the heart	1. Tobacco
2. Malignant neoplasms (cancers)	2. Poor diet and physical inactivity
3. Cerebrovascular diseases (stroke)	3. Alcohol consumption
4. Chronic lower respiratory diseases	4. Microbial agents
5. Accidents (unintentional injuries)	5. Toxic agents
6. Diabetes mellitus	6. Motor vehicles
7. Alzheimer's disease	7. Firearms
8. Influenza and pneumonia	8. Sexual behavior
9. Nephritis, nephrotic syndrome, and nephrosis	9. Illicit drug use
10. Septicemia	

*Miniño, Heron, Smith, & Kochanek (2006).
**Mokdad, Marks, Stroup, & Greberding (2004 & 2005).

Rather, *Healthy People* was important because it summarized the research available up to that point, presented it in a very readable format, and made the information available to the general public. *Healthy People* was then followed by the release of the first set of health goals and objectives for the nation, titled *Promoting Health/Preventing Disease: Objectives for the Nation* (USDHHS, 1980). These goals and objectives, now in their third generation (USDHHS, 2000), have defined the nation's health agenda and guided its health policy since their inception. And, in part, they have kept the importance of good health visible to all Americans.

This focus on good health has given many people in the United States a desire to do something about their health. This desire, in turn, has created a greater need for good health information that can be easily understood by the average person. One need only look at the current best-seller list, read the daily newspaper, observe the health advertisements delivered via the electronic mass media, or consider the increase in the number of health-promoting facilities (not illness or sickness facilities) to verify the interest that American consumers have in health. Because of the increased interest in health, health professionals are now faced with providing the public with the information and the skills needed to make quality health decisions.

Health Education and Health Promotion

In the simplest terms, **health education** is the process of educating people about health. However, two more formal definitions of health education have been frequently cited in the literature. The first comes from the *Report of the 2000 Joint Committee on Health Education and Promotion Terminology* (Joint Committee on Terminology, 2001). The committee defined health education as "Any combination of planned learning experiences based on sound theories that provide individuals, groups, and communities the opportunity to acquire information and the skills needed to make quality health decisions" (p. 99). The second definition was presented by Green and Kreuter (2005), who defined health education as "any planned combination of learning experiences designed to predispose, enable, and reinforce voluntary behavior conducive to health in individuals, groups, or communities" (p. G-4).

Another term that is closely related to health education, and sometimes incorrectly used in its place, is health promotion. *Health promotion* is a broader term than *health education*. The Joint Committee on Terminology (2001) defined **health promotion** as "Any planned combination of educational, political, environmental, regulatory, or organizational mechanisms that support actions and conditions of living conducive to the health of individuals, groups, and communities" (p. 101). However, Green and Kreuter (2005) define *health promotion* slightly different as "any planned combination of educational, political, regulatory and organizational supports for actions and conditions of living conducive to the health of individuals, groups, and communities" (p. G-4).

To help us to further understand and operationalize the term *health promotion,* Breslow (1999) has stated, "Each person has a certain degree of health that may be expressed as a place in a spectrum. From that perspective, promoting health must focus on enhancing people's capacities for living. That means moving them toward the health end of the spectrum, just as prevention is aimed at avoiding disease that can move people toward the opposite end of the spectrum" (p. 1031). According to these definitions of health promotion, health education is an important component of health promotion and firmly implanted in it (see **Figure 1.1**). "Health promotion takes into account that human behavior is not only governed by personal factors (e.g., knowledge, expectancies,

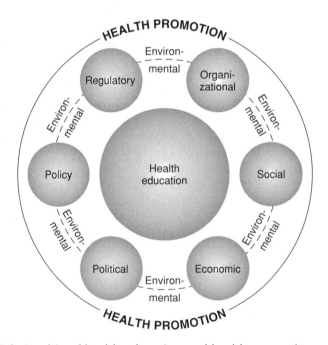

Figure 1.1 Relationship of health education and health promotion

competencies, and well-being), but also by structural aspects of the environment" (Vogele, 2005, p. 272). However, "without health education, health promotion would be a manipulative social engineering enterprise" (Green & Kreuter, 1999, p. 19).

The effectiveness of health promotion programs can vary greatly. However, the success of a program can usually be linked to the planning that takes place before implementation of the program. Programs that have undergone a thorough planning process are usually the most successful. As the old saying goes, "If you fail to plan, your plan will fail."

Health Educators

The individuals best qualified to plan health promotion programs are health educators. A **health educator** is "A professionally prepared individual who serves in a variety of roles and is specifically trained to use appropriate educational strategies and methods to facilitate the development of policies, procedures, interventions, and systems conducive to the health of individuals, groups, and communities" (Joint Committee on Terminology, 2001, p. 100). Today, health educators can be found working in a variety of settings, including schools (K–12, colleges, and universities), community health agencies (governmental and nongovernmental), worksites (business, industry, and other work settings), and health care settings (e.g., clinics, hospitals, and managed care organizations).

The role of the health educator in the United States as we know it today is one that has evolved over time based on the need to provide people with educational interventions to enhance their health. The earliest signs of the role of the health educator appeared in the mid-1800s with school hygiene education, which was closely associated with physical activity. By the early 1900s, the need for health education spread to the public health arena, but it was the writers, journalists, social workers, and visiting nurses who were doing the educating—not health educators as we know them today (Deeds, 1992). As we gained more knowledge about the relationship between health, disease, and health behavior, it was obvious that the writers, journalists, social workers, visiting nurses, and primary caregivers—mainly physicians, dentists, other independent practitioners, and nurses—were unable to provide the needed health education. The combination of the heavy workload of the primary caregivers, the lack of formal training in the process of educating others, and the need for education at all levels of prevention—primary, secondary, and tertiary—(see **Figure 1.2**) created a need for health educators.

As the role of the health educator grew over the years, there was a movement by those in the discipline to clearly define their role so that people inside and outside the profession would have a better understanding of what the health educator did. In January 1979, the **Role Delineation Project** began (National Task Force [on the Preparation and Practice of Health Educators, Inc.], 1985). Through a comprehensive process, this project yielded a generic role for the **entry-level health educator**—that is, responsibilities for health educators taking their first job regardless of their work setting. Once the role of the entry-level health educator was delineated, the task became to translate the role into a structure that professional preparation programs in health

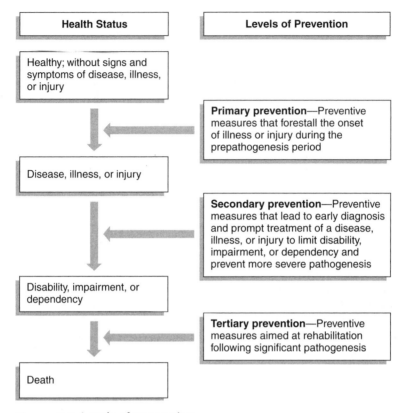

Figure 1.2 Levels of prevention

Source: Adapted from Pickett & Hanlon (1990).

education could use to design competency-based curricula. The resulting document, *A Framework for the Development of Competency-Based Curricula for Entry Level Health Educators* (NCHEC, 1985), and its revised version, *A Competency-Based Framework for the Professional Development of Certified Health Education Specialists* (NCHEC, 1996), provided such a structure. These documents, simply referred to as the *Framework* were comprised of the seven major areas of responsibility, which defined the scope of practice, and several different competencies and subcompetencies, which further delineated the responsibilities.

Even though the seven areas of responsibility defined the role of the entry-level health educator, they did not fully express the work of the health educator with an advanced degree. Thus, over a four-year period beginning in 1992, the profession worked to define the role of an advanced-level practitioner. By July 1997, the governing boards of the National Commission for Health Education, Inc. (NCHEC), the American Association of Health Education (AAHE), and the Society for Public Health Education (SOPHE) had endorsed three additional responsibilities for the advanced-level health educator. Those responsibilities revolved around research, administration, and the advancement of the profession (AAHE, NCHEC, & SOPHE, 1999).

The seven entry-level and three additional advanced-level responsibilities served the profession well, but during the mid- to late-1990s it became obvious that there was a need to revisit the responsibilities and competencies and to make sure that they still defined the role of the health educator. Thus in 1998, the profession launched a six-year multiphase research study known as the *National Health Educator Competencies Update Project* (CUP) to reverify the entry-level health education responsibilities, competencies, and sub-competencies and to verify the advanced-level competencies and sub-competencies (Airhihenbuwa et al., 2005). More specifically, the CUP "addressed the following four research questions:

1. What is the current generic role of the entry-level health education specialist compared with the role previously defined?

2. What are the generic areas of responsibility, competencies, and sub-competencies of advanced-level health education specialists?

3. Are there commonalities in the roles of the entry-level and advanced-level health education specialists across practice settings?

4. Are there differences in the roles of entry-level health educators and advanced-level health education specialists based upon degrees held and years of work experience in health education" (NCHEC, SOPHE, & AAHE, 2006, p. 6).

The four major phases of the CUP included: (1) preliminary research to provide a solid, scientific foundation for the project, (2) pilot research to prepare for the main study, (3) the final project in which a 19-page questionnaire was completed by more than 4,000 practicing health educators from every state in the United States (including the District of Columbia) and from a wide array of work settings (i.e., community, school, college/university, health care, business/industry), and (4) analysis of the resulting data.

What became obvious from the analysis of the CUP data was that the seven responsibilities and many of the competencies and sub-competencies identified in the earlier Role Delineation Project were still valid. However, the wording of the responsibilities was changed slightly, some competencies and sub-competencies were dropped, and a few new ones were added. Also, certain sub-competencies were reported as more important and performed more regularly by health educators who had both more work experience and academic degrees beyond the baccalaureate level. Thus, the CUP model that emerged included responsibilities, competencies, and sub-competencies (see **Box 1.1**), and the development of a three-tiered (i.e., **Entry**, **Advanced-Level 1**, and **Advanced-Level 2**) hierarchical model reflecting the generic role of the health educator (NCHEC, Inc., 2006) (see **Table 1.2** for levels of practice).

In reviewing the seven areas of responsibility, it is obvious that four of the seven are directly related to program planning, implementation, and evaluation and that the other three could be associated with these processes, depending on the type of program being planned. In effect, these responsibilities distinguish health educators from other professionals who try to provide health education experiences.

The importance of the defined role of the health educator is becoming greater as the profession of health promotion continues to mature. This is exhibited by its use in several major professional activities. First, the *Framework* has provided a guide for all

Box 1.1	RESPONSIBILITIES AND COMPETENCIES FOR HEALTH EDUCATORS

The 7 areas of responsibility that provide the structure for the initial and ongoing preparation of health educators are:

Responsibility I: Assess Individual and Community Needs for Health Education

Responsibility II: Plan Health Education Strategies, Interventions, and Programs

Responsibility III: Implement Health Education Strategies, Interventions, and Programs

Responsibility IV: Conduct Evaluation and Research Related to Health Education

Responsibility V: Administer Health Education Strategies, Interventions, and Programs

Responsibility VI: Serve as a Health Education Resource Person

Responsibility VII: Communicate and Advocate for Health and Health Education

Source: NCHEC, SOPHE, & AAHE (2006).

Under these 7 areas of responsibility are 35 competencies and 163 sub-competencies that further define the role of health educators regardless of their work setting. The specific areas of responsibility and competencies associated with the planning, implementing, and evaluating of health promotion programs will be identified in similar boxes throughout this book.

Table 1.2   CUP model hierarchical approach

Level of Practice	Competencies/Sub-competencies
Entry (less than 5 years of experience; baccalaureate or master's degree)	Entry
Advanced 1 (5 or more years of experience; baccalaureate or master's degree)	Entry + Advanced 1
Advanced 2 (doctorate and 5 or more years of experience)	Entry + Advanced 1 + Advanced 2

Source: G. D. Gilmore et al, "Overview of the national health educator competencies update project, 1998–2004," *Health Education & Behavior,* 32(6), pp. 725–737, 2005. Copyright © 2005 Society for Public Health Education. Reprinted by permission of Sage Publications, Inc.

colleges and universities to use when designing and revising their curricula in health education to prepare future health educators. Second, the *Framework* was used by the National Commission for Health Education Credentialing, Inc. (NCHEC) to develop the core criteria for certifying individuals as health educators (Certified Health Education Specialists, or CHES). The first group of individuals (N=1,558) to receive the CHES credential did so between October 1988 and December 1989, during the charter certification period. "Charter certification allowed qualified individuals to be certified based on their academic training, work experience, and references without taking the certification exam" (Cottrell, Girvan, & McKenzie, 2009, p. 177). In 1990, using a criterion-referenced examination based on the *Framework*, the nationwide testing program to certify health educators was begun by NCHEC, Inc. During that first year, 648 passed the examination and received the CHES credential (AAHE, NCHEC, & SOPHE, 1999). As of May 2007, approximately 14,000 individuals have received the CHES credential. Currently, the CHES examination is given twice a year in April and October. **Box 1.2** presents the current eligibility guidelines in order to be able to sit for the examination, whereas **Box 1.3** provides a breakdown of the percentage of questions that come from each Area of Responsibility on the CHES examination.

Box 1.2 ELIGIBILITY GUIDELINES TO SIT FOR THE CHES EXAMINATION

Eligibility to sit for the CHES examination is based exclusively on academic qualifications. An individual is eligible to sit for the examination if he/she has:

A bachelor's, master's, or doctoral degree from an accredited institution of higher education; AND one of the following:

- An official transcript (including course titles) that clearly shows a major in health education, e.g., Health Education, Community Health Education, Public Health Education, School Health Education, etc.

OR

- An official transcript that reflects at least 25 semester hours or 37 quarter hours of course work with specific preparation addressing the Areas of Responsibility of Health Education Specialists.

Source: © The National Commission for Health Education Credentialing, Inc. Reprinted by permission.

Box 1.3 PERCENTAGE OF QUESTIONS FROM EACH AREA OF RESPONSIBILITY ON THE CHES EXAMINATION*

Areas of Responsibility	Percentage of Questions
I. Assess Individual and Community Needs for Health Education	10
II. Plan Health Education Strategies, Interventions, and Programs	15
III. Implement Health Education Strategies, Interventions, and Programs	22
IV. Conduct Evaluation and Research Related to Health Education	13
V. Administer Health Education Strategies, Interventions, and Programs	14
VI. Serve as a Health Education Resource Person	14
VII. Communicate and Advocate for Health and Health Education	12

*Began with the Fall 2007 CHES Exam
Source: D. L. Dennis & J. Rainey, "Percentage of Questions from Each Area of Responsibility on the CHES Examination, "*The CHES Bulletin* 18(1)5, 2007. Copyright © 2007 National Commission for Health Education Credentialing, Inc. Used with permission.

Third, the *Framework* is used by program accrediting and approval bodies to review college and university academic programs in health education. The National Council for the Accreditation of Teacher Education (NCATE) uses the *Framework* to review and accredit teacher preparation programs in health education at institutions of higher education. Also, a joint committee of the Society for Public Health Education, Inc. (SOPHE) and the American Association for Health Education, known as the SOPHE/AAHE Baccalaureate Program Approval Committee (SABPAC), uses the *Framework* to review and approve undergraduate health education programs via self-study and external reviewers.

The use of the *Framework* by the profession to guide academic curricula, provide the core criteria for the health education specialist examination, and form the basis of program approval processes (AAHE, NCHEC, & SOPHE, 1999) has done much to advance the health education profession. "In 1998 the U.S. Department of Commerce and Labor formally acknowledged 'health educator' as a distinct occupation. Such recognition was justified, based to a large extent, on the ability of the profession to specify its unique skills" (AAHE, NCHEC, & SOPHE, 1999, p. 9).

At the time of the writing of this book, the results of the CUP were less than one year old and much discussion was revolving around how the profession would deal with the Advanced Levels 1 and 2 with regard to advanced-level credentialing and the modification and development of health education curricula in graduate programs. Time will tell how well the CUP model will serve the profession.

Assumptions of Health Promotion

So far, we have discussed the need for health, what health education and health promotion are, and the role health educators play in delivering successful health promotion programs. We have not yet discussed the assumptions that underlie health promotion— all the things that must be in place before the whole process of health promotion begins. In the mid-1980s, Bates and Winder (1984) outlined what they saw as four critical assumptions of health education. Their list has been modified by adding several items, rewording others, and referring to them as "assumptions of health promotion." This expanded list of assumptions is critical to understanding what we can expect from health promotion programs. Health promotion is by no means the sole answer to the nation's health care problem or, for that matter, the sole means of getting the smoker to stop smoking or the nonexerciser to exercise. Health promotion is an important part of the health care system, but it does have limitations. Here are the assumptions:

1. Health status can be changed.
2. "Health and disease are determined by dynamic interactions among biological, psychological, behavioral, and social factors" (Pellmar, Brandt, & Baird, 2002, p. 217).
3. Disease occurrence theories and principles can be understood (Bates & Winder, 1984).
4. Appropriate prevention strategies can be developed to deal with the identified health problems (Bates & Winder, 1984).
5. "Behavior can be changed and those changes can influence health" (Pellmar et al., 2002, p. 213).

6. "Individual behavior, family interactions, community and workplace relationships and resources, and public policy all contribute to health and influence behavior change" (Pellmar et al., 2002, p. 217).

7. "Initiating and maintaining a behavior change is difficult" (Pellmar et al., 2002, p. 217).

8. Individual responsibility should not be viewed as victim blaming, yet the importance of health behavior to health status must be understood.

9. For health behavior change to be permanent, an individual must be motivated and ready to change.

The importance of these assumptions is made clearer if we refer to the definitions of health education and health promotion presented earlier in the chapter. Implicit in those definitions was a goal of having program participants voluntarily adopt actions conducive to health. To achieve such a goal, the assumptions must indeed be in place. We cannot expect people to adopt lifelong health-enhancing behavior if we force them into such change. Nor can we expect people to change their behavior just because they have been exposed to a health promotion program. Health behavior change is very complex, and health educators should not expect to change every person with whom they come in contact. However, the greatest chance for success will come to those who have the knowledge and skills to plan, implement, and evaluate appropriate programs.

Program Planning

Since many of health educators' responsibilities are involved in some way with program planning, implementation, and evaluation, health educators need to become well versed in these processes. "Planning an effective program is more difficult than implementing it. Planning, implementing, and evaluating programs are all interrelated, but good planning skills are prerequisite to programs worthy of evaluation" (Breckon, Harvey, & Lancaster, 1998, p. 145). All three processes are very involved, and much time, effort, practice, and on-the-job training are required to do them well. Even the most experienced health educators find program planning challenging because of the constant changes in settings, resources, and priority populations.

Because all three processes—planning, implementing, and evaluating—are very involved, it is not always easy to envision or understand all that will be included in the processes from beginning to end. In order to better understand the "big picture" of how these program processes fit together, it may be helpful to begin with the creation of a logic model. "A logic model attempts to convey visually the connection between program activities and the program's desired outcomes; that is, the *logic* of the program" (Lando, Williams, Sturgis, & Williams, 2006, p. 2). Or stated differently, a **logic model** is a "simplified picture of a program, initiative, or intervention" (University of Wisconsin–Extension, 2002a, p. 2) that "shows the logical relationships among the resources that are invested, the activities that take place, and the benefits or changes that result" (University of Wisconsin–Extension, 2002a, p. 2). Simply put, a logic model is a roadmap (Goldman & Schmalz, 2006).

Logic models can take many different shapes (i.e., linear, circular, lists) and be presented in various levels of detail (i.e., simple, complex) but all provide in a graphic display of boxes and arrows the relationships and linkages of the various components. In its most basic form a logic model includes three components: inputs (or resources), outputs (or activities), and outcomes (or results or effects). Of course, the more detailed the logic model, the more useful it is to those interested in the program being planned. Thus, others (e.g., Goldman & Schmaltz, 2006; University of Kansas, 2007; University of Wisconsin–Extension, 2002b; W. K. Kellogg Foundation, 2004) have suggested that logic models can also include: (1) the purpose or mission of the program, (2) the context, conditions, or situation under which the program will be offered, (3) assumptions associated with the planned program, (4) external factors that could influence the success of the program, and (5) a description of the evaluation of the proposed program. **Box 1.4** provides an example of a logic model that was used in the development of a health promotion program aimed at reducing the incidence of colon cancer.

The remaining chapters of this book present a process that health educators can use to plan, implement, and evaluate successful health promotion programs and will introduce you to the necessary knowledge and skills to carry out these tasks.

Box 1.4   APPLICATION: LOGIC MODEL FOR A COLON CANCER PREVENTION PROGRAM

Inputs	Activities	Short-term Outcomes	Mid-term Outcomes	Long-term Outcomes
Personnel Funding Equipment Supplies Space Educational materials	Educate healthcare providers about program	Change in awareness and knowledge of program	Increase in referral behavior of health care providers	
	Educate public about colon cancer	Change in knowledge, attitudes, beliefs, and motivation	Increase in number of people screened	Colon cancer prevention
				Colon cancer control
	Free colon cancer screenings	Screening sites established		
	Partnerships established among stakeholders	Partners identified and activated		Quality of life of individuals improves

SUMMARY

The increased interest in personal health and the flood of new health information have created a need to provide quality health promotion programs. Individuals are seeking guidance to enable them to make sound decisions about behavior that is conducive to their health. Those best prepared to help these people are health educators who receive appropriate training. Properly trained health educators are aware of the limitations of the discipline and understand the assumptions on which health promotion is based.

REVIEW QUESTIONS

1. Explain the role *Healthy People* played in the relationship between the American people and health.

2. How is *health education* defined by the Joint Committee on Terminology (2001)?

3. What are the key phrases in the definition of health education presented by Green and Kreuter (2005)?

4. What is the relationship between health education and health promotion?

5. Why is there a need for health educators?

6. What is the Role Delineation Project?

7. How is the Competency-Based Framework for Health Educators used by colleges and universities? By NCHEC? By NCATE? By SABPAC?

8. How does one become a Certified Health Education Specialist (CHES)?

9. What are the seven major responsibilities of health educators?

10. What is the National Health Educator Competencies Update Project (CUP)?

11. What assumptions are critical to health promotion?

12. What are logic models? Why are they used? What are the major components of logic models?

ACTIVITIES

1. Based on what you have read in this chapter and your knowledge of the profession of health education, write your own definitions for *health, health education, health promotion*, and *health promotion program*.

2. Write a response indicating what you see as the importance of each of the nine assumptions presented in the chapter. Write no more than one paragraph per assumption.

3. With your knowledge of health promotion, what other assumptions would you add to the list presented in this chapter? Provide a one-paragraph rationale for each.

4. If you have not already done so, go to the government documents section of the library on your campus and read *Healthy People: The Surgeon General's Report on Health Promotion and Disease Prevention (Healthy People,* 1979).

5. Say you are in your senior year and will graduate next June with a bachelor's degree in health education. What steps would you have to take in order to be able to take the CHES exam in April prior to your graduation? (Hint: Check the website for the National Commission for Health Education Credentialing, Inc.).

6. Either on your own or with the help of your professor, locate the written description of a health promotion program. Using this written description, the information you have gained from reading this chapter, and other resources available to you, create a simple logic model for the program described.

WEBLINKS

1. http://www.healthypeople.gov

   Healthy People

   This is the webpage for the U.S. Government's Healthy People initiative including a complete presentation of the three parts of *Healthy People 2010.*

2. http://www.nchec.org/

   The National Commission for Health Education Credentialing, Inc. (NCHEC)

   This is the website for the NCHEC, Inc. It provides the most current information about the CHES credential and the CUP.

3. http://www.uwex.edu/ces/pdande/evaluation/evallogicmodel.html

   The University of Wisconsin–Extension

   This is a website of the University of Wisconsin–Extension that presents information on logic models. This site provides information about logic models, examples of logic models, and PowerPoint® presentations that provide a good overview of logic models.

PART I

PLANNING A HEALTH PROMOTION PROGRAM

The chapters in this section of the book provide the basic information needed to plan a health promotion program. Each chapter presents readers with the tools they will need to develop a successful program in a variety of settings. The chapters and topics presented in this section are:

2

Models for Program Planning in Health Promotion

After reading this chapter and answering the questions at the end, you should be able to:

- Explain the value of the generalized model for program planning.
- Explain the value of using a model in planning a program.
- Identify the models commonly used in planning health promotion programs and briefly explain each.
- Identify the basic components of the planning models presented.
- Apply a model to a program you are planning.

KEY TERMS

administrative and policy
   assessment
APEX-PH
CDCynergy or Cynergy
ecological framework
educational and ecological
   assessment
enabling factors
epidemiological assessment
evaluation
formative research
health communication
Health Communication
   Model

Healthy Communities
Healthy Plan-It
impact evaluation
implementation
intervention alignment
intervention mapping
MAPP
MATCH
message concepts
outcome evaluation
PACE-EH
population-based approach
PRECEDE-PROCEED

predisposing factors
process evaluation
reinforcing factors
SMART
social assessment and
   situational analysis
social marketing
SWOT
A Systematic Approach to
   Health Promotion
Three Fs of Program
   Planning

As noted in Chapter 1, a major portion of the role of the health educator is associated with planning, implementing, and evaluating programs. Good health promotion programs are not created by chance; they are the product of coordinated effort and are usually based on a systematic planning model. Models are the means by which structure and organization are given to the planning process. They provide planners with direction and a framework on which to build. Many different planning models have been developed, some of which are used more frequently than others. Although many of the models have common elements, these elements may have different labels. In fact, "the underlying principles that guide the development of the various models are similar; however, there are important differences in sequence, emphasis, and the conceptualization of the major components that make certain models more appealing than others to individual practitioners" (Simons-Morton, Greene, & Gottlieb, 1995, pp. 126–127). It is important to remember there are no perfect planning models. Planners generally adapt models to fit the needs of the planning situation and the cultural characteristics of the priority population, setting, and health problem (Kline & Huff, 1999).

Most planners will encounter situations where it is not feasible to use a model in its entirety or when it is necessary to combine parts of different models to meet specific needs and situations. What is most critical for any student, practicing health educator, or planner is a working knowledge of the basic steps that most planning models have in common. The Generalized Model for Program Planning (see **Figure 2.1**) outlines these common steps: assessing needs, setting goals and objectives, developing an intervention, implementing the intervention, and evaluating the results.

Developing a working knowledge of the generalized model is significant for a number of reasons; it will: (1) help you better understand all planning models, (2) prepare you to adapt to any planning situation in professional practice, and (3) help you better understand related processes such as grant writing. It is important to realize that new planning models emerge and fade over time in response to professional needs and personal preferences. These models, with their unique steps or phases and terminology, actually come and go quite frequently. What remains constant amidst the change, however, are the guiding principles that are common to most models—the planning principles or steps displayed in the generalized model. Pay special attention to the nature and sequence of these steps and you will quickly comprehend the basic nature of all planning models.

Understanding the generalized model will also help you adapt and respond to complex planning tasks you will experience in professional practice. With planning expertise associated with your working knowledge of the generalized model, you will be able to both lead planning tasks and educate other stakeholders about the basic sequence of the planning process. Even though at first glance most models look linear (i.e., one step leads to the next), they are really more often iterative in nature. In other words, you will most often move back and forth between steps or phases. Thus, knowledge and familiarity with the generalized model will help you quickly assimilate and interpret varying or competing stakeholder preferences for planning into a guiding paradigm that

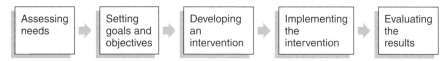

Figure 2.1 Generalized model for program planning

will generally keep you on track. Think of the generalized model as a type of *North Star* for planning. Although there is nothing unique about the model itself, its principles are the building blocks for all other models and actually represent the foundation of health education and health promotion practice.

Another benefit of understanding the generalized model is an increased ability to apply important processes closely related to program planning, such as grant writing. Requirements listed in *requests for applications* (RFAs) or *requests for proposals* (RFPs) related to grant announcements will be developed by the funding agency/organization and include their preferences for language and terminology. But the steps or requirements related to requests for health funding almost always relate back to the steps listed in the generalized model.

Funding requests from the Centers for Disease Control and Prevention (CDC) generally require applicants to organize proposals with the following sections: background and statement of need; work plan; management plan; evaluation; and budget. These sections parallel closely with the generalized model: the background and statement of need relate to the needs assessment; the work plan includes goals and objectives as well as a description of interventions; and the management plan generally includes requirements for program implementation. The Community Tool Box (see WEBLINKS at the end of this chapter), a website designed to assist health professionals with various tasks, outlines a process for writing a grant application. Sections include: introduction; statement of the community problem; project vision, mission, and objectives; methods (interventions); evaluation plan; and budget and budget justification.

Clearly, understanding the basic steps of program planning as presented in the generalized model or the other planning models used in health promotion have broader benefit than just understanding principles related to program planning. A serious study of program planning models in general will help prepare you for work in health promotion and with the skills necessary to perform your work.

Pay particular attention to the models presented in this chapter and see how they integrate these basic steps in one form or another. With an understanding and appreciation for the steps presented in this book, all other planning models will become much easier to use in health promotion settings. Then, when you need to make adjustments in the middle of a planning process, you will be able to identify and preserve the critical planning components.

Selecting a specific planning model to apply will be based on many things: (1) the preferences of stakeholders (e.g., decision makers, program partners, consumers), (2) how much time and funding are available for planning purposes, (3) how many resources are available for data collection and analysis, (4) the degree to which clients are actually involved as partners in the planning process or the degree to which your planning efforts will be consumer-oriented (i.e., planning is based on the wants and needs of consumers), and (5) preferences of a funding agency (in the case of a grant or contract award).

Three important criteria labeled the **Three Fs of Program Planning:** *fluidity, flexibility, and functionality,* should help guide the selection of your model and govern the application of its use. *Fluidity* suggests that steps in the planning process are sequential, or that they build upon one another. It may not be critical if a step is missed, but it is usually a problem if certain steps are performed out of sequence. The appropriate sequence of steps is diagrammed in the Generalized Model for Program Planning. For example, a planner cannot develop goals and objectives until a needs assessment has been performed, and a priority health problem has been identified.

Flexibility means that planning is adapted to the needs of stakeholders. Due to various circumstances, planning is usually modified as the process unfolds. For example, some health problems, such as an outbreak of influenza, require a rapid assessment and scan of the environment. Strict adherence to a model in light of unique circumstances will generally lead to frustration among partners and a less-than-desirable outcome. *Functionality* means that the outcome of planning is improved health conditions, not the production of a program plan itself. A model is only a tool to help planners accomplish their real work—to enhance health and decrease disease and disability.

In addition to the *Three Fs*, when deciding upon a planning model, it is also important to ensure that the model is conducive to planning a *population-based approach* and that it uses an *ecological framework*. Whereas systematic and strategic planning efforts can address smaller populations such as those found in a small-to medium-sized worksite, many planning processes, due to costs and other resources, usually pertain to large population segments of even larger populations—thus the term **population-based approach**.

Planners must understand the interaction between a priority population and the communities in which they live. The **ecological framework** helps planners understand that families, schools, employers, social networks, organizations, communities, and societies exert an influence on individuals and priority populations as they attempt to change health behaviors and improve their health (Bartholomew, Parcel, Kok, & Gottlieb, 2006). Thus, planners must work with priority populations within the context of broad environments.

The remainder of this chapter will present prominent models used by planners in health promotion settings. Four models, PRECEDE-PROCEED, MATCH, CDCynergy, and SMART, will be presented in detail. These models represent a wide range of planning approaches even though they share elements displayed in the Generalized Model. Others, which may be just as good from theoretical or practical perspectives, but used less widely, will be briefly presented and referenced.

Box 2.1 identifies the responsibilities and competencies for health educators that pertain to the material presented in this chapter.

Box 2.1 | RESPONSIBILITIES AND COMPETENCIES FOR HEALTH EDUCATORS

Chapter 2 covers planning models as well as other considerations and criteria necessary to develop a planning sequence from start to finish. Responsibilities and competencies that are connected with the content in this chapter include:

Responsibility II: Plan Health Education Strategies, Interventions, and Programs

Competency A: Involve people and organizations in program planning

Competency B: Incorporate data analysis and principles of community organization

Competency C: Formulate appropriate and measurable program objectives

Competency D: Develop a logical scope and sequence plan for health education practice

Source: NCHEC, SOPHE, & AAHE (2006).

PRECEDE-PROCEED

Currently, the most widely known model in program planning is the **PRECEDE-PROCEED** model. "PRECEDE is an acronym for *predisposing, reinforcing, and enabling constructs in educational/ecological diagnosis and evaluation*" (Green & Kreuter, 2005, p. 9). "PROCEED stands for *policy, regulatory, and organizational constructs in educational and environmental development*" (Green & Kreuter, 2005, p. 9).

PRECEDE-PROCEED has been the basis for many professional projects at the national level. This model is well received professionally because it is theoretically grounded and comprehensive in nature; it combines a series of phases in the planning, implementation, and evaluation process.

PRECEDE-PROCEED was developed over the course of about 20 years and continues to adapt to professional needs. The Precede framework was created in the early 1970s (Green, 1974) and evolved as a planning model during the late 1970s (Green, 1975, 1976; Green, Levine, & Deeds, 1975; Green et al., 1978; Green et al., 1980). The first half of the model, or Precede, "consists of a series of planned assessments that generate information that will be used to guide subsequent decisions" (Green & Kreuter, 2005, p. 8).

The Proceed framework was developed in the 1980s (Green, 1979, 1980, 1981a, 1981b, 1982, 1983a, 1983b, 1984a, 1984b, 1984c, 1984d, 1986a, 1986b, 1986c, 1986d, 1986e, 1987a, 1987b; Green & Allen, 1980; Green & McAlister, 1984; Green, Mullen, & Friedman, 1986; Green, Wilson, & Lovato, 1986; Green, Wilson, & Bauer, 1983) and "is essentially an elaboration and extension of the administrative diagnosis step of PRECEDE, which was the final and least developed link in the PRECEDE framework" (Green & Kreuter, 1991, p. 825). It was influenced by the participation of Green and Kreuter in national policy initiatives and the development of community health promotion programs such as Planned Approach to Community Health (PATCH) (Green & Kreuter, 1992). Proceed, the second half of the model, "is marked by the strategic implementation of multiple actions based on what was learned from the assessments in the initial phase" (Green & Kreuter, 2005, p. 9).

The Eight Phases of PRECEDE-PROCEED

As shown in **Figure 2.2**, PRECEDE-PROCEED is composed of eight phases or steps. At first glance, the model seems complicated, but on close examination, the continuous series of steps reveals a logical sequence for program planning. The underlying approach of this model is to begin by identifying the desired outcome, to determine what causes it, and finally to design an intervention aimed at reaching the desired outcome. In other words, PRECEDE-PROCEED begins with the final consequences and works backward to the causes. Once the causes are known, an intervention can be designed.

Phase 1 in the model is called **social assessment and situational analysis** and seeks to subjectively define the quality of life (problems and priorities) of those in the priority population. The designers of this model suggest that this is best accomplished by involving individuals in the priority population in an assessment of their own needs and aspirations. Some of the social indicators of quality of life include

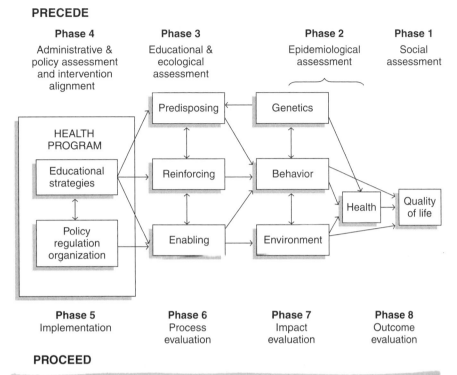

Figure 2.2 PRECEDE-PROCEED model for health promotion planning and evaluation

Source: Lawrence W. Green & Marshall W. Kreuter, *Health Promotion & Planning,* 3/e. Copyright © 1999 Mayfield Publishing. Reprinted by permission of McGraw-Hill Companies, Inc.

achievement, alienation, comfort, crime, discrimination, happiness, self-esteem, unemployment, and welfare.

Phase 2, **epidemiological assessment,** is the step in which the planners use data to identify and rank the health goals or problems that may contribute to or interact with problems identified in Phase 1. These data include traditional vital indicators (e.g., mortality, morbidity, and disability data) as well as genetic, behavioral, and environmental factors (Green & Kreuter, 2005). Genetic factors are a new addition to the model and represent the rapidly expanding relationship between genes and various illnesses, risk factors, and biological conditions (Green & Kreuter). "Behavioral factors refer to the patterns of behavior of individuals and groups that protect or put them at risk for a given health or social problem" (Green & Kreuter, p. 14). Environmental factors exist outside the person and can be changed to support behavior, health, or quality of life (Green & Kreuter). These factors may be related to the economy or the social circumstances of the priority population. They also involve services and resources (or lack thereof) available in the surrounding community. It is important to note that ranking the health problems in this phase is critical, because there are rarely, if ever, enough resources to deal with all or multiple problems. Also, this phase of the model is used to plan health programs. However, a planner may be employed by or associated with an organization that has already collected data related to Phases 1–2 as part of a long-term planning effort. In this case, it may be necessary or even advantageous to skip the first two phases and move directly to Phase 3 (Green & Kreuter, 2005). Note that in Figure 2.2, arrows connect the genetics, behavior, and environment boxes of Phase 2 with the health box of Phase 2 and with Phase 1.

Once identified, the risk factors and/or determinants need to be prioritized. This can be accomplished by first ranking the factors/conditions by importance and changeability and then using the 2×2 matrix presented in **Figure 2.3**.

Phase 3, **educational and ecological assessment**, identifies and classifies the many factors that have the potential to influence a given behavior into three categories: predisposing, reinforcing, and enabling. **Predisposing factors** include knowledge and many affective traits such as a person's attitude, values, beliefs, and perceptions. These factors can facilitate or hinder a person's motivation to change and can be altered through *direct* communication. Barriers or vehicles created mainly by societal forces or systems make up **enabling factors**, which include access to health care facilities, availability of resources, referrals to appropriate providers, enactment of rules or laws, and the development of skills. **Reinforcing factors** comprise the different types of feedback and rewards that those in the priority population receive after behavior change, which may either encourage or discourage the continuation of the behavior. Reinforcing behaviors can be delivered by, but not limited to, family, friends, peers, teachers, self, and others who control rewards. "Social benefits – such as recognition, appreciation, or admiration; physical benefits such as convenience, comfort, relief of discomfort, or pain; tangible rewards such as economic benefits or avoidance of cost; and self actualizing, imagined, or vicarious rewards such as improved appearance, self-respect, or association with an admired person who demonstrates the behavior – all reinforce behavior" (Green & Kreuter, 2005, p. 15).

	More important	Less important
More changeable	High priority for program focus (Quadrant 1)	Low priority except to demonstrate change for political purposes (Quadrant 3)
Less changeable	Priority for innovative program; evaluation crucial (Quadrant 2)	No program (Quadrant 4)

Figure 2.3 Prioritization matrix

Source: Lawrence W. Green & Marshall W. Kreuter, *Health Promotion & Planning,* 3/e. Copyright © 1999 Mayfield Publishing. Reprinted by permission of McGraw-Hill Companies, Inc.

Phase 4 is comprised of two parts: (a) **Intervention Alignment**; and (b) **Administrative and Policy Assessment**. The intent of intervention alignment is to match appropriate strategies and interventions with projected changes and outcomes identified in earlier phases (Green & Kreuter, 2005). In administration and policy assessment, planners determine if the capabilities and resources are available to develop and implement the program. It is between Phases 4 and 5 that PRECEDE (the assessment portion of the model) ends and PROCEED (implementation and evaluation) begins. However, there is not a distinct break between the two phases; they really run together, and planners can move back and forth between them.

The four final phases of the model—Phases 5, 6, 7, and 8—make up the PROCEED portion. In Phase 5— **implementation**—with appropriate resources in hand, planners select the methods and strategies of the intervention, and implementation begins. Phases 6, 7, and 8 focus on the **process, impact,** and **outcome evaluation**, respectively, and are based on the earlier phases of the model, when objectives were outlined in the assessment process. Whether all three of these final phases are used depends on the evaluation requirements of the program. Usually, the resources needed to conduct evaluations of impact (Phase 7) and outcome (Phase 8) are much greater than those needed to conduct process evaluation (Phase 6). (See Chapter 6 for a discussion on the relationship of objectives to evaluation.)

Applying PRECEDE-PROCEED

To assist you in understanding how PRECEDE-PROCEED is used, consider the following hypothetical example using a worksite setting. Remember Phase 1 of the model, social assessment, seeks to define the quality of life of the priority population so that the desired outcomes can be identified. This is best done by including those in the priority population. In a worksite, planners would need to involve both the employer and the employees in the process of assessing needs. Thus, having representation from the various groups within the priority population (labor, management, clerical, etc.) on a planning committee, and letting this committee coordinate a self-study of the priority population would be advised. In this worksite setting, it would not be surprising to find such an assessment identifying that employers are concerned with economic outcomes of the company—or turning a profit. Employees may also be concerned about economic outcomes—their own salary or wages—but also about working conditions. Social indicators that may reflect these desired outcomes include production rates, absenteeism for all reasons (use of personal days, vacation days, and sick days), aesthetics of the work environment, morale of the workers, lack of quality leisure time, and low self-worth as an employee of this company.

In Phase 2 of the model, epidemiological assessment, planners use data to identify and rank health goals or problems that are associated with the economic concerns and working conditions discovered in Phase 1. They also need to identify risk factors or determinants of health in the genetics, behavioral patterns, and environment of the population (Green & Kreuter, 2005). Therefore, planners would want to collect and analyze data that reflect the health status of the workforce. Such sources of data could include reviewing the reasons for the use of sick days, reviewing company safety records, providing health screenings for all employees so that physiological risk factors can be identified, and analyzing the health and disability insurance claims of the company. Once identified, planners need to rank those health concerns as they relate to the quality-of-life issues identified in Phase 1. Common occupational diseases and disorders that arise in work settings include musculoskeletal conditions (e.g., back injuries), dermatological conditions resulting from exposure to chemical or other agents, and lung diseases resulting from the inhalation of toxic substances (McKenzie, Pinger, & Kotecki, 2005). For the purpose of this example, let's assume that back injuries received the highest priority in the epidemiological assessment. Employees with back injuries have both an impact on the economic outcome of the company via lost productivity and on the quality of life of the employee who is off the job.

Having prioritized back injuries as the health concern, planners also want to determine what risk factors or determinants contribute to the back injuries. Is lifting a significant part of the employees' work? If so, are they using good lifting techniques? Are they lifting more weight than they should? Is the work environment conducive to the work the employees are asked to do? Is the work area set up in an ergonomically correct way? Have the workers been provided with appropriate back supports? Answers to these questions will provide the planners with the information they need to conduct the educational and ecological assessment, Phase 3.

The educational and ecological assessment may include (1) surveying the employees to find out what they know about lifting, (2) surveying the employer to find out what kind of training and equipment are provided for new employees and determining what policies are in place to reward injury-free work days, and (3) observing the workers to determine if they are using good lifting techniques. From this assessment, it might be found that the workers know little about appropriate lifting techniques (predisposing factor), they have not been taught any skills for proper lifting, nor have they been provided with back supports (enabling factors), and they are not rewarded for injury-free days (reinforcing factor). Thus, planners decide that an appropriate health promotion intervention would be comprised of an education component to increase knowledge and skills, and the implementation of new corporate polices that require the use of back braces and financial bonuses for a certain number of injury-free work hours.

Through the intervention alignment and administrative and policy assessment (Phase 4), planners must determine what intervention or series of strategies will bring about desired changes and what organizational and administrative support and resources are available to carry out the health promotion intervention. Will the educational component of the intervention be conducted on company time, employee time, or a combination of the two? Can the educational component of the intervention be conducted by a current employee or will a consultant have to be hired? Are there financial resources to buy every employee a back brace or will braces have to be shared between workers on the different shifts?

Once the intervention is identified and availability of program resources is determined, Phase 5, implementation, can begin. The evaluation components (Phases 6, 7, and 8) of this program will be based on the objectives that were created during assessment phases. As each of the objectives were written, it would be important to ensure that criteria (standards of acceptability) noted in each objective were clear. For example, in Phase 6 (process evaluation), planners may be concerned with determining the availability of the educational component of the intervention for each employee. In Phase 7 (impact evaluation), planners would be interested in evaluating changes in the behavior of the employees (e.g., proper lifting technique) and the work environment (e.g., availability of back braces for employees). As for outcome evaluation, Phase 8, planners may be looking for a reduction in the incidence and prevalence of back injuries, or an increase in productivity.

MATCH

MATCH is an acronym for Multilevel Approach to Community Health. This planning model (see **Figure 2.4**) was developed in the late 1980s (Simons-Morton et al., 1988). Like the PRECEDE-PROCEED model, MATCH has also been used in professional practice, including the development of several intervention handbooks created by the Centers for Disease Control and Prevention (Simons-Morton et al., 1995). MATCH is an ecological planning perspective that recognizes that intervention approaches can and should be aimed at a variety of objectives and individuals (B. Simons-Morton, personal communication, October 10, 1999). This is represented in Figure 2.4 by the various levels of influence. The MATCH framework is recognized for emphasizing program implementation (Simons-Morton et al., 1995). "MATCH is designed to be applied when behavioral and environmental risk and protective factors for disease or injury are generally known and when general priorities for action have been determined, thus providing a convenient way to turn the corner from needs assessment and priority setting to the development of effective programs" (Simons-Morton et al,, 1995, p 155).

The Phases and Steps of MATCH

As can be seen in **Box 2.2**, MATCH is comprised of five phases and several steps within each phase. Phase I of MATCH is *goals selection*. In this phase of MATCH, planners select health-status goals based on several different factors, including the prevalence of the health problem, the relative significance of the health problem, the changeability of the problem, and other considerations unique to the setting. Also in this phase, planners need to select the priority population, identify the health behaviors most associated with the health-status goals in order to create health behavior goals, and identify the environmental factors—such as access, availability of resources, enabling practices, and barriers—so that environmental goals can be created (Simons-Morton et al., 1995).

In Phase II of MATCH, *intervention planning*, the planner "matches intervention objectives with the intervention targets and intervention actions" (Simons-Morton et al., 1995, p. 163). This begins with identifying the targets of the intervention actions (TIAs). TIAs are those individuals who exert influence or control over the personal or environmental conditions that are related to the target health and behavior goals (i.e., the level of society at which the intervention will be aimed). The levels include (1) individual level (e.g., persons in the priority population), (2) interpersonal level (e.g., family members, coworkers, friends, teachers, and others close to those in the priority population),

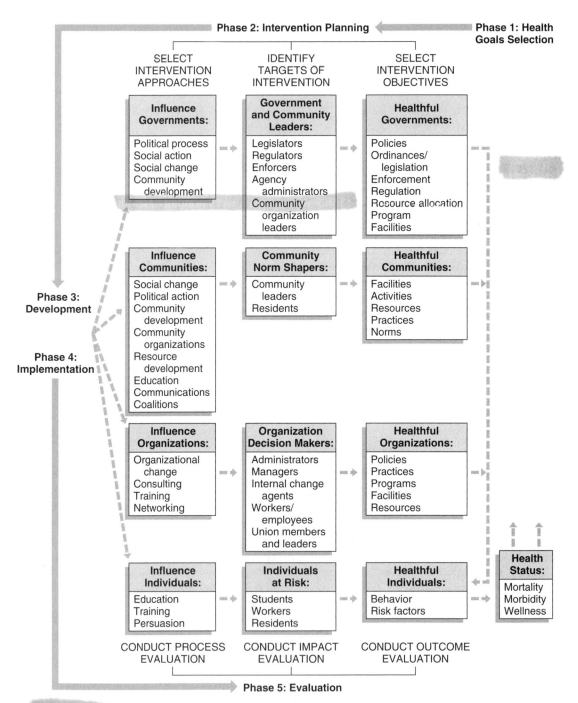

Figure 2.4 MATCH: multilevel approach to community health

Source: B. G. Simmons-Morton et al., *Introduction to Health Education and Health Promotion, 2/e.* Copyright © 1995 Waveland Press, Inc. Reprinted by permission of Waveland Press, Long Grove, IL. All rights reserved.

Box 2.2   MATCH PHASES AND STEPS

Phase 1: Goals Selection

Step 1: Select health-status goals
Step 2: Select high-priority population(s)
Step 3: Identify health behavior goals
Step 4: Identify environmental factor goals

Phase 2: Intervention Planning

Step 1: Identify the targets of the intervention
Step 2: Select intervention objectives
Step 3: Identify mediators of the intervention objectives
Step 4: Select intervention approaches

Phase 3: Program Development

Step 1: Create program units or components
Step 2: Select or develop curricula and create intervention guides
Step 3: Develop session plans
Step 4: Create or acquire instructional materials, products, and resources

Phase 4: Implementation Preparations

Step 1: Facilitate adoption, implementation, and maintenance
Step 2: Select and train implementors

Phase 5: Evaluation

Step 1: Conduct process evaluation
Step 2: Measure impact
Step 3: Monitor outcomes

Source: B. G. Simmons-Morton et al., *Introduction to Health Education and Health Promotion, 2/e.* Copyright ©
1995 Waveland Press, Inc. Reprinted by permission of Waveland Press, Long Grove, IL. All rights reserved.

(3) organizational level (e.g., a decision maker in an organization), (4) societal level
(e.g., community leaders), and (5) governmental level. After identifying the TIAs, they
are matched with the health behavioral and environmental factors identified in Phase I.
Once this match is made, the planner selects an intervention action(s) to be used. Intervention actions commonly used by health educators include teaching, training, counseling, policy advocacy, consulting, community organization, social marketing, and social
action. If the TIAs are individuals, planners need to consider those mediating factors
causally associated with target behaviors, such as knowledge, attitudes, skills, experiences, and reinforcements (Simons-Morton et al., 1995).

The third phase of MATCH is *program development* and begins with the creation of
the program units or components. Components are frequently organized according to a
priority population subgroup (e.g., males, females, minority or age groups), proposed
objectives (e.g., smoking, diet, physical activity), intervention target and level, setting and
structural unit (e.g., classroom, food service, health services), or intervention approach

or channel (e.g., interpersonal, media) (Simons-Morton et al., 1995). After the creation of the program components, planners either select from already developed curricula or develop their own guides. This would include the development of individual session or lesson plans, and the acquisition or creation of instructional materials, products, and resources (Simons-Morton et al., 1995).

In Phase IV, *implementation preparations,* planners prepare for implementation and conduct the interventions. To achieve effective implementation, planners must (1) develop a specific proposal and advocate for the adoption of change; (2) develop the need, readiness, and environmental supports for change; (3) provide evidence that the intervention works; (4) identify and select change agents and opinion leaders and convince them of the need for change; and (5) establish good working relationships with the decision makers (Simons-Morton et al., 1995). In addition, depending on who will implement the program, there may be a need to select, train, support, and monitor those who perform the implementation (Simons-Morton et al., 1995).

Phase V of MATCH is *evaluation.* Like the PRECEDE-PROCEED model, MATCH's evaluation also includes process, impact, and outcome components. "Process evaluation is concerned with the utility of the implementation plan and procedures, the extent and quality of implementation, and the effects of implementation on immediate learning outcomes" (Simons-Morton et al., 1995, p. 183). Impact evaluation is concerned with measuring the targeted mediators (usually knowledge, attitudes, and practices), health behaviors, and environmental factors (Simons-Morton et al., 1995). Outcome evaluation is typically focused on health behaviors but may also monitor long-term maintenance of changes in behavior or environmental factors. However, because of the time it takes for some outcomes to develop, there are often occasions in program planning when there is not enough time or resources to do outcome evaluation (Simons-Morton et al., 1995).

Applying MATCH

To help you understand the phases and steps of MATCH, consider this implementation example. As you read through this example, it will help if you refer to a diagram of the model in Figure 2.4. As is common when using MATCH, let's assume that the needs assessment is complete and that heart disease is the focus of the program we are planning. The behavioral risk factors that are apparent are lack of exercise and poor eating habits, and the environmental risk factors we are concerned with are the lack of exercise facilities in the community and meals served in the school lunch program. See **Table 2.1** for a presentation of the program focus.

We begin our planning with goals selection (Phase I). Based on the epidemiological data available to us, it is obvious that heart disease is the leading cause of death in our

Table 2.1   Behavioral and environmental risk factors for MATCH example

Health Problem	Behavioral Risk Factors	Environmental Risk Factors
Heart disease	**1.** Lack of exercise **2.** Poor eating habits	**1.** Lack of exercise facilities **2.** School lunch program

community and that the heart disease death rate is much greater than the national rate. We also know that several of the behaviors associated with the disease are changeable. Therefore, our health-status goal will be to reduce the prevalence of heart disease. We have decided to focus on elementary school children for the program because they are accessible, they possess a number of the behavioral risks, and the school administration is interested in seeing such a program in the school. The health behavior goals chosen will be to decrease sedentary lifestyle and to improve eating habits. These were chosen because of their prevalence in the children, their association with heart disease, and their changeability. Environmental goals will focus on available exercise facilities, the school's curriculum with regard to physical activity and nutrition, and school policies that can influence physical activity and eating habits.

For Phase II, intervention planning, we need to identify the levels of society at which we plan to intervene, what our intervention objectives will be, the mediators with which we will be concerned, and what intervention approaches we will take (see **Table 2.2**). It is decided that we will intervene at the (1) individual level, with the fifth- and sixth-graders, to influence their exercise and eating behaviors with an educational approach aimed at knowledge, attitudes, skills, and behaviors; (2) organizational level, with the members of the board of education, school administrators, teachers, and school cafeteria workers, to change the physical education and nutrition curricula and policies related to the creation of school lunch menus via organization change and training approaches; and (3) governmental level, with the city parks and recreation division, to lobby for enhanced resources by better equipping the recreational areas within the city.

Phase III, program development, will focus on several program components, including (1) the training of teachers for classroom instruction for the fifth- and sixth-graders in physical activity and nutrition, (2) the training of cafeteria workers to create healthier

Table 2.2   MATCH Phase II—objectives, mediators, and intervention approaches by societal level

Step 1 **Focus of the Intervention**	Step 2 **Objectives**	Step 3 **Mediators**	Step 4 **Intervention Approaches**
Individual Students • 5th-graders • 6th-graders	Health behaviors • Exercise • Eating habits	Knowledge Attitudes Skills Behavior	*Educational* • Teaching • Positive reinforcement
Organizational Board of education School administrators Teachers School cafeteria workers	Programs Practices Policies Resources	Knowledge Attitudes Skills Behavior	*Organizational Change* • Curricula change • School lunch menu policy • In-service training
Governmental City council City parks and recreation board City parks and recreation workers	Programs Practices Policies Resources	Knowledge Attitudes Skills Behavior	*Political Action* • Lobbying • Policy advocacy • Interest-group pressure

school lunches, and (3) lobbying the city parks and recreation board for better equipped parks. The training for the teachers will include the selection or development of a curriculum, scheduled in-service sessions, and the acquisition of the materials to support the curriculum development. A similar approach will be taken with the cafeteria workers by conducting in-service sessions aimed at planning and preparing nutritious meals. In preparation for the lobbying, policy advocacy, and interest-group pressure of city council and the parks and recreation board, sessions will need to be planned with appropriate resources to training advocates in political action techniques.

With the program components in place, Phase IV, implementation preparations, can begin. Planners will next facilitate the adoption, implementation, and maintenance of their program components by preparing those impacted by the program for change. This will mean selling them on the need for change. This can be done by showing those who are affected the possible consequences of no change, that many of the opinion leaders in the community support the change, and that similar programs have been successful in other communities. Of course, with implementation, planners will need to select and, if necessary, train the implementors so they can conduct the in-service sessions for the teachers and cafeteria workers, and prepare those who will be lobbying the city parks and recreation board.

Finally, the planners will need to plan for program evaluation (Phase V). Process evaluation will examine the success of the implementation of the various program components. How was the quality of the in-service sessions? What was good about them? How could they be improved? What were the immediate learning outcomes for the teachers, cafeteria workers, and those learning lobbying skills? What was the quality of the curriculum offered for the fifth- and sixth-graders? How did the implementation go with the school lunches using the new menu? The impact evaluation will measure the knowledge, attitudes, and health practices of the fifth- and sixth-graders with regard to physical activity and nutrition. It will also include an examination of changes that may have occurred at the city parks. Since the health goal of the program was to reduce the prevalence of heart disease in the community and aimed at students in grades 5 and 6, the resources would not be available to track these students for a long period of time. Thus, outcome evaluation would not be conducted.

Consumer-Based Planning

PRECEDE-PROCEED and MATCH are examples of planning models that have been used successfully in many health promotion settings. It is important for planners to understand and be able to apply these models. Although these and other planning models presented in this chapter may incorporate data from the consumer (priority population) in the planning process, in *consumer-based planning*, most, if not all program decisions are based on consumer input and made with consumers in mind. In other words, consumer-based planning includes consumers throughout the entire planning process. Data are collected to understand the wants, needs, and preferences of consumers themselves, then used to continually test all aspects of intervention and communication strategies. There is some evidence to suggest that this planning approach may be more effective than traditional approaches used in health promotion (Neiger & Thackeray, 2002).

Two methodologies that typically apply a consumer-based planning strategy are health communication and social marketing. Social marketing, in particular, is defined and characterized by its consumer orientation. Though they are generally considered distinct approaches, they both craft communication strategies, develop interventions, and perform evaluations to improve programs only after they identify who their consumers are, what they need, and how they will respond and change most effectively.

Health Communication

Health communication is the use of strategies to inform and influence individual and community decisions to enhance health (NCI, 2002). It can also be defined by the form it takes in health promotion programs (i.e., mass media, media advocacy, risk communication, public relations, entertainment education, print material, electronic communication). The effective use of health communication principles can be used narrowly to design an intervention such as a brochure or website, or it can be used broadly to design a multidimensional communication campaign.

The sophistication with which health information is communicated has changed dramatically over the last few decades (USDHHS, 2000). The private sector, in particular, has been successful in designing communication and marketing campaigns that combine cutting-edge technology with segmentation approaches and tailored messages. For example, consumers increasingly receive health information from nontraditional sources including downloads to devices such as MP3 players, personal digital assistants (PDAs), and cell phones, as well as technologies such as pod casts and Internet-based blogs and webinars. To compete for the attention and participation of consumers, those who plan health promotion programs must either develop a working knowledge of these communication technologies or have the foresight to access those who can provide the necessary expertise. Research indicates that effective health communication campaigns adapt audience-centered approaches (USDHHS, 2000). This requires that planners understand consumer tendencies, needs, and preferences before designing campaigns and messages.

Planners must also avoid attaching unrealistic expectations to their health communication campaigns. For example, health communication alone is rarely sufficient to change behavior and reduce the risk of disease. It can, however, influence attitudes, perceptions, awareness, knowledge, and social norms, which all tend to act as precursors to behavior change. A one-dimensional approach to health promotion that relies solely on mass media without proper program support strategies or interventions has been shown to be insufficient (USDHHS, 2000).

Planners must also be able to communicate with multiple audiences using multiple channels. In addition to the primary population of interest, secondary and tertiary audiences such as health promotion partners, health care providers, the news media, and policymakers, must receive appropriate health communication to support the basic objectives of a campaign (Nelson, Brownson, Remington, & Parvanta 2002).

Although the use of health communication alone is usually insufficient to change behaviors or impact health status, it does play an important role in influencing health knowledge, beliefs, and attitudes. During the next 10 years, the application of new technologies in health communication will provide cost-effective applications that can be more easily tailored to large numbers of people (Suggs, 2006). In response, health promotion planners and practitioners must be ready to adapt to the rapidly evolving communication environment in which they work.

Social Marketing

Social marketing applied to health campaigns has been used successfully in domestic settings for nearly 40 years and even longer in international settings. **Social marketing** is "the application of commercial marketing technologies to the analysis, planning, execution, and evaluation of programs designed to influence the voluntary behavior of target audiences in order to improve their personal welfare and that of their society" (Andreasen, 1995, p. 7).

A frequent misinterpretation of social marketing is that it is limited to narrow interventions, such as communication or advertising strategies. Used correctly, social marketing is best viewed as a planning framework that positions consumers at the core of all activity. Although it is not necessarily a complicated process, it can represent a time-consuming and resource-intense process.

Early international social marketing interventions focused primarily on immunizations, family planning, agricultural reforms, and nutrition (Walsh et al., 1993). Social marketing activity in the United States has focused on diverse issues, including the prevention of AIDS and cardiovascular disease, low-fat eating, the Five-a-Day Campaign, prevention and treatment of drug use, and breast cancer screening (Neiger et al., 2001).

Based on the results of a Delphi survey conducted among leading social marketing authorities (Maibach, Shenker, & Singer, 1997), 10 key elements displayed in **Box 2.3** probably best characterize social marketing. What becomes most apparent is that social

---

Box 2.3 KEY ELEMENTS THAT BEST CHARACTERIZE THE PRACTICE OF SOCIAL MARKETING

- Audience-centered program development
- Promotion of voluntary behavior change
- Audience segmentation and profiling
- Formative research to develop and test programs
- A range of product development based on audience research
- Product distribution based on audience research
- Program promotion through channels identified in audience research
- Process evaluation
- Outcome evaluation
- Audience and community involvement in the planning process

Source: Maibach, Shenker, and Singer (1997).

marketing attempts to strategically understand the consumer and ensure that interventions are based not only on consumer input but also tested with consumers before being implemented. This is different from traditional health promotion practice. In fact, the hallmark of social marketing is a continual focus on the consumers who will eventually participate in the health promotion program. Therefore, consumers should be placed at the center of all program planning and implementation by addressing not only their wants and needs, but also their concerns. The most critical responsibility of social marketers is an assurance that what is finally offered in the form of an intervention satisfies consumer wants and needs.

Two models that capture the critical characteristics of health communication and social marketing are CDCynergy and SMART, respectively. They both focus on priority audiences, rely heavily on consumer data for decision making, and attempt to continually return to the consumer for feedback and program improvement.

CDCynergy

Perhaps the most comprehensive and theoretically based health communication planning model is **CDCynergy**, or **Cynergy** for short, developed by the Office of Communication at the Centers for Disease Control and Prevention (CDC) in the mid-1990s. Although it is an interactive CD-ROM tool, its contents resemble most planning models and contain the basic components outlined in the generalized model (see Figure 2.1), and included in both the PRECEDE-PROCEED and MATCH models.

CDCynergy was developed primarily for public health professionals at the CDC with responsibilities for health communication. However, because of widespread interest in the model, CDC made it available to other health professionals who found the model useful for health promotion in community, worksite, school, and health care (including managed care) settings. Currently, *CDCynergy* is considered public domain (meaning restrictions are not placed on copying or general use). A copy of *CDCynergy* can be obtained via training by the Society for Public Health Education (SOPHE), or directly from the Public Health Foundation.

The basic edition of CDCynergy (3.0) presents a general methodology for health communication planning, a step-by-step guide, a reference library, and links to templates that allow tailored plans to be created (CDC, 2003). In addition, CDC and its partners have produced tailored editions of Cynergy to meet the specific needs of planners addressing various health problems. These editions include: cardiovascular disease, immunizations, micronutrients, diabetes, tobacco prevention and control, emergency risk communication, and social marketing. CDC has also produced an abbreviated edition of the model entitled *CDCynergy Lite* (see **Box 2.4**) to help practitioners expedite the health communication planning process when necessary.

The Phases of CDCynergy   Cynergy uses six phases involving multiple steps to help planners acquire a thorough understanding of a health problem and who it affects; explore a wide range of possible strategies for influencing the problem; systematically select the strategies that show the most promise; understand the role communication can play in planning, implementing, and evaluating selected strategies; and develop a comprehensive communication plan (CDC, 2003). Box 2.4 displays the six sequential and interrelated phases.

Box 2.4   *CDCYNERGY LITE*—AN ABRIDGED VERSION OF THE CDCYNERGY HEALTH COMMUNICATION MODEL

Phase 1: Describe Problem

- Identify and define health problems that may be addressed by your program interventions.
- Examine and/or conduct necessary research to describe the problems.
- Assess factors and variables that can affect the project's direction, including strengths, weaknesses, opportunities, and threats (SWOT).

Phase 2: Analyze Problem

- List causes of each problem you plan to address.
- Develop goals for each problem.
- Consider strengths, weaknesses, opportunities, threats, and ethics of health: (1) engineering, (2) communication/education, (3) policy/enforcement, and (4) community service intervention options.
- Select the types of intervention(s) that should be used to address the problem(s).

Phase 3: Plan Intervention

- Decide whether communication is needed as a dominant intervention and/or as support for other intervention(s).
  - If communication is used as a dominant intervention, list possible audiences.
  - If communication is to be used to support community services, engineering, and/or policy/enforcement interventions, list possible audiences to be reached in support of each selected intervention.
- Conduct necessary audience research to segment intended audiences.
- Select audience segment(s) and write communication objectives for each audience segment.
- Write a creative brief to provide guidance in selecting appropriate concepts/ messages, settings, activities, and materials.

Phase 4: Develop Intervention

- Develop and test concepts, messages, settings, channel-specific activities, and materials with intended audiences.
- Finalize and briefly summarize a communication implementation plan. The plan should include:
  - Background and justification, including SWOT and ethics analyses
  - Audiences
  - Communication objectives
  - Messages
  - Settings and channels for conveying your messages
  - Activities (including tactics, materials, and other methods)
  - Available partners and resources

Box 2.4   CONTINUED

- ♦ Tasks and timeline (including persons responsible for each task, date for completion of each task, resources required to deliver each task, and points at which progress will be checked)
- ♦ Internal and external communication plan
- ♦ Budget
- Produce materials for dissemination.

Phase 5: Plan Evaluation

- Determine stakeholder information needs.
  - Decide which types of evaluation (e.g., implementation, reach, effects) are needed to satisfy stakeholder information needs.
  - Identify sources of information and select data collection methods.
  - Formulate an evaluation design that illustrates how methods will be applied to gather credible information.
  - Develop a data analysis and reporting plan.
    - ♦ Finalize and briefly summarize an evaluation implementation plan. The plan should include:
    - ♦ Stakeholder questions
    - ♦ Intervention standards
    - ♦ Evaluation methods and design
    - ♦ Data analysis and reporting
    - ♦ Tasks and timeline (including persons responsible for each task, date for completion of each task, resources required to deliver each task, and points at which progress will be checked)
    - ♦ Internal and external communication plan
    - ♦ Budget

Phase 6: Implement Plan

- Integrate, execute, and manage communication and evaluation plans.
- Document feedback and lessons learned.
- Modify program components based on feedback.
- Disseminate lessons learned and evaluation findings.

Source: Centers for Disease Control and Prevention. (2003).

The first phase of CDCynergy is called *Describe Problem*. Like other planning models, CDCynergy initially relies on good epidemiologic data and professional expertise to identify a primary health problem or contributing factor that merits attention and resources. Although programs and interventions are not generally implemented in a consumer-based model before obtaining adequate consumer input, an initial focus based on epidemiology or other good information is important to set the planning process in the right direction. Phase 1 requires the planner to state the problem and determine if the organization has the authority, capacity, and justification to address the problem (CDC, 2003).

A short written problem statement assesses the difference between what is occurring and what should occur in relation to the identified health problem. Using epidemiologic data, the problem is described in terms of who is affected and to what extent, where the problem exists geographically, when it occurs, and any related trends that may be evident. The problem statement also determines and describes distinct subgroups affected by the health problem.

In addition to describing the scope and magnitude of the problem, Phase 1 examines whether the organization is in a good position to address the problem. To help make this determination, Cynergy encourages planners to answer several questions related to current strengths, weaknesses, opportunities, and threats.

Finally, the organization assesses whether it has the capacity to address the problem. It does this by analyzing things such as human resources, including knowledge and expertise, technology resources, and the political climate in general. If the organization cannot adequately respond to these issues, it is important to stop the Cynergy planning process and either identify a more appropriate problem or use a more appropriate planning approach.

At the conclusion of Phase 1, program planners end up with a brief description of the problem, a rationale for why the organization is addressing the problem, and a list of factors that justify the organization's involvement with the problem (CDC, 1999a). This problem definition and description can then provide a rationale to justify a program to supervisors, funding agencies, decision makers, the public, the press, constituents, or program partners. It gives program planners confidence in decision making and provides a clear direction and foundation for subsequent phases.

Whereas Phase 1 identifies the problem and provides a rationale for why an organization is doing something about the problem, Phase 2, *Analyze Problem*, guides program planners in describing the problem in more detail. The first task in this phase is identification of factors that directly or indirectly contribute to the problem, including biology, behavior, the environment, policies (or lack of policies), other barriers, and resources. A thorough understanding of contributing factors allows the planners to more effectively identify appropriate interventions.

For example, let's assume that the problem statement in Phase 1 pertained to a lack of physical activity among older adults. Contributing factors could include a lack of awareness among older adults of the relationship between physical activity and chronic diseases. Perhaps older adults experience discomfort during and after exercise, or maybe adequate walking paths or other resources do not exist for physical activity.

A direct cause is a factor representing an immediate cause of the health problem whereas an indirect cause is something that exerts an effect on the direct cause (CDC, 2003). Following the example of lack of physical activity among older adults, a direct cause may be lack of safe and convenient walking paths. An indirect cause may be unwillingness by political leaders to spend public funds to provide these walking paths. In this sense, Cynergy helps planners step back from the primary cause and address secondary causes as well.

During Phase 2, planners also prioritize the importance of subproblems. In part, priority setting will be influenced by the complexity or difficulty of the direct and indirect causes leading to the health problem. Other criteria for priority setting may include: size and seriousness of the problem, effectiveness of interventions, community concern, and lost productivity. The process of setting priorities helps planners avoid overcommitting scarce resources and addressing too many problems. Stakeholders will ultimately decide how much time, money, personnel, and energy can be devoted to multiple populations and problems. Generally though, it is best to do fewer things well.

Once a manageable number of subproblems have been selected, goals are developed for each. These goals will merely identify general outcomes and time frames to help planners further examine relevant theories and possible interventions. Program planners consider strengths, weaknesses, opportunities, and threats (SWOT), as well as ethics related to each of the potential interventions. Phase 2 then requires planners to actually select the intervention(s) that will be implemented for each subproblem and develop a corresponding logic model that displays a sequence of all relevant steps in the planning process. Finally, given the selection of interventions, Phase 2 examines the need for new partners and resources and pursues appropriate funding.

Phase 3 is titled *Plan Intervention*. In this phase, planners must determine whether communication will play a dominant or supportive role for each intervention. For example, a dominant role might involve a community-wide media campaign that includes television and radio spots and paid advertising in newspapers to promote physical activity among older adults. A supportive communication role may be interpersonal communications with city planners to create more opportunities for physical activity in the community.

In order to identify actual audiences for interventions, segmentation is performed. This process narrows a large population to a more manageable size based on common characteristics. To do so, CDCynergy recommends that the audience segment, at a minimum, be large enough and unique enough to justify a separate communication intervention (CDC, 2003). Planners decide which segments are appropriate for interventions based on these criteria and how they intend to reach and influence these audiences with communication efforts. As in Phase 2, goals are developed, but these pertain only to communication. Relevant communication theories are considered in order to gain insight into ways to reach communication goals and direction to perform formative research (CDC, 2003).

In general, formative research is the sum of all preparation activities that occur before a program is implemented. It includes literature reviews and other research needed to develop and achieve communication and program goals. Most significantly, formative research involves research with intended audiences to understand wants, needs, and preferences before interventions are developed and implemented. This information can be collected through surveys, focus groups, in-depth interviews, public hearings, and community forums. After formative research is completed, planners should be able to develop profiles for each of the subgroups or audiences previously identified. These profiles include relevant theories and models pertaining to the audience, key data, or information on the audience that relate to its preferences, and preliminary ideas for communication concepts, messages, settings, channels, and support materials (CDC, 2003).

With the completion of audience profiles, Phase 3 requires planners to transform communication goals into specific and measurable communication objectives that specify what measurable impact and change will be experienced within the audience segments. Accompanying the communication objectives are creative briefs which are two-to four-page summaries used to guide the process of developing, testing, and tailoring communication components (i.e., messages, channel-specific activities, materials, settings) of the communication interventions produced in Phase 4 (CDC, 2003). Finally, plans are confirmed with stakeholders and partners discuss evaluation of all significant program components.

Phase 4, *Develop Intervention*, guides planners to test all concepts in the creative briefs with the intended audiences. Most often, this means holding focus groups or performing theater testing with members of the audience segment to assess their reactions. Theater testing involves large groups providing feedback on messages or audiovisual materials either electronically or via questionnaires (NCI, 2002). Adjustments are then made before production and implementation occur.

In Phase 4, planners must also decide upon settings (where the audience segment will receive or be exposed to the communication messages and interventions). Identifying an appropriate setting requires planners to determine where and when the audience is most receptive to communication. Examples include a worksite where employees might see a poster, schools where public announcements may be broadcast, or homes where television may be viewed (CDC, 2003). Other important communication variables addressed in Phase 4 include exploring possible channels and activities. A channel is the route of message delivery (i.e., interpersonal, small group, organizational, community, mass media). An activity is used within a channel to deliver a message (e.g., holding training classes to help older adults start their own walking clubs). Once activities are identified, planners must also develop necessary supporting materials (i.e., print material, curriculum, posters, public service announcements).

Before communication messages, activities and materials are implemented within appropriate channels, they are pretested (i.e., surveys, interviews, focus groups) with the audience segment. After appropriate feedback is received and incorporated, communication materials are produced for dissemination.

Phase 5, *Plan Evaluation*, follows CDC's *Framework for Program Evaluation in Public Health* (CDC, 1999c). This model, a six-step approach includes (1) engaging stakeholders, (2) describing the program, (3) focusing the evaluation design, (4) gathering credible evidence, (5) justifying conclusions, and (6) ensuring use and sharing lessons learned (see Chapter 13 for more on this framework). Planners develop a data analysis and reporting plan, formalize agreements, develop internal and external communication plans with staff and partners, and create timetables and a budget (CDC, 2003).

In specific terms, Phase 5 addresses both formative and summative evaluation (see Chapter 14 for more information on both types of evaluation). This means that those who perform evaluation are examining how well the program is being implemented and how well the consumers are responding to the communication strategies. Evaluators also determine whether changes in direct and indirect causes are being made as a result of accomplishing the communication objectives. Phase 5 includes measurements of the reach and exposure of communications, cost analysis, and relevance of theories that are linked with the communication strategies.

The final phase in Cynergy, Phase 6, is *Implement Plan*. The important components of this phase involve working with partners to (a) integrate, execute, and manage communication and evaluation plans; (b) document feedback; and (c) modify program components based on this feedback. This phase also addresses issues such as lessons learned during the course of program implementation and delivery, how these lessons can be shared with others, and how this new discovery can be directed back to the program. This includes the creation of a dissemination plan for key findings.

Careful observance and completion of all steps and phases in the Cynergy model will result in a strategic communication plan that is both science- and audience-based. This will increase the likelihood of achieving program goals and objectives and, more importantly, enhancing health among priority populations.

SMART

Although social marketing has been used to improve health for nearly 40 years, relatively few social marketing planning frameworks exist. Bryant (1998) and Andreason (1995) have outlined sequential processes to facilitate social marketing activity. Existing social marketing models were synthesized by Walsh and colleagues (1993) into a useful systematic planning framework. **SMART** (Social Marketing Assessment and Response Tool) (Neiger & Thackeray, 1998), influenced primarily by Walsh and colleagues (1993), is also a composite of these planning frameworks but differs in the sequence of steps, certain content areas, and consistency with models most often used in health promotion settings. Unlike other models, SMART has been used from start to finish on multiple occasions in successful social marketing interventions (Neiger & Thackeray, 2002). A careful review of the model provides an excellent overview of social marketing in general.

As displayed in **Box 2.5**, SMART is composed of seven phases. Like other social marketing planning models, the central focus of SMART is consumers. The heart of this model, composed of Phases 2 through 4, pertains to acquiring a broad understanding of the consumers who will be the recipients of a program and its interventions. These three phases seek to understand consumers before interventions are developed or implemented. Though these phases (2–4) are displayed in linear fashion, and for clarity will be described in sequence, they are typically performed simultaneously with members of the priority population.

The Phases of SMART   *Preliminary Planning* is critical for any type of health promotion program. It is also the first phase of SMART. Preliminary planning allows program planners to objectively assess all health problems and determine which one is most appropriate to address. This is most often accomplished through analysis of epidemiologic data, including various mortality and morbidity rates and associated risk factor data. It also includes objective priority setting with predetermined criteria. Sometimes planners do not undergo a process to select a priority health problem because the decision has already been made or the organization is dedicated to a specific health problem (e.g., the American Heart Association). Once a single health problem is determined, it is defined in terms of behaviors. Risk factors, or contributing factors, then become the focus of the social marketing process. This is similar to most health promotion programs.

Although goals are outlined in Phase 1, objectives are not. This makes sense from a social marketing perspective, since consumer research has not yet been performed. The goals are general statements of intent or direction, but they do not specify program components or direct the planner into specific courses of action.

Box 2.5	THE SMART MODEL

Phase 1: Preliminary Planning

- Identify a health problem and name it in terms of behavior.
- Develop general goals.
- Outline preliminary plans for evaluation.
- Project program costs.

Phase 2: Consumer Analysis

- Segment and identify the priority population.
- Identify formative research methods.
- Identify consumer wants, needs, and preferences.
- Develop preliminary ideas for preferred interventions.

Phase 3: Market Analysis

- Establish and define the market mix (4Ps).
- Assess the market to identify competitors (behaviors, messages, programs, etc.), allies (support systems, resources, etc.), and partners.

Phase 4: Channel Analysis

- Identify appropriate communication messages, strategies, and channels.
- Assess options for program distribution. Determine how channels should be used.
- Identify communication roles for program partners.

Phase 5: Develop Interventions, Materials, and Pretest

- Develop program interventions and materials using information collected in consumer, market, and channel analyses.
- Interpret the marketing mix into a strategy that represents exchange and societal good.
- Pretest and refine the program.

Phase 6: Implementation

- Communicate with partners and clarify involvement.
- Activate communication and distribution strategies.
- Document procedures and compare progress to time lines.
- Refine the program.

Phase 7: Evaluation

- Assess the degree to which the priority population is receiving the program.
- Assess the immediate impact on the priority population and refine the program as necessary.
- Ensure that program delivery is consistent with established protocol.
- Analyze changes in the priority population.

Source: Adapted from Walsh et al., (1993) by Neiger & Thackeray (1998).

Another task in Phase 1 is to develop preliminary plans for evaluation. Theoretically, it will make sense to most planners to consider evaluation early in the planning process. In reality, evaluation is too often an afterthought. Preliminary decisions regarding evaluation outcomes must be made up front in order to account for personnel, time, and budget requirements. Therefore, it is also important to determine how preprogram (pretest or baseline) and postprogram (posttest) data will be collected and to identify valid survey or data collection instruments. Planners can also control for various kinds of bias or error in data collection if these basic evaluation concepts are considered before the program is implemented.

Finally, program costs need to be projected before the social marketing project begins. Social marketing can be an expensive proposition in terms of staff costs and direct expenses. When performed correctly, a social marketing project can easily take a year before implementation even begins. Program planners and organizations must decide if they are ready to make these kinds of time and financial commitments. Planning for both cost-benefit and cost-effectiveness analyses, outlined in Chapter 14, are appropriate in this phase.

At the end of Phase 1, the social marketing planners have (1) identified the focus of interest in terms of modifiable behaviors, (2) developed goals that provide general direction, (3) outlined preliminary plans for evaluation, and (4) estimated total project costs. Based on this information, the planners and organizations can make an informed decision about the potential costs and benefits of the project.

Phase 2 of SMART is *Consumer Analysis*. In social marketing language, the process of performing consumer analysis is formative research. **Formative research**, as defined in social marketing, is a process that identifies differences among subgroups within a population, identifies a subgroup, determines the wants and needs of the subgroup, and identifies factors that influence its behavior, including benefits, barriers, and readiness to change (Bryant, 1998).

As discussed in CDCynergy, it is important to narrow a large and perhaps unwieldy population into smaller segments that make a project more manageable. Segmentation also allows a planner to focus on a subpopulation that is either at highest risk or, for other important reasons, is the most appropriate focus for social marketing interventions. At times, and perhaps too often, health promotion programs are extended to anyone and everyone in the population. Dismal program results are then discouraging and perplexing. In contrast, programs that segment populations based on factors such as readiness to change, interest, learning style, support, self-efficacy, and locus of control hold more promise for successful outcomes (Albrecht & Bryant, 1996).

Segmentation can be performed with geographic, demographic, psychographic, attitudinal, or behavioral criteria. Attitudinal variables involve judgments about products and services, benefits sought, and readiness to change. Behavioral variables include rationale for purchase decisions, product use, user status, and loyalty level (Albrecht & Bryant, 1996). (See Chapter 11 for more information on segmentation.)

Once a priority audience has been segmented, and only after segmentation has occurred, does the bulk of formative research occur—that is, actually talking to consumers in the priority population about their wants, needs, and preferences. A commonly used method is focus groups. In-depth interviews, key informant interviews, public hearings, opinion polls, and a variety of other survey techniques can also be used to collect information about the priority population. The purpose of these techniques is to find out what consumers think about the health problem that has been identified as well as its related behaviors or contributing factors. (See Chapter 4 for different techniques of data collection.)

It is important to remember that no single type of data collection technique is necessarily best in performing formative research. To the contrary, it is helpful to use multiple methods to gain a better perspective of the priority population. It is a mistake for those who engage in social marketing to perform one or two focus groups in the name of consumer analysis and allege they understand their consumers.

At the conclusion of Phase 2, a priority population is identified. Adequate formative research has been performed yielding data about major themes, directions, and consumer preferences related to the health problem and related interventions. Although Phases 2 through 4 are often performed simultaneously, information collected in Phase 2 can provide context for the other two phases. For example, knowing about consumer preferences related to some type of behavior change allows planners to more effectively understand consumer preferences related to the market mix and communication strategies.

Phase 3, *Market Analysis,* examines the fit between the focus of interest (desired behavior change) and important market variables within the priority population. *Marketing mix* is a term that is often used in both commercial and social marketing. It is composed of four components, also known as the 4Ps: product, price, place, promotion. (See Chapter 11 for a discussion of the 4Ps.)

All of the factors in the market mix are analyzed in context of the priority population and provide additional issues that should be addressed in the formative research process. Market analysis also analyzes the marketplace to identify competitors and allies. For example, a competitor in social marketing may be anything that vies for the necessary resources to engage in the behavior as prescribed. If the product is an exercise program that combines strength training and cardiovascular endurance, a competitor may be a toning program that focuses on different approaches. A busy schedule may be a competitor. An ally may be a supportive workplace that encourages and even promotes exercise behavior.

At the conclusion of this phase, consumer analysis is enriched by a better understanding of important market variables that influence consumers. Combined with consumer analysis and channel analysis, market analysis provides a powerful combination of useful information about consumers, the environment they live in, and strengths and weakness associated with potential social marketing interventions.

The fourth phase of SMART is *Channel Analysis.* Although communication may not be the focal point of a social marketing campaign, it will play a secondary role in communicating important messages about the product. In addition to messages and related strategies, formative research includes specific questions about the type of communication channels consumers believe are most appropriate for the behavior change in question. As described in CDCynergy, communication channels include interpersonal, small group, organizational, community, and mass media channels. Channels also relate to place in the market mix or how the product is accessed. In other words, the channel must be appropriate for the way the product is distributed. For example, if the product is increased vegetable consumption and the place is the worksite cafeteria, an appropriate channel might be an organizational newsletter.

In most cases, the use of multiple channels increases the likelihood that the messages will be heard and acted upon. However, if the message is not consumer oriented and is not adequately supported by an effective market mix, the channel itself is relatively unimportant. That is why all these factors are planned in unison.

Finally, Phase 4 considers which potential partners, if any, might collaborate in sharing the burden of communication. For example, if mass media is an appropriate channel, and consumer-oriented public service announcements are used in the communication strategy, perhaps television and radio stations would be willing to donate air time. One problem frequently experienced in social marketing is that multiple organizations with similar missions communicate competing, albeit only slightly different, messages. In extreme cases, the messages can be nearly polar opposites. For this reason alone, it is important to develop communication partners. At the conclusion of Phase 4, communication channels are identified that are consistent with preliminary messages, and product distribution points and potential communication and intervention partners are identified.

Phase 5 of SMART consists of *Developing Interventions, Materials, and Pretesting.* Once formative research is performed, it is critical that the data are transferred or infused adequately into the design of programs, interventions, and communication strategies. To do this, data must be analyzed and categorized appropriately to assure that planners understand what they have seen, heard, and observed. As planners meet to design programs and materials, they should keep formative research data in front of them and refer to them often. Discussion and decisions should reflect all data and represent a consensus among all planners. In other words, materials and methods should represent what was learned in formative research.

Once a program prototype is developed, it is imperative to return to the priority population and test the concepts before implementing a widespread campaign. In fact, social marketing represents a process of continually returning to the consumers until the program and all its support mechanisms are consistent with their views and preferences. Several mechanisms are available to perform pretesting. One example is a pilot test where the program can be implemented with the priority population on a smaller, less expensive scale. Theater testing or focus groups can also be used to test communication messages, key components of interventions, and program formats and sequences.

Phase 6 of SMART is *Implementation.* Implementation in social marketing is closely related to the implementation factors addressed in CDCynergy. This phase is concerned with clarifying everyone's role, including external partners. This means that procedures are communicated and documented, and that time lines are developed and followed. In this phase, the communication and distribution plans are activated and the actual program and its interventions are offered. In addition, the program is refined continually, based on consumer feedback.

The seventh and final phase of SMART is *Evaluation.* The preliminary evaluation strategies that were identified in Phase 1 now take effect. Evaluation always has at least two major objectives: improve the quality of the program and determine the effectiveness of the program. With respect to quality, program planners assess the degree to which the priority population, within the larger population, is actually receiving the program or interventions. Planners also assess the immediate impact the program is having and whether the interventions and related support strategies are acceptable and engaging to the priority population. Planners also ensure that program delivery is consistent with program protocol or at least consistent with developed time lines.

Ultimately, social marketing, and all its related work, is of little value unless behavior change occurs and health is improved. Evaluation also concerns itself with measuring these outcomes. Effective planners and evaluators also make sure that evaluation results are folded back into the program so that it can be improved before it is too late. This requires communicating evaluation results effectively to stakeholders.

Other Planning Models

As noted at the beginning of this chapter, other planning models are available to planners in addition to the PRECEDE-PROCEED, MATCH, CDCynergy, and SMART models. If you are interested in learning more about these models, check the original sources provided in the reference section at the back of the book.

A Systematic Approach to Health Promotion (*Healthy People 2010*)

A Systematic Approach to Health Promotion is the planning model that was used to develop *Healthy People 2010* and is composed of four key elements: (1) goals, (2) objectives, (3) determinants of health, and (4) health status. Whether used for planning activities at the national, state, or local community levels, these four elements remain the same.

As in other planning models, goals provide general direction for this approach and serve to guide the development of objectives which specify outcomes as well as time frames (USDHHS, 2000). The two general goals associated with *Healthy People 2010* are (1) increasing quality and years of healthy life, and (2) eliminating health disparities.

A total of 467 objectives involving 28 focus areas are included in *Healthy People 2010*. As in other planning initiatives, objectives specify who will be effected, what will change, where it will occur, when change will occur, and how much change will occur (see Chapter 6 for more information on goals and objectives).

The *Healthy People 2010* model clearly addresses the key determinants of health (risk or protective factors that lead to illness or well-being, respectively). Determinants in this model include behaviors (i.e., physical activity, wearing safety belts, healthy diet), biology (a person's genetic predisposition to health or disease, family history), social environment (i.e., interactions with family, friends, colleagues, and others in the community), physical environment (e.g., that which is seen, touched, heard, smelled, and tasted), policies and interventions, and access to quality health care. Collectively, these determinants have a complete effect on the health and well-being of individuals, communities, and the nation. More importantly, they represent the focus of health promotion interventions identified throughout *Healthy People 2010*. In order to change the health status of a community, planners must ultimately address and modify key determinants.

Finally, health status (i.e., death rates, life expectancy, quality of life, morbidity from specific diseases), the ultimate standard of success by which health promotion can be evaluated, is determined as a baseline measure and later as a target measurement.

Mobilizing for Action through Planning and Partnerships (MAPP)

Mobilizing for Action through Planning and Partnerships (**MAPP**) was developed by the National Association of County and City Health Officials (NACCHO). As such, it represents a planning approach common to city or county health departments (also known as local health departments). The vision for implementing the MAPP approach involves improving health and quality of life through mobilized partnerships and taking strategic action (NACCHO, 2001). **Figure 2.5** displays the six phases of MAPP as well as the four MAPP assessments.

MAPP is composed of multiple steps in six general phases. In the first phase of MAPP, *Organizing for Success and Partnership Development,* core planners assess whether or not the MAPP process is timely, appropriate or even possible. This involves assessing resources, including budgets, the expertise of available personnel, support of key decision makers and other stakeholders, and general interest of community members. If resources are not in place, the process is delayed. If the decision is made to undertake a MAPP process, the following work groups are created: (1) a core support team, which prepares most, if not all of the material needed for the process; (2) the MAPP Committee, composed of key sponsors (usually influential figures from the private sector who lend support and other resources) and stakeholders who guide and oversee the process; and (3) the community itself, which provides input, representation, and decision making. This phase answers basic questions about the general feasibility, resources, and appropriateness of the MAPP process.

Phase 2 of the MAPP process, *Visioning,* guides the community through a process that results in a shared vision (what the ideal future looks like) and common values (principles and beliefs that will guide the remainder of the planning process) (NACCHO, 2001). Generally, a facilitator conducts the visioning process and involves anywhere from

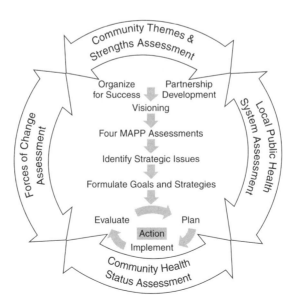

Figure 2.5 Displays the six phases of MAPP as well as the four MAPP assessments

Source: Courtesy of National Association of County & City Health Officials from *Achieving Healthier Communities through MAPP: A User's Handbook.*

50–100 participants including the advisory committee, the MAPP committee, and key community leaders.

Phase 3, the *Four MAPP Assessments,* represents the defining characteristic of the MAPP model. The four assessments include (1) the community themes and strengths assessment (community or consumer opinion), (2) the local public health assessment (general capacity of the local health department), (3) the community health status assessment (measurement of the health of the community by use of epidemiologic data), and (4) the forces of change assessment (forces such as legislation, technology, and other environmental or social phenomenon that do or will impact the community). Collectively, the MAPP assessments provide insight on the gaps that exist between current status in the community and what was learned in the visioning phase as well as strategic direction for goals and strategies (NACCHO, 2001).

In Phase 4 of MAPP, *Identify Strategic Issues,* a prioritized list of the most important issues facing the health of the community is developed. Only issues that jeopardize the vision and values of the community are considered. Important tasks in this phase include consideration of what would happen if certain issues were not addressed, understanding why an issue is strategic, consolidating overlapping issues, and identifying a prioritized list. Phase 5, *Formulate Goals and Strategies,* creates goals related to the vision and priority strategic issues. It also selects and adopts strategies. This phase is not unlike similar phases in the models that have already been discussed in this chapter. Finally, Phase 6, *The Action Cycle,* is similar to implementation and evaluation phases in other planning models. In this phase, implementation details are considered, evaluation plans (gathering credible evidence) are developed, and plans for disseminating results are made (NACCHO, 2001).

Assessment Protocol for Excellence in Public Health (APEX-PH)

Assessment Protocol for Excellence in Public Health (**APEX-PH**), a planning and assessment process also developed by NACCHO, was introduced in 1991 after extensive collaboration and testing with many public health partners (NACCHO, 1991). APEX-PH was developed initially to help county or local health departments respond to the Institute of Medicine's (IOM) report "The Future of Public Health," where it was stated that every public health agency should regularly and systematically collect, assemble, and analyze information on community health needs (IOM, 1988). Although APEX-PH has been largely subsumed by the MAPP model, some local health departments still use APEX-PH, particularly because of its first phase, the organizational assessment, which is familiar and flexible to those responsible for planning efforts.

APEX-PH is promoted by NACCHO as a planning model for local health officials to assess the organization and management of the health department, provide a framework for working with community members and other organizations in assessing the health status of the community, and establish a leadership role for the health department in the community. It is considered a flexible tool that can be easily integrated with other planning tools (NACCHO, 1991).

The APEX-PH process involves three steps. The first, *Organizational Capacity Assessment,* requires the local health department to perform an internal assessment of administrative capacity including strengths, weaknesses, resources, and expertise. Because the second step in the APEX-PH process involves a community assessment, health directors and their teams will also need to assess internal capacity to conduct a comprehensive data collection and analysis process.

The second step in APEX-PH is *The Community Process*. During this step, health data are collected and analyzed in addition to community opinion data. One challenge to this approach is finding a balance between data that are often in conflict. For example, epidemiologic data in the United States will most often dictate that chronic diseases such as heart disease, cancer, or stroke (or their determinants) be the focus of a program activity. Consumer opinion data, on the other hand, often focus on social or environmental problems such as violence, drug use, teen pregnancy, or neighborhood safety. When both types of data are collected, planners must inevitably compromise and identify multiple priorities using multiple interventions. During this step, problems are analyzed and priorities are developed.

The final step in APEX-PH, *Completing the Cycle,* is similar to the final steps in most planning models. That is, this step guides the development of policies, services, and other interventions, creates an implementation plan, and assures that all programs are monitored and evaluated.

APEX-PH has established a track record of success within local health departments. It has also spawned the development of **PACE-EH**, which is a planning protocol used by local health departments for environmental health planning. Lessons learned from APEX-PH have been successfully transferred to the MAPP model, which carries forward the tradition and promise of sequential and meaningful planning efforts within counties and cities across the United States.

SWOT (Strengths, Weaknesses, Opportunities, Threats) Analysis

The **SWOT** analysis has historically been associated with strategic planning efforts in the business and marketing sectors. In simple terms, it is an analysis of an organization's internal strengths and weaknesses, as well as opportunities and threats in the operating environment. Technically, its use should be limited to the preliminary stages of decision making in preparation for more comprehensive strategic planning (Johnson, Scholes, & Sexty, 1989; Bartol & Martin, 1991).

In health promotion practice, SWOT analyses are common among planners who want to minimize planning time and move quickly to action steps. Generally, a facilitator helps a planning group identify issues or problems, set or clarify goals, and create a plan. Common to SWOT analyses is the use of a 2×2 matrix that lists strengths and weaknesses along the horizontal axis and opportunities and threats along the vertical axis. The organization can then decide if it prefers to build on strengths or improve upon weaknesses in context of environmental opportunities and threats.

A SWOT analysis requires planners to examine their organization's strengths. This may include an assessment of what the organization does well or what it does differently or better than similar organizations, existing resources (i.e., funds, equipment, supplies, materials), expertise of personnel, quality of partnerships in the community, or track record of successful working relationships. Conversely, the SWOT analysis also examines weaknesses which may pertain to the same factors cited under strengths. In addition, weaknesses may involve a poor reputation among stakeholders, including clients. It may involve an inability to address certain health problems or determinants because of codes, regulations, policy, or management decisions that give authority to another entity.

Whereas strengths and weaknesses assessed in a SWOT analysis pertain to the organization's internal environment, opportunities and threats relate to the external environment. Opportunities may involve unfulfilled consumer needs, loosening or removal of administrative or legislative barriers that finally allow the development of a new program, a new funding stream made available by a government agency or other granting agency, or a newly organized coalition formed to address an emerging health problem. Threats may involve shifts in consumer trends, organizational or ideological competition, or private industry that promotes products or services that are harmful to the health of a community (i.e., the tobacco or alcohol industry, fast food corporations), or changing technology.

The SWOT analysis differs substantially from other models discussed in this chapter. It truly represents rapid internal and external scans that allow planners to implement interventions in a much shorter time frame. Building upon strengths or addressing specific weaknesses while taking advantage of opportunities in the environment is an advantage of the SWOT analysis. Certainly this approach can lead to challenges if consumer input is not received, problems are not analyzed thoroughly, relevant determinants are not addressed, or interventions are identified and implemented without adequately understanding of the underlying theory or rationale. In fact, poorly planned programs can be more harmful than no programs at all. However, the SWOT analysis has its place in planning methodology and its simplicity is appealing to many planners.

Healthy Communities

Healthy Communities (or Healthy Cities) is a movement that began in the 1980s in Canada and, with the assistance of the World Health Organization, spread to various locations throughout Europe. As a result, organizations like California Healthy Cities and Indiana Healthy Cities were created in the United States. The movement is characterized by community ownership and empowerment and driven by the values, needs, and participation of community members with consultation from health professionals. Another characteristic of Healthy Communities is diverse partnership. It is not uncommon to see partners from business or labor, transportation, recreation, public safety, or even politicians participate in the Healthy Communities process.

Although various models are used in Healthy Communities, the Department of Health and Human Services has produced a guide entitled, *Healthy People in Healthy Communities* (USDHHS, 2001) that provides a five-step framework for the Healthy Communities process in general. Step 1, *Mobilize Key Individuals and Organizations*, identifies and organizes people who care about the health of their community. These people have more than passing interest in their community; they are passionate and willing to work. It does require a process of canvassing the community (e.g., businesses, religious organizations, charities) to find these special people. This step also involves creating a vision for a healthy community among this core group of individuals that reflects their values and personalities. Eventually, this small core group expands into a larger coalition of individuals and organizations who share in the established vision.

The second step in the process, *Assessing Community Needs, Strengths, and Resources*, involves gathering and evaluating a wide range of data about the community and setting priorities. The third step, *Plan for Action,* requires the coalition to plan an approach to address the priorities that were analyzed earlier. As with other models, this involves creating objectives, identifying appropriate interventions, assigning specific responsibilities to individuals or organizations and developing timelines. Step 4, *Implement the Action Plan,* and Step 5, *Track Progress and Outcomes,* follow patterns associated with planning models discussed earlier in this chapter. Coalition members must understand their roles and responsibilities, communicate effectively, follow up meticulously, and track and measure the success of all program components.

Although many of the steps associated with Healthy Communities appear quite similar to the Generalized Model, this approach is characterized by community ownership more so than any other planning approach. While organizing community groups and getting people involved requires patience, the model has been implemented widely throughout the world. Lessons learned from Healthy Communities include the idea that the pursuit of shared values in the context of ownership and empowerment is a viable approach to improving health in the community.

The Health Communication Model

The National Cancer Institute (NCI) has produced a document that is essential to any planner engaged in health communication planning entitled, *Making Health Communications Work* (NCI, 2002). The NCI model for health communication is presented in four phases: (1) Planning and Strategy Development; (2) Developing and Pretesting Concepts, Messages, and Materials; (3) Implementing the Program; and (4) Assessing Effectiveness and Making Refinements.

Planning and Strategy Development involves several steps including: assessing the health issue or problem and identifying potential solutions; defining communication objectives; defining potential audiences and learning about them; investigating appropriate settings, channels, and activities best suited for the identified audiences; and developing a communication strategy for each potential audience (NCI, 2002). Like all planning models, the NCI model begins by identifying the most significant health problems facing a community and assessing who in the community may be most vulnerable to the problem, or who, for other reasons, may be the most appropriate audience for communication interventions. Unlike other models, objectives and intervention strategies are developed early in the NCI model. Although consumer data are described as one component of assessment, they are not a central or integral component of early decision making in the model.

Developing and Pretesting Concepts, Messages, and Materials direct planners to review existing materials for appropriateness. Often times, print material, public service announcements, and other resources may be available and appropriate with few, if any, modifications. Still, it may be necessary to create new concepts, messages, and materials to meet the needs of a specific audience. In this phase, **message concepts** (messages or visuals in early stages) are developed and tested. These will eventually evolve into messages and materials that become the basis of the communication campaign. In this phase, planners develop and pretest the finished messages and materials in the manner outlined in CDCynergy.

The third phase, *Implementing the Program,* usually begins with a kickoff event that draws positive attention to the campaign and related programs and interventions. This is generally associated with a press conference which brings partners together to formally introduce a new program. Appropriate spokespeople are selected and special attention is given to framing issues to maximize coverage, interest, and participation. Developing strategies for ongoing media relationships and coverage are also designed in this phase. As with other planning models, communication, reinforcement of partnerships, and adherence to planned timelines are characteristics of this phase.

Finally, *Assessing Effectiveness and Making Refinements* involves refining the communication plan as immediate feedback is received through process **evaluation** and evaluating the effectiveness of the campaign in terms of changes in determinants and health status. Planners must determine what information the evaluation must provide, define the data to collect, decide upon data collection methods, collect and process the data, analyze the data, write an evaluation report, and disseminate the evaluation report (NCI, 2002).

Because health communication is becoming an increasingly important method and discipline within the field of health promotion, use of the NCI model or CDCynergy is imperative if planners are to implement such communication campaigns appropriately. The models themselves share many characteristics. Both have been designed and tested by a range of health professionals in a variety of settings.

Intervention Mapping

Intervention mapping was designed to fill a gap in health promotion practice by translating data collected in the Precede phases of PRECEDE-PROCEED (i.e., social, epidemiological, educational, ecological, administrative, organizational, and policy assessments) into theoretically based and otherwise appropriate interventions (Green & Kreuter, 2005). Once planners identify program objectives, they are guided by diagrams and matrices that incorporate outputs of the assessment process with relevant theory (Green & Kreuter). These diagrams and matrices are perhaps the defining strength of intervention mapping.

Intervention mapping is comprised of six steps. The first step, *needs assessment*, is conducted by using the Precede phases of the PRECEDE-PROCEED model and includes two major components: (1) scientific, epidemiologic, behavioral, and social analysis of a priority population or community; and (2) an effort to understand the character of the priority population or community (Bartholomew et al., 2006). Step 2, *matrices of change objectives*, specifies who and what will change as a result of the intervention (Bartholomew et al., 2006). Although the identification of goals and objectives is common to all planning models, intervention mapping makes a unique contribution in this regard. In this step, planners "create a matrix of change objectives for each level of intervention planning (individual, interpersonal, organizational, community, and societal) by crossing performance objectives with determinants and writing change objectives (Bartholomew et al., 2006, p. 19). In this regard, planners can more clearly see who and what will change as a result of the intervention.

Step 3, *theory based methods and practical strategies*, guides the planner through a process of selected theory-based interventions and strategies that hold the greatest promise to change the health behavior(s) of individuals in the priority population. Although planners search for theory-based methods, they also ensure that practical strategies are selected and that final strategies match the change objectives from the matrices. Step 4, *program*, describes the scope and sequence of the intervention, the completed program materials, and program protocols (Bartholomew et al., 2006). In addition, program materials are pretested with the priority population prior to implementation.

Step 5 of intervention mapping is *adoption and implementation*. This step requires the same development of matrices as in step 2, except in these matrices, the focus is on adoption and implementation of performance objectives (Bartholomew et al., 2006). In other words, instead of focusing on who and what will change within the priority population, the focus is on what will be done by whom among planners or program partners. Finally, step 6 is *evaluation planning*. In this step, planners decide if determinants were well specified, if strategies were appropriately matched to methods, what proportion of the priority population was reached, and whether or not implementation was complete and executed as planned (Bartholomew et al., 2006).

As with all planning models, intervention mapping follows a logical sequence of steps or phases that are common to the generalized model of planning. However, this model holds promise for linking interventions with theory, with identified objectives related to various personal and external determinants, and with the professionals who are responsible for specific tasks and assignments.

Healthy Plan-It

Healthy Plan-It was developed by the Sustainable Management Development Program at the Centers for Disease Control and Prevention (CDC, 2000) to strengthen in-country management training capacity in the health sector of developing countries. The Health Analysis for Planning Prevention Services (HAPPS), a planning model that was commonly used in the 1980s, is the basis for Healthy Plan-It (CDC, 2000). The model itself consists of six steps: (1) priority setting, (2) establishing goals, (3) outcome objectives, (4) strategy, (5) evaluation, and (6) budget.

The first step, *Priority Setting*, involves participatory planning and consensus building, as well as priority setting, using the Basic Priority Rating Process (see Chapter 4). Participatory planning and consensus building requires broad representation from the community, a facilitation process that promotes empowerment, and nurturing respect for all those involved in the planning process. This phase builds a foundation of trust within an atmosphere of flexibility (CDC, 2000). Priority setting examines the size and seriousness of health problems, effectiveness of interventions, and the propriety, economic feasibility, acceptability, resources, and legality associated with all potential health problems. The result is a ranked list of priorities.

The second step, *Establishing Goals*, follows the pattern outlined in previous models. Goals are generalized statements of the result or achievement to which your effort is directed (CDC, 2000). At times funding or other resources for different program emphases become available. Other times, partners may come forward and invite your participation on unrelated initiatives. When these types of opportunities present themselves, goals help planners stay focused on the program emphasis.

The third step in Healthy Plan-It develops *Outcome Objectives*. These are related to the program goal(s), are usually long-term in nature, and are always measurable. Outcome objectives also relate to the actual health problem (the specific disease or injury).

The basis for program success is generally linked to the degree to which objectives are accomplished. The fourth step, *Strategy*, involves developing the methods or interventions that will be implemented to accomplish outcome objectives. Strategies are designed to affect the determinants and contributing factors that lead to the health problem and will vary depending upon program goals and objectives.

The final phases, *Evaluation* and *Budget,* identify ways to measure the success of outcome objectives as well as program impacts related to determinants and contributing factors (impact objectives). The process of evaluating program delivery, as well as changes in behaviors and actual health problems, is designed and implemented. Development of program budgets involves planning for physical resources, personnel, facilities, and equipment. Although initial budgetary planning may be performed prior to step one to identify planning parameters, actual project costs are analyzed and distributed in the final step.

Still Other Planning Models

The models discussed in this chapter are either some of the more well-known models or most widely used models within health promotion. However, still other models are available to planners. These include the Planning, Program Development, and Evaluation Model (Timmreck, 2003); the Model for Health Education Planning (Ross & Mico, 1980); the Comprehensive Health Education Model (Sullivan, 1973); the Model for Health Education Planning and Resource Development (Bates & Winder, 1984); and the Generic Health/Fitness Delivery System (Patton, Corey, Gettman, & Graff, 1986). These models, all useful and instructive in their own right, share common themes, steps, and phases with the models that have been reviewed in this chapter.

What should now be evident is that although various planning models exist, they are more similar than they are different or unique. These models all generally seek to assess needs, set goals and objectives, develop an intervention, implement the intervention, and evaluate the results as outlined in the Generalized Model. The remainder of the text focuses on the steps outlined in the Generalized Model. As you identify and understand these key steps, planning models and the planning process in general will become much easier to understand and implement.

SUMMARY

A model can provide the framework for planning a health promotion program. Several different planning models have been developed and revised over the years. The planning models for health promotion presented in this chapter are the following:

1. PRECEDE-PROCEED (Predisposing, Reinforcing, and Enabling Constructs in Educational/Environmental Diagnosis and Evaluation; Policy, Regulatory, and Organizational Constructs in Educational and Environmental Development)

2. MATCH (Multilevel Approach To Community Health)

3. CDCynergy

4. SMART (Social Marketing Assessment and Response Tool)

5. A Systematic Approach to Health Promotion *(Healthy People 2010)*

6. MAPP (Mobilizing for Action through Planning and Partnerships)

7. APEX-PH (Assessment Protocol for Excellence in Public Health)

8. SWOT (Strengths, Weaknesses, Opportunities, Threats)

9. Healthy Communities (or Healthy Cities)

10. The Health Communication Model

11. Intervention Mapping

12. Healthy Plan-It

To date, probably the best-known model and the one most often used in health promotion is the PRECEDE-PROCEED model. MATCH has also been a time-honored model. The newer models of CDCynergy and SMART are starting to take hold and are being used more and more. And finally, several others have made and continue to make valuable contributions (see **Table 2.3**).

REVIEW QUESTIONS

1. How does an understanding of the Generalized Model for Program Planning help you understand all planning models?

2. Why is it important to use a model when planning?

3. Name the 12 models presented in this chapter, and list one distinguishing characteristic of each.

4. Of the models presented, which one has been most commonly used? Name the different phases of this model.

5. How are the CDCynergy and SMART models different from the others presented in this chapter?

6. What components seem to be common to all the models? (Note that the names of the components may not be the same, but the concepts are.)

ACTIVITIES

1. After reviewing the models presented in this chapter, create your own model by identifying what you think are the common components of the models. Provide a rationale for including each component. Then draw a diagram of your model so that you can share it with the class. Be prepared to explain your model.

2. In a one-page paper, defend what you believe is the best planning model presented in this chapter.

Table 2.3   Summary of health education/promotion planning models (by author and year)

PRECEDE-PROCEED (Green & Kreuter, 2005)	MATCH (Simons-Morton et al., 1988)	CDCynergy (2003)	SMART (Neiger & Thackeray, 1998)	A Systematic Approach to Health Promotion (USDHHS, 2000)
Phase 1 Social assessment	**Phase 1** Goals selection	**Phase 1** Describe problem	**Phase 1** Preliminary planning	**Phase 1** Goals
Phase 2 Epidemiological assessment	**Phase 2** Intervention planning	**Phase 2** Analyze problem	**Phase 2** Consumer analysis	**Phase 2** Objectives
Phase 3 Educational and ecological assessment	**Phase 3** Program development	**Phase 3** Plan intervention	**Phase 3** Market analysis	**Phase 3** Determinants of health
Phase 4 Administrative and policy assessment and intervention alignment	**Phase 4** Implementation preparations	**Phase 4** Develop intervention	**Phase 4** Channel analysis	**Phase 4** Health status
Phase 5 Implementation	**Phase 5** Evaluation	**Phase 5** Plan evaluation	**Phase 5** Develop interventiors, materials, and pretest	
Phase 6 Process evaluation		**Phase 6** Implement plan	**Phase 6** Implementation	
Phase 7 Impact evaluation			**Phase 7** Evaluation	
Phase 8 Outcome evaluation				

(Table 2.3 continues)

Table 2.3   *(continued)*

MAPP (NACCHO, 2001)	APEX-PH (NACCHO, 1991)	SWOT	Healthy Communities (USDHHS, 2001)	NCI Model (NCI, 2002)	Healthy Plan-It (CDC, 2000)	Intervention Mapping (Bartholomew, Parcel, Kok, & Gottlieb, 2006)
Phase 1 Organizing for success and partnership development	**Phase 1** Organizational capacity assessment	**Phase 1** Strengths	**Phase 1** Mobilize key individuals and organizations	**Phase 1** Planning and strategy development	**Phase 1** Priority setting	**Step 1** Needs assessment
Phase 2 Visioning	**Phase 2** Community process	**Phase 2** Weaknesses	**Phase 2** Assessing community needs, strengths, and resources	**Phase 2** Developing and pretesting concepts, messages, and materials	**Phase 2** Establishing goals	**Step 2** Matrices of change objectives
Phase 3 Four MAPP assessments	**Phase 3** Completing the cycle	**Phase 3** Opportunities	**Phase 3** Plan for action	**Phase 3** Implementing the program	**Phase 3** Outcome objectives	**Step 3** Theory-Based methods and practical strategies
Phase 4 Identify strategic issues		**Phase 4** Threats	**Phase 4** Implement the action plan	**Phase 4** Assessing effectiveness and making refinements	**Phase 4** Strategy	**Step 4** Program
Phase 5 Formulate goals and strategies			**Phase 5** Track progress and outcomes		**Phase 5** Evaluation	**Step 5** Adoption and implementation plan
Phase 6 The action cycle					**Phase 6** Budget	**Step 6** Evaluation plan

3. Using a hypothetical health problem for a specific priority population, write a paper explaining the steps/phases for one of the models presented in this chapter.

4. List and describe any potential advantages and disadvantages of using a consumer-based planning model in health promotion. How do these advantages and disadvantages compare with more traditional planning models used in health promotion? Be prepared to discuss your ideas in class.

5. Identify a public service announcement on television or radio, or obtain a copy of one from a nearby health agency. Analyze factors such as messages, settings, and channels. Based on your analysis, was the public service announcement developed appropriately for the intended audience? Summarize your comments in a one-page paper.

6. Using either the CDCynergy or SMART model, identify a relevant health problem or a specific audience, perform or gather appropriate consumer research, and develop ideas for appropriate intervention and communication strategies. Summarize your findings in a three-page paper.

WEBLINKS

1. **http://www.healthypeople.gov/document/**

   Healthy People 2010 (U.S. Department of Health and Human Services)

   At this website, A Systematic Approach to Health Promotion may be viewed in its entirety, including all objectives, focus areas, and leading indicators associated with *Healthy People 2010*. It is a site with which planners in health promotion should be familiar.

2. **http://www.healthypeople.gov/state/toolkit/default.htm**

   Healthy People 2010 Tool Kit: A Field Guide to Health Planning

   This tool kit provides valuable resources to implement both A Systematic Approach to Health Promotion (*Healthy People 2010*) as well as Healthy Communities. The site includes information on building a leadership structure; identifying and securing resources; identifying and engaging community partners; setting health priorities; obtaining baseline measures, setting targets, and measuring progress; managing and sustaining the process; and communicating health goals and objectives.

3. **http://ctb.ku.edu/**

   Community Tool Box

   This website is an indispensable tool for all planners in health promotion. According to the website itself, "the Tool Box involves over 6,000 pages of practical skill-building information on over 250 different topics" related to planning steps and phases discussed in this chapter. "Topic sections include step-by-step instruction, examples, checklists, and related resources."

4. http://mapp.naccho.org/mapp_introduction.asp

   National Association of County and City Health Officials

   At this website, the MAPP Model is comprehensively diagrammed and explained. The Four MAPP Assessments are described, including how they are implemented, how to use subcommittees for each assessment, and how to make linkages between assessments.

5. http://www.communityhlth.org/communityhlth/resources/hlthycommunities.html

   Association for Community Health Improvement

   This website provides helpful information on the Healthy Communities Initiative including current projects and links.

6. http://www.cdc.gov/communication/cdcynergy.htm

   Communication at the Centers for Disease Control and Prevention

   This website provides an overview of CDCynergy, news and updates, information on all editions, current campaigns, practice areas, and resources.

7. http://www.cancer.gov/pinkbook

   Making Health Communications Work (National Cancer Institute, 2002)

   At this website, the entire document (2002 edition) is available, including the Health Communication Model. This is arguably the most comprehensive document available on health communication planning.

3

Starting the Planning Process

After reading this chapter and answering the questions at the end, you should be able to:

- Develop a rationale for planning and implementing a health promotion program.
- Explain the importance of gaining the support of decision makers.
- Identify the individuals who could make up a planning committee.
- Explain what planning parameters are and the impact they have on program planning.

KEY TERMS

advisory board	influencers	planning parameters
doers	institutionalized	priority population
evidence	literature	program ownership
evidence-based practice	organizational culture	stakeholders
Guide to Community	planning committee	steering committee
Preventive Services		

Planning a health promotion program is a multi-step process. "To *plan* is to engage in a process or a procedure to develop a method of achieving an end" (Breckon, Harvey, & Lancaster, 1998, p. 145). However, because of the many different variables and circumstances of any one setting, the multi-step process of planning does not always begin the same way. There are times when the need for a program is obvious and that a new program should be put in place. For example, if a community's immunization rate for its children is less than half the national average, a program should be created. There are other times when a program has been successful in the past but needs to be changed or reworked slightly before being implemented again. And, there are situations where planners have been given the independence and authority to create the programs that are needed in a community in order to improve the health and quality of life. However, when the need is not so obvious, or when there has not been successful health promotion programming in the past, the planning process often begins with the planners creating a rationale to gain the support of key people in order to obtain the necessary resources to ensure that the planning process and the eventual implementation proceeds as smoothly as possible.

This chapter presents the steps of creating a program rationale to obtain the support of decision makers, identifying those who may be interested in helping to plan the program, and establishing the parameters in which the planners must work. **Box 3.1** identifies the responsibilities and competencies for health educators that pertain to the material presented in this chapter.

Box 3.1   RESPONSIBILITIES AND COMPETENCIES FOR HEALTH EDUCATORS

The content of Chapter 3 includes information on several tasks that occur early in the program planning process. These tasks are not associated with a single area of responsibility, but rather *five different areas* of responsibility of the health educator:

Responsibility I: Assess Individual and Community Needs for Health Education
Competency A: Access existing health-related data

Responsibility II: Plan Health Education Strategies, Interventions, and Programs
Competency A: Involve people and organizations in program planning

Responsibility V: Administer Health Education Strategies, Interventions, and Programs
Competency D: Obtain acceptance and support for programs

Responsibility VI: Serve as a Health Education Resource Person
Competency A: Use health-related information resources

Responsibility II: Communicate and Advocate for Health and Health Education
Competency A: Analyze and respond to current and future needs in health education

Source: NCHEC, SOPHE, & AAHE (2006).

The Need for Creating a Rationale to Gain the Support of Decision Makers

No matter what the setting of a health promotion program—whether a business, an industry, the community, a clinic, a hospital, or a school—it is most important that the program have support from the highest level (the administration, chief executive officer, church elders, board of health, or board of directors) (Chapman, 1997, 2006; Wolfe, Slack, & Rose-Hearn, 1993) of the "community" for which the program is being planned. It is the individuals in these top-level decision-making positions who are able to provide the necessary resource support for the program.

"Resources" usually means money, which can be turned into staff, facilities, materials, supplies, utilities, and all the myriad number of things that enable organized activity to take place over time. "Support" usually means a range of things: congruent organizational policies, program and concept visibility, expressions of priority value, personal involvement of key managers, a place at the table of organizational power, organizational credibility, and a role in integrated functioning. (Chapman, 1997, p. 1)

There will be times when the idea for, or the motivating force behind, a program comes from the top-level people. When this happens, it is a real boon for the program planners because they do not have to "sell" the idea to these people to gain their support. However, this scenario does not occur frequently.

Often, the idea or the big push for a health promotion program comes from someone other than one who is part of the top level of the "community." The idea could start with an employee, an interested parent, a health educator within the organization, a member of the parish or congregation, or a concerned individual or group from within the community. The idea might even be generated by an individual outside the "community," such as one who may have administrative or oversight responsibilities for activities in a community. An example of this arrangement may be an employee of a state health department who provides consultative services to those in a local health department. Or it may be an individual from a regional level agency who is partnering with a group within the community to carry out a collaborative project. When the scenario begins at a level below the decision makers, those who want to create a program must "sell" it to the decision makers. In other words, in order for resources and support to flow into health promotion programming, decision makers need to clearly perceive a set of values or benefits associated with the proposed program (Chapman, 1997). Without the support of decision makers, it becomes more difficult, if not impossible, to plan and implement a program. Behrens (1983) has stated that health promotion programs in business and industry have a greater chance for success if all levels of management, including the top, are committed and supportive. This is true of health promotion programs in all settings, not just programs in business and industry.

If they need to gain the support of decision makers, program planners should develop a rationale for the program's existence. Why is it necessary to "sell" something that everyone knows is worthwhile? After all, does anyone doubt the value of trying to help people gain and maintain good health? The answer to these and similar questions is that few people are motivated by health concerns alone. Decisions by top-level management to develop new programs are based on a variety of factors, including finances, policies, public image, and politics, to name a few. Thus to "sell" the program to those at the top, planners need to develop a rationale that shows how the new program will help decision makers to meet the organization's goals and, in turn, to carry out its mission. In other words, planners need to position their program rationale politically, in line with the organization.

Steps in Creating a Program Rationale

Planners must understand that gaining the support of the decision makers is one of the most important steps in the planning process and it should not be taken lightly. Many program ideas have died at this stage because the planners were not well prepared to "sell" the program to decision makers. Thus, before making an appeal to decision makers, planners need to have a sound rationale for creating a program that is supported by evidence that the proposed program will benefit those for whom it is planned.

There is no formula or recipe for writing a rationale, but through experience, the authors have found a logical format for putting ideas together to help guide planners (see **Figure 3.1**). Note that Figure 3.1 is presented as an inverted triangle. This

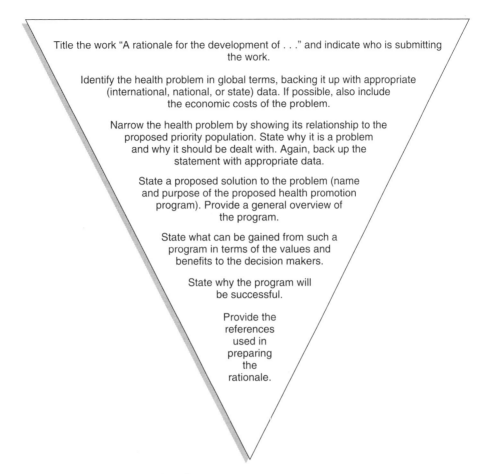

Title the work "A rationale for the development of . . ." and indicate who is submitting the work.

Identify the health problem in global terms, backing it up with appropriate (international, national, or state) data. If possible, also include the economic costs of the problem.

Narrow the health problem by showing its relationship to the proposed priority population. State why it is a problem and why it should be dealt with. Again, back up the statement with appropriate data.

State a proposed solution to the problem (name and purpose of the proposed health promotion program). Provide a general overview of the program.

State what can be gained from such a program in terms of the values and benefits to the decision makers.

State why the program will be successful.

Provide the references used in preparing the rationale.

Figure 3.1 Creating a rationale

inverted triangle is symbolic in design to reflect the flow of a program rationale beginning at the top by identifying a health problem in global terms and moving toward a more focused solution at the bottom of the triangle.

Step 1: Identify Appropriate Background Information

Before planners begin to write a program rationale, they need to identify appropriate sources of information and data that can be used to "sell" program development. The place to begin the process of identifying appropriate sources of information and data to support the development of a program rationale is to conduct a search of the existing literature. The **literature** includes the articles, books, government publications, and other documents that explain the past and current knowledge about a particular topic. By conducting a search, planners will gain a better understanding of the health problem(s) of concern, approaches to reducing or eliminating the health problem, and an understanding of the people for whom the program is intended (these individuals are referred to as the **priority population**). There are a number of different ways that planners can carry out a review of the literature. In Chapter 4, we present a process for doing so.

In general, the types of information and data that are useful in writing a rationale include those that (1) express the needs and wants of the priority population, (2) describe the status of the health problem(s) within a given population, (3) show how the potential outcomes of the proposed program align with what the decision makers feel is important, (4) show compatibility with the health plan of a state or the nation, (5) provide evidence that the proposed program will make a difference, and (6) show how the proposed program will protect and preserve the single biggest asset of most organizations—the people. Though many of these types of information and data are generated through a review of the literature, the first one discussed below—needs and wants of the priority population—is not.

Information and data that express the needs and wants of the priority population can be generated through a needs assessment. A *needs assessment* is the process of identifying, analyzing, and prioritizing the needs of a priority population. Needs assessments are carried out through a multiple-step process in which data are collected and analyzed. The analysis generates a prioritized list of needs of the priority population (see Chapter 4 for a detailed explanation of the needs assessment process). Even though information and data that express the needs and wants of the priority population can be very useful in generating a rationale for a proposed program, more than likely at this point in the planning process, a formal needs assessment will not have been completed. Often, a complete needs assessment does not take place until decision makers give permission for the planning to begin. However, the review of literature may generate information about a needs assessment of another related or similar program. If so, it can provide valuable information and data that can help to develop the rationale.

Information and data that describe the status of a health problem within a population can be obtained by analyzing epidemiological data. Epidemiological data are those that result from the process of epidemiology, which has been defined as "the study of the distribution and determinants of health-related states or events in specific populations, and the application of this study to control health problems" (*Dictionary of Epidemiology* as cited in Last, 2007, p. 111). Epidemiological data are available from a number of different sources and include but are not limited to the *U.S. Census,* the *Statistical Abstract of the United States,* the *Monthly Vital Statistics Report, Morbidity and Mortality Weekly Report,* the *National Health Interview Survey,* the *National Health and Nutrition Examination Survey,* the *Behavioral Risk Factor Surveillance System (BRFSS),* the *Youth Risk Behavior Surveillance System (YRBSS),* the *National Hospital Discharge Survey,* and the *National Hospital Ambulatory Medical Care Survey.*

Epidemiological data gain additional significance when it can be shown that the described health problem(s) is/are the result of modifiable health behaviors and that spending money to promote healthy lifestyles and prevent health problems makes good economic sense. For example, we know that smoking causes almost $170 billion "in annual health-related economic costs, including adult mortality-related productivity costs, adult medical expenditures, and medical expenditures for newborns" (ACS, 2007, p. 37). Examples of another 18 commonly seen health problems (e.g., breast cancer, cervical and colorectal cancer, coronary heart disease, HIV/AIDS transmission, low birth weight, and tuberculosis) in the United States and their related economic impact are presented in a publication titled *An Ounce of Prevention . . . What Are the Returns?* (CDC, 1999a). However, it should be noted that "proving" the economic impact of many health promotion programs is not easy. Research conducted to date suggest that the economic impact of health promotion programs is modest (Golaszewski, 2001).

There are a number of reasons for this including the multi-causation of many health problems, the complex interventions needed to deal with them, and the difficulty of carrying out rigorous research studies. Additionally, McGinnis and colleagues (2002) feel that part of the problem is that health promotion programs are held to a different standard than medical treatment programs when cost-effectiveness is being considered.

> "In a vexing example of double standards, public investments in health promotion seem to require evidence that future savings in health and other social costs will offset the investments in prevention. Medical treatments do not need to measure up to the standard; all that is required here is evidence of safety and effectiveness. The cost-effectiveness challenge often is made tougher by a sense that the benefits need to accrue directly and in short term to the payer making investments. Neither of these two conditions applies in many interventions in health promotion" (p. 84).

For those planners interested in using economic impact and cost-effectiveness of health promotion programs as part of a program rationale, we recommend that the work of the following authors be reviewed: Aldana (2001), Chapman (2003, 2006), Edington (2001), Golaszewski (2001), Riedel (1999), and USDHHS (2003). For those planners specifically interested in worksite health promotion, a series of articles is presented in the May/June 2001 issue of the *American Journal of Health Promotion* in which 10 managers in corporate settings reflect on what matters to them and the decision makers they report to in determining if health promotion is a good investment for their organization.

Other information and data that are useful in creating a rationale are those that show how the potential outcomes of the proposed program align with what the decision makers feel is important. Planners can often get a hint of what decision makers value by reviewing the organization's mission statement and/or annual report. More specific methods of determining the values and benefits that could be included in a rationale are noted in **Box 3.2.** Chapman (1997) outlines the values and benefits

---

Box 3.2	METHODS FOR DETERMINING THE VALUES AND BENEFITS THAT SHOULD BE EMPHASIZED

1. Examine recent or past meeting minutes, decisions, or comments that are relevant to the value placed on health and prevention.

2. Find out from the individuals in a position to know, why past decisions related to budget or employee benefits were made by the managers involved.

3. Review past formal reports or evaluations of health programs and benefits that have been commissioned or carried out on behalf of the decision makers.

4. Conduct an informal survey of the most influential decision makers to get some sense of their own as well as their perception of the value priorities of the other decision makers involved.

5. Conduct a formal survey of all or a portion of the key decision makers involved to determine what is the most important to them.

6. Analyze the implementation questions that have been raised in the past on similar programs or topics.

Source: Chapman, "Securing Support from Top Management," *The Art of Health Promotion* 1(2), 1997, p. 2. Copyright © 1997.

associated with health promotion programs in which supporting data and/or documentation exist or can be collected. Further, the values and benefits he presents focus on four different types of programming: for worksites, communities, individuals, and managed care organizations. Chapman's work is presented in **Table 3.1**.

Table 3.1   Values or benefits associated with health promotion programming

Focus	Value or Benefit Statement	Supporting Data and/or Documentation
Worksite	Increased worker morale	Studies using survey instruments that measure employee morale, industry or trade association data, human resource annual surveys with carefully selected questions
	Potentially greater employer loyalty	Survey results and patterns over time, use of loyalty proxy questions, survey or focus group findings
	Improved employee resiliency and decision making quality	Studies from the psychological and exercise physiology literature
	Positive public and community relations	Recognition awards for local or peer employers, coalition or community consortium activities, industry and trade showcase or write-ups
	Increased worker productivity	Business and industrial management studies, selected studies from the worksite health promotion literature, local or trade data using collective productivity indicators
	Informed, health care cost-conscious workforce	Studies and anecdotal articles about consumer activism, scores from consumer health knowledge surveys, survey results on self-efficacy and consumerism
	Recruitment tool	Social psychology literature and business survey literature, selected labor market survey data
	Retention tool	Social psychology literature and business survey literature, selected labor market survey data
	Opportunity for cost savings via: Reduced sick leave absenteeism	A large number of worksite health promotion studies that address sick leave absenteeism effects, survey data from National Institutes of Occupational Health & Safety (*NIOSH*) and from trade and industry associations
	Opportunity for cost savings via: Reduced short- and long-term disability claims	A few articles on worksite health promotion programs and their impact on disability days, benefits and business surveys, risk management literature
	Opportunity for cost savings via: Decreased health care utilization	A moderate number of articles on the evaluation of worksite health promotion programs and their impact on health care costs, the medical care research literature and the managed care research literature, which also contain a variety of references; another major set of references are the actuarial studies that have been done on the relationship of health risks to health costs

(Table 3.1 continues)

Table 3.1   *(continued)*

Focus	Value or Benefit Statement	Supporting Data and/or Documentation
	Opportunity for cost savings via: Reduced premature retirement	Studies of early medical or disability retirement from the benefits, disability management, and actuarial literature
	Opportunity for cost savings via: Decreased overall health benefit costs	Worksite health promotion evaluation costs literature, business and benefits management literature, trade or competitor information
	Opportunity for cost savings via: Fewer on-the-job accidents	Worksite health promotion evaluation literature, risk management literature, safety literature, NIOSH publications, publications of the Bureau of Labor Statistics
	Opportunity for cost savings via: Lower casualty insurance costs	Casualty underwriter's publications and risk management literature
	Opportunity for cost savings via: Smaller total workforce	Business literature plus projections at various sick leave and disability reduction levels, review of personal replacement cases that have occurred in the last 2 to 5 years
	Opportunity for cost savings via: Reduced medical leave time	Occupational health literature and payroll system coding data
	Opportunity for cost savings via: Reduced occupational medical costs	Occupational health literature and occupational health unit data
Community	Provides a model for other local organizations	Community health promotion literature and community organization literature plus Robert Wood Johnson Community Snapshots Project
	Contributes to establishing good health as a norm	Community health promotion literature and cultural change literature plus Centers for Disease Control and Prevention publications
	Complements and reinforces national and local public health initiatives	Office of Disease Prevention and Health Promotion publications and Objectives for the Nation: 2000 plus local public health reports and plans
	Improves quality of life of citizenry	Community Health Care Forum materials and National League of Cities publications
	Helps control (and possibly reduce) the economic and social burden on all taxpayers from premature mortality and morbidity	Compression of morbidity literature and community health promotion literature plus Health Care Financing and Agency for Health Services Research publications and studies
	Helps improve the general economic well-being of communities through the improvement in general health status and productivity	Community health promotion literature and national econometric studies and analyses
Individual	Increased morale via employer's, provider's, or community's interest in their health and well-being	Social psychological and psychological literature
	Increased knowledge about the relationship between lifestyle and health	Attitude and correlated research within the health promotion and health education literature

(Table 3.1 continues)

Table 3.1   *(continued)*

Focus	Value or Benefit Statement	Supporting Data and/or Documentation
	Increased opportunity to take control of their health and medical treatment	Consumer satisfaction surveys and national market research studies plus self-efficacy literature
	Improved health and quality of life through reduction of risk factors	Literature surrounding the use of SF12 and SF36 and self-reported perception of health status
	Increased opportunity for support from co-workers and environment	Social psychological literature, health education research literature, cultural change literature
	Reduced work absences	Attitude and correlated research within the health promotion and health education literature
	Reduced out-of-pocket and premium costs for medical care	Attitude and correlated research within the health promotion and health education literature plus Bureau of Commerce and Census publications
	Reduced pain and suffering from illness and accidents	Attitude and correlated research within the health promotion and health education literature
Managed Care Organizations	Greater member satisfaction	Perceived value of health benefit literature, Health Plan Employer Data Information Set (HEDIS) literature
	Increased market share through differentiation	Managed care marketing literature and strategic planning literature for the managed care industry
	More appropriate utilization by consumers and patients	Medical self-care literature, case management literature, medical care literature, and demand management literature
	Reduced utilization and cost through improvements in morbidity	Compression of morbidity literature, epidemiology literature, managed care and demand management literature
	Improved price competitiveness	Managed care literature, financial analysis of managed care industry literature, benefit survey literature
	Improved HEDIS performance	National Committee on Quality Assurance publications and particularly HEDIS Version 3.0

Source: Chapman, "Securing Support from Top Management," *The Art of Health Promotion* 1(2), 1997, p. 2. Copyright © 1997. Reprinted by permission.

A fourth source of information for a rationale is a comparison between the proposed program and the health plan for the nation or a state. Comparing the health needs of the priority population with those of other citizens of the state or of all Americans, as outlined in the goals and objectives of the nation (USDHHS, 2000), should enable planners to show the compatibility between the goals of the proposed program and those of the nation's health plan. A discussion of these national health goals and objectives is presented in Chapter 6.

A fifth source of information and data is *evidence* that the proposed program will be effective and make a difference if implemented. By **evidence** we mean the body of data that can be used to make decisions when planning a program. Such data can come from needs assessments, knowledge about the causes of a health problem, research that has tested the effectiveness of an intervention, and evaluations conducted on other health promotion programs. When program planners systematically find, appraise, and use evidence as the basis for decision making when planning a health promotion program, it is referred to as **evidence-based practice** (Cottrell & McKenzie, 2005). A most useful source of evidence-based practice is the ***Guide to Community Preventive Services*** (simply referred to as the *Community Guide*) (Zara, Briss, & Harris, 2005). "The *Community Guide* summarizes what is known about the effectiveness, economic efficiency, and feasibility of interventions to promote community health and prevent disease" (CDC, 2007a, ¶ 1), and includes evidence on topics such as alcohol, cancer, physical activity, obesity, and tobacco to name a few. The *Community Guide* was developed and is continually updated by the nonfederal Task Force on Community Preventive Services, which is comprised of public health experts who are appointed by the Director of the CDC. The Task Force is charged with reviewing and assessing the quality of available evidence and developing appropriate recommendations. (See the weblinks at the end of this chapter for the online version of the *Community Guide*.)

Finally, when preparing a rationale to gain the support of decision makers, planners should not overlook the most important resource of any community—the people who make up the community. Promoting, maintaining, and in some cases restoring human health should be at the core of any health promotion program. Whatever the setting, better health of those in the priority population provides for a better quality of life. For those planners who end up practicing in a worksite setting, the importance of protecting the health of employees (i.e., protecting human resources) should be noted in developing a rationale. "Labor costs typically represent 60% to 70% of total annual operating costs for most organizations" (Chapman, 2006, p. 10); thus people are a company's single biggest asset. "Fit and healthy people are more productive, are better able to meet extraordinary demands and deal with stress, are absent less, reflect better on the company or community as exemplars, and so forth" (Chapman, 1997, p. 6).

Step 2: Titling the Rationale

Once the planners have identified and are familiar with the sources of information and data that can be used to "sell" program development, they are ready to begin the process of putting a rationale together. Thus, the next step is giving a title to the rationale. This can be very simple in nature, such as "A Rationale for (title of program): A Program to Enhance the Health of (name of priority population)." Immediately following the title should be a listing of who contributed to the authorship of the rationale.

Step 3: Writing the Content of the Rationale

The first paragraph or two of the rationale should identify the health problem in global terms. This is where epidemiological and other needs assessment data can be used. If possible, also include the economic costs of such a problem; it will strengthen the rationale. Most local health problems are also present on the international, national, and/or state levels. Presenting the problem at these higher levels shows decision makers that dealing with the health problem is consistent with the concerns of others.

Showing the relationship of the local health problem to the "bigger problem" at the international, national, and/or state levels is the next logical step in presenting the rationale. Thus the next portion of the rationale should identify the local health problem and state *why* it is a problem and *why* it should be dealt with. If the information is available, include the needs and wants of the priority population.

At this point in the rationale, propose a solution to the problem. The solution should include the name and purpose of the proposed health promotion program, and a general overview of what the program may include. Since the writing of a program rationale often precedes much of the formal planning process, the general overview of the program is often based upon the "best guess" of those creating the rationale. For example, if the purpose of a program is to improve the immunization rate of children in the community, a "best guess" of the eventual program might include interventions to increase awareness and knowledge about immunizations, and the reduction of the barriers that limit access to receiving immunizations. Following such an overview, include statements indicating what can be gained from the program. Do your best to align the potential values and benefits of the program with what is important to the decision makers.

Next, state why this program will be successful. This is the place to use the results of *evidence-based practice* to support the rationale. It can also be helpful to point out the similarity of the priority population to others with which similar programs have been successful. And finally, using the argument that the "timing is right" for the program can also be useful. By this we mean that there is no better time than now to work to solve the problem facing the priority population.

Step 4: Listing the References Used to Create the Rationale

The final step in creating a rationale is to include a list of the references used in preparing the rationale. Having a reference list shows decision makers that you studied the available information before presenting your idea. (See the examples of rationales presented in the Activities section at the end of the chapter.)

Planning Committee

The number of people involved in the planning process is determined by the resources and circumstances of a particular situation. "One very helpful method to develop a clearer and more comprehensive planning approach is to establish a committee" (Gilmore & Campbell, 2005, p. 27). Identifying individuals who would be willing to serve as members of the **planning committee** (sometimes referred to as a **steering committee** or **advisory board**) becomes one of the planner's first tasks. The number of individuals on a planning committee can differ depending on the setting for the program and the size of the priority population. For example, the size of a planning committee for a safety belt program in a community of 50,000 people would probably be larger than that of a committee planning a similar program for a business with 50 employees. There is no ideal size for a planning committee, but the following guidelines, which have been presented earlier (McKenzie, 1988) and are given here in a modified form, should be helpful in setting up a committee.

1. The committee should be comprised of individuals who represent a variety of sub-groups within the priority population. To the extent possible, the committee should have representation from all segments of the priority population (e.g., administrators/students/teachers, age groups, health behavior participants/nonparticipants, labor/management, race/ethnic groups, different genders, socioeconomic groups, union/nonunion members, etc.). The greater the number of individuals who are represented by committee members, the greater the chance of the priority population's developing a feeling of **program ownership**. With program ownership there will be better planned programs, greater support for the programs, and people who will be willing to help "sell" the program to others because they feel it is theirs (Strycker et al., 1997).

2. The committee should be comprised of willing individuals who are interested in seeing the program succeed. Select a combination of **doers** and **influencers**. Doers are people who will be willing to roll up their sleeves and do the physical work needed to see that the program is planned and implemented properly. Influencers are those who with a single phone call or signature on a form will enlist other people to participate or will help provide the resources to facilitate the program. Both doers and influencers are important to the planning process.

3. The committee should include an individual who has a key role within the organization sponsoring the program—someone whose support would be most important to ensure a successful program and institutionalization.

4. The committee should include representatives of other **stakeholders** (people who have a stake in the program being planned) not represented in the priority population. For example, if health care providers are needed to implement a health promotion program they need to be represented on the planning committee.

5. The committee membership should be reevaluated regularly to ensure that the composition lends itself to fulfilling program goals and objectives.

6. If the planning committee will be in place for a long period of time, new individuals should be added periodically to generate new ideas and enthusiasm. It may be helpful to set a term of office for committee members. If terms of office are used, it is advisable to stagger the length of terms so that there is always a combination of new and experienced members on the committee.

7. Be aware of the "politics" that are always present in an organization or priority population. There are always some people who bring their own agendas to committee work.

8. Make sure the committee is large enough to accomplish the work, but small enough to be able to make decisions and reach consensus. If necessary, subcommittees can be formed to handle specific tasks.

The actual means by which the committee members are chosen varies according to the setting. Commonly used techniques include:

1. Asking for volunteers by word of mouth, a newsletter, a needs assessment, or some other widely distributed publication

2. Holding an election, either throughout the community or by subdivisions of the community

3. Inviting people to serve

4. Having members formally appointed by a governing group or individual

Once the planning committee has been formed, someone must be designated to lead it. This is an important step (Strycker et al., 1997). The leader (chairperson) "should be interested and knowledgeable about health education programs, and be organized, enthusiastic, and creative" (McKenzie, 1988, p. 149). One might think that most planners, especially health educators, would be perfect for the committee chairperson's job. However, sometimes it is preferable to have someone other than the program planners serve in the leadership capacity. For one thing, it helps to spread out the workload of the committee. Planners who are not good at delegating responsibility may end up with a lot of extra work when they serve as the leaders. Second, having someone else serve as the leader allows the planners to remain objective about the program. And third, the planning committee can serve in an advisory capacity to the planners, if this is considered desirable. **Figure 3.2** illustrates the composition of a balanced planning committee.

Once the planning committee has been organized and a leader is selected, for the committee to be effective it needs to be well organized and run. The committee should meet regularly, have a formal agenda for each meeting, and keep minutes of the meetings (Hunnicutt, 2007). Further, the committee meetings should be efficient, not long and boring (Johnson & Breckon, 2007). In other words, the meeting should be productive and a good use of the committee members' time. In addition, it is important for the committee to communicate frequently with both the decision makers and those in the priority population so that all can be kept informed. By communicating regularly, the committee has the unique opportunity to educate and inform others about health and the specific priorities of the program (Hunnicutt, 2007).

Parameters for Planning

Once the support of the decision makers has been gained and a planning committee formed, the committee members must identify the **planning parameters** within which they must work. There are several questions to which the committee members should have answers before they become too deeply involved in the planning process. In an earlier work (McKenzie, 1988), six such questions were presented, using the example of school-site health promotion programs. The six questions are modified for presentation here. It should be noted, however, that not all of the questions would be appropriate for every program because of the different circumstances of each setting.

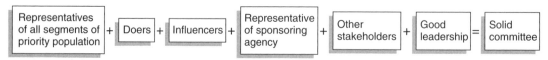

Figure 3.2 Make-up of a solid planning/steering committee

1. What is the decision makers' philosophical perspective on health promotion programs? What are the values and benefits of the programs to the decision makers? (Chapman, 1997). Do they see the programs as something important or as "extras"?

2. What type of commitment to the program are the decision makers willing to make? Are they interested in the program becoming **institutionalized?** That is, are they interested in seeing that the "program becomes imbedded within the host organization, so that the program becomes sustained and durable" (Goodman et al., 1993, p. 163)? Or are they more interested in providing a one-time or pilot program? (*Note:* Goodman and colleagues [1993] have developed a scale for measuring institutionalization.)

3. What type of financial support are the decision makers willing to provide? Does it include personnel for leadership and clerical duties? Released/assigned time for managing the program and participation? Space? Equipment? Materials?

4. Are the decision makers willing to consider changing the **organizational culture?** For example, are they interested in "well" days instead of sick days? Are they as interested in *presenteeism*— that is, showing up for work even if one is too ill, stressed, or distracted to be productive—as much as they are interested absenteeism? Would they like to create employee nonsmoking and safety belt policies? Change vending machine selections to more nutritious foods? Set aside an employee room for meditation? Develop a health promotion corner in the organization's library?

5. Will all individuals in the priority population have an opportunity to take advantage of the program, or will it be available to only certain subgroups?

6. What is the authority of the planning committee? Will it be an advisory group or a programmatic decision making group? What will be the chain-of-command for program approval?

After the planning parameters have been defined, the planning committee should understand how the decision makers view the program, and should know what type and amount of resources and support to expect. Identifying the parameters early will save the planning committee a great deal of effort and energy throughout the planning process.

SUMMARY

Creating a program rationale to gain the support of the decision makers is an important initial step in program planning. Planners should take great care in developing a rationale for "selling" the program idea to these important people. A planning committee can be most useful in helping with some of the planning activities and in helping to "sell" the program to the priority population. Therefore, the committee should be composed of interested individuals, doers and influencers, who are representative of the priority population. If the planning committee is to be effective, it will need to work efficiently and to know the planning parameters set for the program by the decision makers.

REVIEW QUESTIONS

1. What is the reason for creating a program rationale?

2. Why is the support of the decision makers important in planning a program?

3. What kinds of reasons should be included in a rationale for planning and implementing a health promotion program?

4. How important is "selling" the idea of a program to decision makers?

5. What items should be addressed when creating a program rationale?

6. Who should be selected as the members of a planning committee?

7. What are *planning parameters?* Give a few examples.

8. Why is it important to know the planning parameters at the beginning of the planning process?

ACTIVITIES

1. Write a two-page rationale for "selling" a program you are planning to decision makers, using the guidelines presented in this chapter.

2. Write a two-page rationale for beginning an exercise program for a company with 200 employees. A needs assessment of this priority population indicates that the number one cause of lost work time of this cohort is back problems and the number one cause of premature death is heart disease.

3. For a program you are planning, write a two-page description of the individuals (by position/ job title, not name) who will be asked to serve on the planning committee, and provide a rationale for asking each to serve.

4. Provide a list (by position/job title, not name) and a rationale for each of the 10 individuals you would ask to serve on a communitywide safety belt program. Use the town or city in which your college/university is located as the community.

5. Following are two program rationales written by former students at Ball State University. Read each of the rationales and then select one to critique using the guidelines presented in this chapter. Critique by describing the following: (a) the strengths of the rationale, (b) the weaknesses, and (c) how you would change the rationale to make it stronger. Be critical! Closely examine the content, reasoning, and references.

Example 1

A rationale for "No Butts About It": A campaign to create a smoke-free ordinance in the restaurants of Delaware County, Indiana.*

The global tobacco use pandemic is responsible for 4.9 million deaths a year worldwide (WHO, 1998). The United States ranks as the second highest consumer of cigarettes in the world with 451 billion consumed each year (WHO, 1998). Tobacco use has been labeled the single most important preventable cause of death and disease in the United States, causing more than 440,000 deaths and resulting in more than $75 billion in direct medical costs annually. Nationally, smoking results in more than 5.6 million years of potential life lost each year.

In the United States, approximately 80% of adult smokers started smoking before the age of 18. That means that each day nearly 5,000 young people under the age of 18 try their first cigarette (USDHHS, 2000). It is clear that years of cigarette smoking vastly increase the risk of developing several fatal conditions. Cigarette smoking is responsible for one-third of all cancers. It is the leading cause of lung cancer contributing to 90% of all lung cancers. It is also associated with cancers of the mouth, pharynx, larynx, esophagus, stomach, pancreas, uteri cervix, kidney, bladder, and colon (USDHHS, 1994). Smoking also increases the risk of cardiovascular disease including stroke, heart attack, vascular disease, and aneurysm (USDHHS, 1994).

Environmental tobacco smoke (ETS) is a mixture of the smoke given off by the burning end of a cigarette (sidestream smoke) and the smoke emitted at the mouthpiece and exhaled from the lungs of smokers (main stream smoke). ETS, also known as second hand smoke, is a major source of indoor air pollution. In the United States, approximately 38,000 deaths are attributable to ETS exposure each year (NCI, 2000). When a cigarette is smoked, only 15% of the smoke is inhaled by the smoker, the other 85% goes directly into the air. Cigarette smoke contains more than 4,000 substances, and 40 of these are classified as carcinogens (cancer causing agents). Nearly nine out of ten nonsmoking Americans are exposed to ETS, as measured by the levels of cotinine, a chemical the body metabolizes from nicotine, in their blood. Eighty-eight percent of all nontobacco users had measurable levels of cotinine in their blood according to a study conducted by the CDC. The presence of cotinine is documentation that a person has been exposed to ETS. Serum cotinine levels can be used to estimate nicotine exposure over the last two to three days.

ETS is estimated to cause approximately 3,000 lung cancer deaths per year among nonsmokers and contributes to 40,000 deaths related to cardiovascular disease (USDHHS, 1994). These deaths are all due to breathing the smoke of others' cigarettes and make ETS the third leading preventable cause of death in the United States. Some of the highest reported exposures to concentrations of ETS are found in food service establishments (EPA, 1992).

Approximately, one out of every four adults in Indiana smokes making it the fourth highest in the nation (27% compared to the U.S. median of 23.3%) (CDC, 2002). The number of adults between ages 18 to 24 who smoke has risen due to the tobacco companies targeting that age group since 1996 (SFI, 2003). The results of the Indiana Youth Tobacco Survey show that 9.8% of middle school students and 31.6% of high school students are current cigarette smokers (SFI, 2000). The smoking attributable mortality

---

*This rationale was written by Peggy Chute, Fariba Mirzaei, and Joe Turner while they were graduate students at Ball State University, Muncie, IN. Reprinted with permission.

rate (SAM) in Indiana is also higher (341.4/100,000) compared to the median for the United States (295.5/100,000) (CDC, 2002).

The five leading causes of death in Delaware County are cardiovascular disease, malignant neoplasm, chronic obstructive pulmonary disease, and unintentional injuries (Synergy, 1998). Lung and bronchial cancer had higher incidence of death when compared to other cancers. "Residents of Delaware County are clearly at risk for cigarette smoking, with 3 in 10 claiming to smoke and having smoked 100 or more cigarettes in their entire lives" (Synergy, 1998, p. 17). Delaware County residents were significantly higher when compared to the national average and the percentage of smokers increased from 1989 (27%) to 1998 (30%). Currently, Delaware County has no ordinance to prohibit smoking in public, including restaurants. This allows ETS to have effects on their nonsmoking clients, smoking clients, and workers of the restaurants.

One of the national health objectives for 2010 is to reduce public exposure to ETS (USDHHS, 2000). Objective 27-13c is specifically related to laws on smokefree air in restaurants. The base line measure for this objective was only 3 states and the target for 2010 is 51 states (50 states and the District of Columbia).

To reduce public exposure to ETS, the Centers for Disease Control and Prevention recommends smoking bans and restrictions in public places to reduce exposure to second-hand smoke. The Task Force on Community Prevention Services, a nonfederal public health panel, which conducted in-depth systematic reviews on selected tobacco interventions concluded that smoking bans and restrictions are the most effective measures to reduce exposure to second-hand smoke (CDC, 2002).

Local ordinances requiring restaurants to be smokefree have spread rapidly. Over 230 U.S. municipalities in different states, among these states Massachusetts, Texas, Colorado, Wisconsin, New York, Oregon, North Carolina, and Arizona, have smokefree ordinances in some of their cities. Fort Wayne is a good example in the state of Indiana, where a smokefree ordinance was passed in 1998. Additionally, the states of California, Maine, Maryland, Vermont, and Utah have smokefree restaurant laws. Several Canadian jurisdictions also have restaurant smoking bans.

Contrary to popular belief, restaurants that implement smokefree policies do not see a decline in profits. Studies in cities that have implemented such policies have shown sales to remain constant and in some cases sales have increased (Americans for Nonsmokers' Rights, 2002).

In addition to stable economic conditions, health care costs decline due to a decrease in worker's compensation claims, decrease in absenteeism, and an increase in worker productivity (CDC, 2002).

After reviewing national, state and local data it is clear that there is a significant health problem in regards to ETS in Delaware County. It is important to "think globally and act locally." This community problem provides a need for action at the local level. In order to succeed in a local campaign to prohibit smoking in restaurants it is important to mobilize grassroots activities. Educating the citizens regarding the health risks of ETS, and mobilizing local advocates will empower the Tobacco Free Coalition of Delaware County's activities in executing a smokefree ordinance campaign. A significant and active grassroots base of support is the most potent weapon to counter the relentless and well-funded opposition from the tobacco industry. Tobacco control advocates have the expertise to draft sound smokefree policies based on successes and lessons learned from other clean indoor air campaigns across the country, while policymakers often lack tobacco control knowledge or expertise.

The above rationale adds up to the conclusion that the Tobacco Free Coalition of Delaware County can succeed in advocating for and passing a smokefree ordinance in

Delaware County if it obtains active grassroots support from the community. Passage of an ordinance in turn will decrease the dangers of ETS exposure in Delaware County. Therefore the *No Butts About It* program can be a means to achieving these goals.

References

Americans for Nonsmoker's Rights Foundation (2002). *Smokefree advertising examples.* Retrieved March 25, 2003, from http://www.no-smoke.org/ads.html

Centers for Disease Control and Prevention (CDC). (2002). Strategies for reducing exposure to environmental tobacco smoke: Increasing tobacco-use cessation, and reducing initiation in communities and health care systems. *Morbidity and Mortality Weekly Report, 49* (RR-12). Retrieved April 6, 2003, from http://www.cdc.gov/mmwr/preview/mmwrhtml/rr4912a1.htm

Centers for Disease Control and Prevention (CDC). (2001). *Clean Indoor Air Regulations, Fact Sheet.* Retrieved March 26, 2003, from http://www.cdc.gov/tobacco/sgr/sgr_2000/factsheets/factsheet_2002clean.htm

Centers for Disease Control and Prevention (CDC). (2002). *Indiana Highlights.* Retrieved April 15, 2003, from http://www.cdc.gov/tobacco/statehi/html_2002/indiana.htm

National Cancer Institute (NCI). (2000). *Cancer Facts, Environmental Tobacco Smoke.* Retrieved April 5, 2003, from http://cis.nci.nih.gov/fact/3_9.htm

Smokefree Indiana (SFI). (2000). *Indiana Youth Tobacco Survey Report.* Retrieved April 5, 2003, from http://www.smokefreeindiana.org/pdf/IYTSExecSumm.pdf

Smokefree Indiana (SFI). (2003, March 3). Indiana smoking rate ranks high. *The Sublink.* Indianapolis, IN: Author.

Synergy. (1998). *Let's Talk Health '98.* Indianapolis, IN: Synergy.

U.S. Department of Health and Human Services (USDHHS). (2000). *Healthy People 2010 (CD-ROM Version).* Washington, DC: Author.

United States Department of Health and Human Services (USDHHS). (1994). *Preventing tobacco use among young people: A report of the Surgeon General.* Atlanta, GA: Author.

World Health Organization (WHO). (1998). *Tobacco Free Initiative.* Retrieved March 26, 2003, from http://www.who.int/tobacco/repsitory/stp84/30%20Map%206%20Cig.%20Consumption.pdf

Example 2

A Rationale for "Mind, Body, and Soul": A Health Education Program at First Presbyterian Church, Muncie, IN*

The health status of Americans has improved greatly in the last 50 years as evidenced by the decrease in the number of cases of communicable disease, increased life expectancy, and the declining death rates (NCHS, 1997). However, the health status of Americans could be further improved if Americans were willing to make additional changes. We now know that better control of behavioral risk factors alone—such as lack of exercise, poor diet, use of tobacco and other drugs, and alcohol abuse—could prevent between 40% and 70% of all mature deaths, one-third of all acute disabilities, and two-thirds of chronic disabilities (USDHHS, 1990).

---

*This rationale was written by the undergraduate students enrolled in the program planning classes at Ball State University, Muncie, Indiana.

Closer to home, recent data also indicate that the health status of Hoosiers has improved but they too could do more to improve their health. In 1996, 32% of the adults (>17 years of age) in Indiana were overweight, 29% were current smokers, and 66% were classified as having a sedentary lifestyle (ISDH, 1998). The data from Indiana are also consistent with the data that were collected from the members of the adult education class, the Mariners, at First Presbyterian Church in Muncie, IN. The data collected using a health risk appraisal (HRA) (Healthier People Software, no date) and a health and spirituality questionnaire (developed by health science students from Ball State University) indicated that the Mariners were interested in educational programs on faith and its relationship to health, humor and healing, and stress management (including prayer as a means of stress reduction). In addition, there appears to be a need for or an interest in programs associated with aging (including Alzheimer's disease), the family, nutrition, weight control, and exercise.

It seems logical to try to address some of the health needs and interests of those in the Mariners class through the Christian Education program of the church. For a long time, religious organizations have functioned as "healing" institutions as evidenced by the mental health issues addressed through pastoral counseling (Ransdell & Rehling, 1996). The idea of addressing the health needs and interests of a priority population in combination with spiritual practices has been encouraged. "In recent years, both the validity of spiritual and religious practices as well as the potential to the overall health and well-being have not only been acknowledged by modern medicine, but encouraged as mechanisms for health enhancement" (Droege, 1996, p. 7). And further, it makes good sense to offer health related programs at church since the Bible "provides a very powerful foundation for the development of health programs within the spiritual framework of the church" (Jackson, 1991, pp. 8–9). In a more practical sense, religious organizations have a number of important potential advantages for involvement in health education/promotion programs because religious organizations (1) tend to involve large numbers of entire families, (2) are often the center of the neighborhood and a natural gathering place, (3) have a long history of outreach and helping others, (4) often have a talented and multi-disciplinary membership, (5) have been found to be receptive to the efforts of primary prevention, and (6) have the facilities to accommodate such programs (Lasater, Carleton, & Wells, 1991). In addition, religious organizations are good settings for health education/promotion programs because when people attend they do so with the expectation of learning; religious organizations are accepted as educational institutions (Lasater, Carleton, & Wells, 1991). Consequently, the church is a natural community arena for health education/promotion programs that focus on behaviors which are then reinforced by the social support and social networks that exist in churches (Levin, Larson, & Puchalski, 1997; Thomas, Quinn, Billingsley, & Caldwell, 1994).

Several benefits can be anticipated from the Mind, Body, and Soul program offered at First Presbyterian Church. First and foremost, it should be expected that the Mariners class members will increase their knowledge about the topics presented. Such knowledge will be beneficial to both the Mariners class members and the people—family and friends—with whom they come in contact. Second, such a program will introduce participants to topics that have not been addressed before in the class. Third, the program will provide participants with an opportunity to apply spiritual and religious concepts to everyday living. And fourth, such a program may attract other members of the congregation to the Mariners class that have not attended in the past.

The Mind, Body, and Soul program for the First Presbyterian Church Mariners class has great potential for being successful for several reasons. First, as noted earlier, the Bible provides a solid base on which to build a health education/promotion program (Jackson, 1991). A number of the scriptures support the healing power of faith (Lloyd, 1994). Class members are interested in learning more about the Bible. Second, the majority of similar other church-based health promotion programs have been highly successful (Cook, 1993). And finally, the program will be well planned and will meet the needs and interests of the class members. Ransdell and Rehling (1996) have indicated that such programs have a better chance of being successful.

References

Cook, D. A. (1993). Research in African American churches: A mental health imperative. *Journal of Mental Health Counseling, 17:* 320–333.

Droege, T. (1996). Spirituality and healing. *Faith and Health,* Summer: 7.

Healthier People Software. (no date). *Healthier People: Health Risk Appraisal Program.* Memphis, TN: Author.

Indiana State Department of Health (ISDH). (1998). *Indiana Health Behavior Risk Factors.* Indianapolis, IN: Author.

Jackson, C. (1991). Healthy spirits, souls, and bodies. *Spirit of Truth,* June: 8–9.

Lasater, T. M., Carleton, R. A., & Wells, B. L. (1991). Religious organizations and large-scale health related lifestyle change programs. *Journal of Health Education, 22:* 233–239.

Levin, J. S., Larson, D. B., & Puchalski, C. M. (1997). Religion and spirituality in medicine: Research and Education. *The Journal of the American Medical Association, 278:* 792–793.

Lloyd, J. J. (1994). Collaborative health education training for African American health ministers and providers of community services. *Educational Gerontology, 20:* 265–276.

National Center for Health Statistics (NCHS). (1997). *Health, United States, 1996–97 and Injury Chartbook* (DHHS pub. no. PHS 97 1232). Hyattsville, MD: Author.

Ransdell, L. B., & Rehling, S. L. (1996). Church-based health promotion: A review of the current literature. *American Journal of Health Behavior, 20*(4): 195–207.

Thomas, S. B., Quinn, S. C., Billingsley, A., & Caldwell, C. (1994). The characteristics of northern black churches with community outreach programs. *American Journal of Public Health, 84:* 575–579.

U.S. Department of Health and Human Services (USDHHS). (1990). *Prevention '89/'90.* Washington, D.C.: U.S. Government Printing Office.

WEBLINKS

1. http://www.thecommunityguide.org/index.html

   Guide to Community Preventative Services

   This is the webpage for the *Guide to Community Preventive Services* that includes evidence-based recommendations for programs and policies to promote population-based health.

2. http://www.astho.org

   Association of State and Territorial Health Officials (ASTHO)

   This is the website for the ASTHO. ASTHO is the national nonprofit organization representing the state and territorial public health agencies of the United States, the U.S. Territories, and the District of Columbia. This website has links to all the state and territorial health departments. If you are planning a program for the community setting, this site contains a lot of information that could help you develop a rationale for your program.

3. http://www.census.gov/compendia/statab

   The U.S. Census Bureau

   This page at the U.S. Census Bureau website provides information about the national data book called *Statistical Abstract of the United States*. The data book contains a collection of statistics on social and economic conditions in the United States. Selected international data are also included. The *Abstract* is also your Guide to Sources of other data from the Census Bureau, other Federal agencies, and private organizations.

4. http://www.welcoa.org/

   The Wellness Councils of America (WELCOA)

   This is the website for the WELCOA. WELCOA was founded in 1987 as a national nonprofit membership organization dedicated to promoting healthier life styles for all Americans, especially through health promotion initiatives at the worksite. If you are planning a program for the worksite setting, this site contains a lot of information that could help you develop a rationale for your program.

Assessing Needs

After reading this chapter and answering the questions at the end, you should be able to:

- Define need and needs assessment.
- Explain why a needs assessment is an important part of the planning process.
- Explain what should be expected from a needs assessment.
- Differentiate between primary and secondary data sources.
- Locate secondary data sources that are in print and on the World Wide Web.
- Explain how a needs assessment can be completed.
- Conduct a needs assessment within a given population.

KEY TERMS

action research	need	proxy measure
basic priority rating (BPR)	needs assessment	random-digit dialing
bias	networking	secondary data
categorical funds	nominal group process	self-assessments
community empowerment	observation	self-report
community forum	obtrusive observation	significant others
Delphi technique	opinion leaders	single-step survey
focus group	participatory data	unobtrusive
health assessments (HAs)	collection	observation
HIPAA	participatory research	walk-through
key informants	photovoice	windshield tour
mapping	primary data	

Once the planning committee is in place, the next step in the planning process is to identify the needs of those in the priority population. Gilmore and Campbell (2005) have defined **need** as "the difference between the present situation and a more desirable one" (p. 6). These needs can be expressed in many different ways. For example, there may be a need for better health, or a need for more knowledge, or a need to possess a certain skill, to name a few. Whether a need of the priority population is actual (*true* need) or perceived (*reported* need) does not matter (Gilmore & Campbell, 2006). What matters is being able to identify all needs, actual and perceived, so that they can be addressed through appropriate program planning.

The process of identifying, analyzing, and prioritizing needs of a priority population is referred to as a **needs assessment**. Other terms that have been used to describe the process of determining needs include *community analysis, community diagnosis,* and *community assessment.* Conducting a needs assessment may be the most critical step in the planning process because it "provides objective data to define important health problems, set priorities for program implementation, and establish a baseline for evaluating program impact" (Grunbaum et al., 1995, p. 54).

There are many reasons why a needs assessment should be completed before the other steps of the planning process begin. First, it is a logical place to start (Gilmore & Campbell, 2005). Before a need can be met, it first must be identified and measured. Second, a needs assessment can help insure the appropriate use of planning resources. Without determining and prioritizing needs, resources can be wasted on unsubstantiated programming. Third, failure to perform a needs assessment may lead to a program focus that prevents or delays adequate attention directed to a more important health problem. For example, a health problem that tends to create a high emotional response, particularly among parents, is the trauma associated with bicycle injuries in children. Of course, it is a tragedy when a preventable death occurs. In 2005, 16% of the 784 bicyclists killed in the United States were children ages 14 and under (NHTSA, 2007). But an even more significant determinant of childhood injury and death in the United States is the inadequate use of safety belts or car seats involved with motor vehicle crashes. In fact, motor vehicle injuries are the leading cause of death among children at every age after their first birthday and are the greatest public health threat to children in the United States today (CDC, 2006). A needs assessment that examined both bicycle and motor vehicle crashes would lead planners to determine in most locations, in most instances, that restraining children in motor vehicles with safety belts or approved car seats is an even more important problem.

Fourth, a needs assessment can determine the internal capacity of a community to address specific needs. That is, what are the strengths, resources, and assets within the community to deal with the need? Fifth, a needs assessment can provide a focus for developing an intervention to meet the needs of the priority population. And finally, knowing the needs of a priority population provides a reference point to which future assessments can be compared.

Having just stated several reasons why a needs assessment should be completed, it may seem odd that there are a few planning scenarios where a needs assessment would not be used. The first would be if another needs assessment had been conducted recently, possibly for another related program, and the funding or other resources to conduct a second needs assessment in such a short period of time were not available. A second scenario where a needs assessment may not be used is one where the program planners are employed by an agency that deals only with a specific need that is already known (e.g., cancer and the American Cancer Society), or the agency for which they work has received **categorical funds** that must be used for dealing with a specific disease (e.g., HIV/AIDS) or program (e.g., immunization) (Bartholomew et al., 2006).

The remaining portions of this chapter will present discussions on what to expect from a needs assessment, the types and sources of data used to conduct a needs assessment, and a suggested process for conducting a needs assessment. **Box 4.1** identifies the responsibilities and competencies for health educators that pertain to the material presented in this chapter.

Box 4.1 RESPONSIBILITIES AND COMPETENCIES FOR HEALTH EDUCATORS

The content of Chapter 4 is associated with a single area of responsibility. That responsibility and related competencies include:

Responsibility I: Assess Individual and Community Needs for Health Education

Competency A: Access existing health-related data

Competency B: Collect health-related data

Competency C: Distinguish between behaviors that foster or hinder well-being

Competency D: Determine factors that influence learning

Competency E: Identify factors that foster or hinder the process of health education

Competency F: Infer needs for health education from obtained data

Source: NCHEC, SOPHE, & AAHE (2006).

What to Expect From a Needs Assessment

By examining the needs assessment definitions presented by others, planners can get an idea of what to expect from a needs assessment. Gilmore and Campbell (2005) defined needs assessment as "a planned process that identifies the reported needs of an individual or group" (p. 7). The National Commission for Health Education Credentialing, Inc., along with two professional health education organizations, have defined needs assessment as a "systematic, planned collection of information about the health knowledge, perceptions, attitudes, motivation, and practices of individuals or groups and the quality of the socioeconomic environment in which they live" (NCHEC, SOPHE, & AAHE, 2006, p. 20). A third definition of needs assessment states that it is the process of collecting and analyzing information to develop an understanding of the issues, resources, and constraints of the priority population, as related to the development of health promotion programs (Anspaugh et al., 2000). Altschuld and Witkin (2000) provided a more encompassing definition when they defined a needs assessment as a "process of determining, analyzing, and prioritizing needs, and in turn, identifying and implementing solution strategies to resolve high-priority needs" (p. 253).

Other authors have indicated that a needs assessment should answer certain questions. Peterson and Alexander (2001) have suggested that a needs assessment should answer the following questions: (1) Who is the priority population? (2) What are the needs of the priority population? (3) Which subgroups within the priority population have the greatest need? (4) Where are these subgroups located geographically? (5) What is currently being done to resolve identified needs? and (6) How well have the identified needs been addressed in the past?

No matter how needs assessment is defined, the concept embedded in the definitions is the same: identifying the needs of the priority population and determining the degree to which the needs are being met.

Acquiring Needs Assessment Data

Two types of data are generally associated with a needs assessment: primary data and secondary data. **Primary data** are those data you collect yourself (e.g., a survey, a focus group, in-depth interviews, etc.) which answer unique questions related to your specific needs assessment. Most methods of collecting primary data are ones in which those collecting the data interact with (e.g., interviewing) those from whom the data are being collected. Such methods have been labeled as *interactive contact methods* (Marti-Costa & Serrano-Garcia as cited in Minkler, 2005). **Secondary data** are those data already collected by somebody else and available for your immediate use. Thus, the methods to collect these data have been labeled as *no contact methods* (Marti-Costa & Serrano-Garcia as cited in Minkler, 2005). The advantages of using secondary data are that (1) they already exist, and thus collection time is minimal, and (2) they are usually fairly inexpensive to access. Both of these advantages are important to planners because programs are often planned when both time and money are limited. However, a drawback of using secondary data is that the information might not identify the true needs of the priority population—perhaps because of how the data were collected, when they were collected, what variables were considered, or from whom the data were collected. A good rule is to move cautiously and make sure the secondary data are applicable to the immediate situation before using them.

Primary data have the advantage of directly answering the questions planners want answered by those in the priority population. However, collecting primary data can be expensive and when done correctly, take a great deal of time.

An overview of the means of acquiring primary and secondary data are presented in the following pages.

Sources of Primary Data

Primary data can be collected using a variety of methods. Those most commonly used in planning health promotion programs are presented (see **Table 4.1**).

Single-Step or Cross-Sectional Surveys   Single-step surveys, or as they are often called, *cross-sectional surveys*, are a means of gathering primary data in which the data collectors gather the data from the individuals or groups with a single contact—thus, the term

Table 4.1   Sources of primary data

Single-Step or Cross-Sectional Surveys
    From priority population—self-report
        written questionnaires
        telephone interviews
        face-to-face interviews
        electronic interviews
        group interviews
    Proxy measures
    From significant others
    From opinion leaders
    From key informants
Multi-Step Survey: Delphi Technique
Community Forum (Town Hall Meeting)
Meetings
Focus Group
Nominal Group Process
Observation
    Direct observation
    Indirect observation (proxy measures)
    "Windshield" or walk-through (walking tours)
    Photovoice
Self-Assessments

single-step. Such surveys often take the form of written questionnaires and interviews. When individuals or groups (also sometimes called *respondents*) are answering questions about themselves, the information that is provided is referred to as **self-report** data. Thus, respondents are asked to recall ("When was your last visit to your dentist?") and report accurate ("On average, how many minutes do you exercise each day?") information. Self-report measures are essential for many needs assessments and evaluations because of the need to obtain subjective assessments of experiences (e.g., feelings about available programs, self-assessments of health status, and health behavior, such as eating patterns) (Bowling, 2005) and even marketing data (i.e., the best location for a program, the best time to offer a program, and willingness to pay for a program). In addition, self-report measures have a broad appeal to those who need to collect data, because "they are often quick to administer and involve little interpretation by the investigator" (Bowling, 2005, p. 15). However, planners should be aware that self-report data do have limitations. One such limitation is **bias** (those data that have been distorted because of the way they have been collected). (See the section in Chapter 5 on bias data.) To overcome some of these limitations and to maximize the usefulness of self-report, Baranowski (1985) has developed eight steps to increase the accuracy of this method of data collection:

1. Select measures that clearly reflect program outcomes.

2. Select measures that have been designed to anticipate the response problems and that have been validated.

3. Conduct a pilot study with the priority population. (See Chapter 5 for pilot studies).

4. Anticipate and correct any major sources of unreliability.

5. Employ quality-control procedures to detect other sources of error.

6. Employ multiple methods.

7. Use multiple measures.

8. Use experimental and control groups with random assignment to control for biases in self-report.

By following these steps, planners can enhance the accuracy of self-report, making this a more effective method of data collection.

For a variety of reasons, there are times when those in the priority population cannot respond for themselves or do not want to respond. In such situations, planners will have to collect the data indirectly. Such a method is referred to as a proxy (or indirect) measure. A **proxy measure** is an outcome measure that provides evidence that a behavior has occurred. Or as Dignan (1995) states, "indirect measures are unmistakable signs that a specific behavior has occurred" (p. 103). Examples of proxy or measures may include (1) lower blood pressure for the behavior of medication taking, (2) body weight for the behaviors of exercise and dieting, (3) cotinine in the blood for tobacco use, (4) empty alcoholic beverages in the trash for consumption of alcohol, or (5) a spouse reporting on the compliance of his/her partner (Cottrell & McKenzie, 2005). Proxy measurements of skills or behavior usually require more resources and cooperation to obtain than self-report or direct observation (Dignan, 1995). The greatest concern associated with proxy measures is making sure that the measure is both valid and reliable (Cottrell & McKenzie, 2005).

In addition to surveying the priority population, there are other groups of individuals who are commonly asked to respond to single-step surveys for the purpose of collecting primary needs assessment data. They include significant others of the priority population, community opinion leaders, and key informants. **Significant others** may include family members and friends. Collecting data from the significant others of a group of heart disease patients is a good example. Program planners might find it difficult to persuade the heart disease patients themselves to share information about their outlook on life and living with heart disease. A survey of spouses or other family members might help elicit this information so that the program planners could best meet the needs of the heart disease patients.

Opinion leaders are individuals who are well respected in a community and who can accurately represent the views of the priority population. These leaders are:

1. Discriminating users of the media

2. Demographically similar to the priority group

3. Knowledgeable about community issues and concerns

4. Early adopters of innovative behavior (see Chapter 11 for an explanation of these terms)

5. Active in persuading others to become involved in innovative behavior

Opinion leaders include political figures, chief executive officers (CEOs) of companies, union leaders, administrators of local school districts, and other highly visible and respected individuals. (See **Figure 4.1** for a form for tallying opinion leader survey data.)

Key informants are strategically placed individuals who have knowledge and ability to report on the needs of those in the priority population. They may or may not be in positions with formal authority, but they are often respected by others in the community and thus possess informal authority. Because they may be biased, planners need to be careful not to base an entire needs assessment on the data generated from a key informant survey.

Single-step surveys of those in the priority population, significant others, opinion leaders, and key informants can be administered, as noted earlier, several different ways. The primary means of collecting data from these individuals include written questionnaires, telephone interviews, face-to-face interviews, electronic interviews, and group interviews. A discussion of each follows.

Written Questionnaires. Probably the most often used method of collecting self-reported data is the written questionnaire. It has several advantages, notably the ability to reach a large number of respondents in a short period of time, even if there is a large geographic area to be covered. This method offers low cost with minimum staff time needed. However, it often has the lowest response rate.

With a written questionnaire, each individual receives the same questions and instructions in the same format, so that the possibility of response bias is lessened. The corresponding disadvantage, however, is the inability to clarify any questions or confusion on the part of the respondent.

Data collection method				Number of interviewers	
Total number of people interviewed				From: _____ To: _____	
				Date Collected _____	

Rank	Health Problem	Number of Persons Identifying Problem	Percentage of Persons Identifying Problem
1.			
2.			
3.			
4.			
5.			
6.			
7.			
8.			
9.			
10.			

Source: U.S. Department of Health and Human Services, Centers for Disease Control and Prevention (no date), p. A3-12.

Figure 4.1 Form to tally opinion leader survey data

As mentioned, the response rate for mailed questionnaires tends to be low especially if respondents cannot remain anonymous, but there are several ways to overcome this problem. One way is to include with the questionnaire a postcard that identifies the person in some way (such as by name or identification number). The individual is asked to return the questionnaire in the envelope provided and to send the postcard back separately. Anonymity is thus maintained, but the planner/evaluator knows who returned a questionnaire. The planner/evaluator can then send a follow-up mailing (including a letter indicating the importance of a response and another copy of the questionnaire with a return envelope) to the individuals who did not return a postcard from the first mailing. The use of incentives also can increase the response rate. For example, some hospitals offer free health risk appraisals to those who return a completed needs assessment instrument.

The appearance of the questionnaire is also extremely important when collecting data. It should be attractive, easy to read, and offer ample space for the respondents answers. It should also be easy to understand and complete, because written questionnaires provide no opportunity to clarify a point while the respondent is completing the questionnaire. In addition, all mailed questionnaires should be accompanied by a cover letter, to help clarify directions for completion.

Short questionnaires that do not take a long time to complete and questionnaires that clearly explain the need for the information are more likely to be returned. Planners/evaluators should give thought to designing a questionnaire that is as easy to complete and return as possible.

Face-to-Face Interviews. At times, it is advantageous to administer the instrument to the respondents in a face-to-face interview setting. This method is time consuming, since it may require not only time for the actual interview but also travel time to the interview site and/or waiting time between interviews. As with telephone interviews, the interviewer must be carefully trained to conduct the interview in an unbiased manner. It is important to explain the need for the information in order to conduct the needs assessment/evaluation and to accurately record the responses. Methods of probing, or eliciting additional information about an individual's responses, are used in the face-to-face interview, and the interviewer must be skilled at this technique.

This method of self-report allows the interviewer to develop rapport with the respondent. The flexibility of this method, along with the availability of visual cues, has the advantage of gaining more complete evaluation data from respondents. Smaller numbers of respondents are included in this method, but the rate of participation is generally high. It is important to establish and follow procedures for selecting the respondents. There are also several disadvantages to the face-to-face interview. It is more expensive, requiring more staff time and training of interviewers. Variations in the interviews, as well as differences between interviewers, may influence the results.

Telephone Interviews. Compared to mailed surveys or face-to-face interviews, the telephone interview offers a relatively easy method of collecting self-reported data at a moderate cost. The planner/evaluator must choose a way of selecting individuals to participate in this type of data collection: this method will reach only those individuals who have access to a telephone. One possibility is to call a randomly selected group of people who have completed a health promotion program. Another method is to select telephone numbers at random from a telephone directory—for example, a local telephone book, student directory, church directory, or employee directory. This method will not reach all the population, since some people have unlisted telephone numbers and cell phones. One way to overcome this problem is a method known as **random-digit dialing**, in which telephone number combinations are chosen at random. This method would include businesses as well as residences and nonworking as well as valid numbers, making it more time consuming. The numbers may be obtained from a table of random numbers or generated by a computer. The advantage of random-digit dialing is that it includes the entire survey population with a telephone in the area, including people with unlisted numbers and cell phones. Drawbacks to this method include some peoples' resistance to answer questions over the telephone or resentment in being interrupted with an unwanted call. This later reason seems to be more of a problem with the increase in telemarketing. Those conducting the interviews may also have difficulty reaching individuals because of unanswered phones or answering machines.

Telephone interviewing requires trained interviewers; without proper training and use of a standard questionnaire, the interviewer may not be consistent during the interview. Explaining a question or offering additional information can cause a respondent to change an initial response, thus creating a chance for interviewer bias. The interviewer does have the opportunity to clarify questions, which is an advantage over the written questionnaire, but does not have the advantage of visual cues that the face-to-face interview offers.

Electronic Interviews.   With more and more individuals having access to the Internet, email has been explored (Kittleson, 1995, 1997, 2003) as a means of collecting data. Advantages to this type of data collection is that is low in cost and almost instantaneous (McDermott & Sarvela, 1999). However, it has several drawbacks, including (1) access to a limited population, (2) lack of anonymity for respondents, and (3) easily ignored (McDermott & Sarvela, 1999). Until the drawbacks are overcome, this means of data collection will be used sparingly.

Group Interviews.   Interviewing individuals in groups provides for economy of scale. That is, data can be collected from several people in a short period of time. But there are some drawbacks of such data collection that primarily revolve around one or more group members influencing the response of others. A specific form of group interview discussed later in this chapter is focus groups. Focus groups are useful in collecting information for a needs assessment, but can also be used to determine if programs are being implemented effectively or determine program outcomes.

Multistep Survey   As its title might suggest, a multistep survey is one in which those collecting the data contact those who will provide the data on more than one occasion. The technique that uses this process is called the **Delphi technique**. It is a process that generates consensus through a series of questionnaires, which are usually administered via the mail or electronic mail. The process begins with those collecting the data asking the priority population to respond to one or two broad questions. The responses are analyzed, and a second questionnaire, with more specific questions, is developed and sent to the priority population. The answers to these more specific questions are analyzed again, and a new questionnaire is sent out, requesting additional information. If consensus is reached, the process may end here; if not, it may continue for another round or two (Gilmore & Campbell, 2005). Most often, this process continues for five or fewer rounds.

Community Forum The **community forum**, also sometimes referred to as a *town hall meeting*, approach brings together people from the priority population to discuss what they see as their group's problems/needs. It is not uncommon for a community forum to be organized by a group representing the priority population, in conjunction with the program planners. Such groups include labor, civic, religious, or service organizations, or groups such as the Parent Teacher Association (PTA). Once people have arrived, a moderator explains the purpose of the meeting and then asks those from the priority population to share their concerns. One or several individuals from the organizing group, called *recorders*, are usually given the responsibility for taking notes or taping the session to ensure that the responses are recorded accurately. However, when moderating a community forum, it is important to be aware that the silent majority may not speak out and/or a vocal minority may speak too loudly. For example, an individual parent's view may be wrongly interpreted to be the view of all parents.

At a community forum, participants may also be asked to respond in writing (1) by answering specific questions or (2) by completing some type of instrument. **Figure 4.2** is an example of an instrument that could be used to collect data from participants in a community forum.

Meetings Meetings are a good source of information for a preliminary needs assessment or various aspects of evaluation. For example, if a health department is planning to conduct a needs assessment and would like some direction on what health topics to key in on, planners may meet with a small group from the priority population to find out what they see as health issues in the community.

Directions: Please rank the need for each program in the community by placing a number in the space to the left of the programs. Use 1 to rank the program of greatest need, 2 for the next greatest need, and so forth, until you have ranked all seven programs. The program with the highest number next to it should be the one that, in your opinion, least needed. If you feel that a program should not be considered for implementation in our community, please place an X in the space to the left of the program instead of a number. Please note that the number you place next to each program represents its need in the community, not necessarily your desire to participate in it. After ranking the program, place an X to the right of the program in the column(s) that represent the age group(s) to which you feel the program should be targeted.

Program	All ages	Children 5–12	Teens 13–19	Adults 20–64	Older adults 65+
_____ Alcohol education:	_____	_____	_____	_____	_____
_____ Exercise/fitness:	_____	_____	_____	_____	_____
_____ Nutrition education:	_____	_____	_____	_____	_____
_____ Safety belt use:	_____	_____	_____	_____	_____
_____ Smoking cessation:	_____	_____	_____	_____	_____
_____ Smoking education:	_____	_____	_____	_____	_____
_____ Weight loss:	_____	_____	_____	_____	_____

Figure 4.2 Instrument for ranking program need

Source: Modified from a form developed by Amy L. Bernard, Ph.D., CHES; Associate Professor, University of Cincinnati. Adapted by permission.

The meeting structure can be flexible to avoid limiting the scope of the information gained. The cost of this form of data collection is minimal. Possible biases may occur when meetings are used as the sole source of data collection. Those involved may give "socially acceptable" responses to questions rather than discussing actual concerns. There also may be limited input if relatively few participants are included, or if one or two participants dominate the discussion.

Focus Group   The **focus group** is a form of qualitative research that grew out of group therapy. Focus groups are used to obtain information about the feelings, opinions, perceptions, insights, beliefs, misconceptions, attitudes, and receptivity of a group of people concerning an idea or issue. Focus groups are rather small, compared to community forums, and usually include only 8 to 12 people. If possible, it is best to have a group of people who do not know each other so that their responses are not inhibited by acquaintance. Participation in the group is by invitation. People are invited about one to three weeks in advance of the session. At the time of the invitation, they receive general information about the session but are not given any specifics. This precaution helps ensure that responses will be spontaneous yet accurate.

Once assembled, the group is led by a skilled moderator who has the task of obtaining candid responses from the group to a set of predetermined questions. In addition to eliciting responses to the questions, the moderator may ask the group to prioritize the different responses. As in a community forum, the answers to the questions are recorded through either written notes and/or audio or video recordings, so that at a later date the interested parties can review and interpret the results.

Focus groups are not easy to conduct. Special care must be given to developing the questions that will be asked. Poorly written questions will yield information that is less than useful. In addition, the moderator should be one who is skilled in leading a group. As might be surmised, the level of skill needed to conduct a focus group increases as the topic of discussion becomes more controversial.

Although focus groups have been shown to be an effective way of gathering data, they do have one major limitation. Participants in the groups are usually not selected through a random-sampling process. They are generally selected because they possess certain attributes (e.g., individuals of low income, city dwellers, parents of disabled children, or chief executive officers of major corporations). Participants may not be representative of the priority population. Therefore, the results of the focus group are not generalizable. "Findings [of focus groups] should be interpreted as suggestive and directional rather than as definitive" (Schechter, Vanchieri, & Crofton, 1990, p. 254). For more detail and information about preparing for and conducting focus groups, see Gilmore and Campbell (2005) and National Cancer Institute (2002).

Nominal Group Process   The **nominal group process** is a highly structured process in which a few knowledgeable representatives of the priority population (five to seven people) are asked to qualify and quantify specific needs. Those invited to participate are asked to record their responses to a question without discussing it among themselves. Once all have recorded a response, participants share their responses in a round-robin fashion. While this is occurring, the facilitator is recording the responses on a chalkboard or flipchart for all to see. The responses are clarified through a discussion. After the discussion, the participants are asked to rank-order the responses by importance to the priority population. This ranking may be considered either a preliminary or a final vote. If it is preliminary, it is followed with more discussion and a final vote.

Observation   Observation, defined as "notice taken of an indicator" (Green & Lewis, 1986, p. 363), can also be an effective means of collecting data. Not only can people be observed, but the environment (i.e., those things around the priority population) can be observed as well. Because those doing the observation can "see" but do not interact with those in the priority, observation has been labeled a *minimal-contact method of data collection.*

Observation can be direct or indirect. *Direct observation* means actually seeing a situation or behavior. For example, direct observation may include watching the eating patterns of children in a school lunchroom, observing workers on an assembly line to see if they are wearing their protective glasses, checking the smoking behavior of employees on break, and observing drivers for safety belt use. This method is somewhat time consuming, but it seldom encounters the problem of people refusing to participate in the data collection, resulting in a high response rate.

Observation is generally more accurate than self-report, but the presence of the observer may alter the behavior of the people being observed. For example, having someone observe smoking behavior may cause smokers to smoke less out of self-consciousness due to their being under observation. When people know they are being observed it is referred to as **obtrusive observation. Unobtrusive observation** means just the opposite; the persons being studied are not aware they are being measured, assessed, or tested. Typically, unobtrusive observation provides less biased data, but some question whether or not unobtrusive observation is ethical.

Differences among observers may also bias the results, because different observers may not observe and report behaviors in the same manner. Some behaviors, such as safety belt use, are very easy to observe accurately. Others, such as a person's degree of tension, are more difficult to observe. This method of data collection requires a clear definition of the exact behavior to observe and how to record it, in order to avoid subjective observations. Observer bias can be reduced by providing training and by determining rater reliability. If the observers are skilled, observation can provide accurate evaluation data at a moderate cost.

As noted earlier in this chapter, *indirect observation* (or proxy measure) can also be used to determine whether or not a behavior has occurred. This can be completed by either "observing" the outcomes of a behavior or by asking others (e.g., spouse) to report on such outcomes (see the earlier discussion on proxy measures). In addition, these measures can be used to verify self-reports when observations of the actual changes in behavior cannot be observed.

Some specific methods of observation that have been useful in collecting data for health promotion programs are *windshield tours* or *walk-throughs* and *photovoice.* When using a **windshield tour** or **walk-through,** the person(s) doing the observation "walks or drives slowly through a neighborhood, ideally on different days of the week and at different times of the day, on the lookout for a variety of potentially useful indicators of community health and well-being" (Hancock & Minkler, 2005, p. 150). Potentially useful indicators may include: "A) Housing types and conditions, B) Recreational and commercial facilities, C) Private and public sector services, D) Social and civic activities, E) Identifiable neighborhoods or residential clusters, F) Conditions of roads and distances must travel, G) Maintenance of buildings, grounds and yards" (Eng & Blanchard, 1990–1991, p. 96–97).

Photovoice (formerly called photo novella) is the creation of Wang and Burris (1994, 1997). It is a form of **participatory data collection** (i.e., those in the priority population participate in the data collection) in which those in the priority population are provided with cameras and skills training, then use the cameras to convey their own images of the community problems and strengths (Minkler & Wallerstein, 2005). "Photovoice has three goals. It enables people to record and reflect their community's strengths and problems. It promotes dialogue about important issues through group discussion and photographs. Finally, it engages policymakers" (Wang, 2005, ¶ 2).

Self-Assessments   Data can also be collected by those in the priority population through self-assessments. "A majority of these approaches address primary prevention issues, such as the assessment of risk factors in one's lifestyle pattern and the secondary prevention process of the early detection of disease symptoms" (Gilmore & Campbell, 2005, p. 143). Examples of such assessments include breast self-examination (BSE), testicular self-examination (TSE), self-monitoring for skin cancer, and **health assessments (HAs)**. "Health assessments include instruments known as health risk appraisals or health risk assessments (HRAs), health status assessments (HSAs), various lifestyle-specific (e.g., nutrition, stress, and physical activity) assessment instruments, wellness and behavioral/habit inventories" (SPM Board of Directors, 1999, p. xxiii), and disease/condition status assessments (e.g., chances of getting heart disease or diabetes).

Of the different self-assessments, it is the HAs that have been most useful in the needs assessment process, because from such assessments planners can obtain "group data which summarize major health problems and risk factors" (Alexander, 1999, p. 5). And of the HAs, it is the HRAs that are most often included in the needs assessment process. HRAs are instruments that estimate "the odds that a person with certain characteristics will die from selected causes within a given time span" (Alexander, 1999, p. 5). Even though HRAs are used as part of needs assessments, this was not their original intent. The original purpose of HRAs was to engage family physicians and their patients in conversation about risks of premature death and preventive health behaviors (Robbins & Hall, 1970).

To use an HRA as part of a needs assessment, planners would have those in the priority population complete a questionnaire. The instruments include questions about health behavior (e.g., smoking, exercise), personal or family health history of diseases (e.g., cancer, heart disease), demographics (e.g., age, gender), and usually some physiological data (e.g., height, weight, blood pressure, cholesterol). The resulting risk appraisals, in most cases, are calculated by computers, but some HRAs are hand-scored by the participant or health professional (Alexander, 1999). Most HRAs generate both individual and group reports. Thus planners can use the individual reports as part of an educational program for the priority population and use the group reports as another source of primary needs assessment data.

There are many HA instruments on the market. An excellent source for examining the different HAs available is the *SPM Handbook of Health Assessment Tools* (Hyner et al., 1999). This volume not only physically presents many of the HAs available today but it also includes information on (1) theoretical models associated with health assessment; (2) the use and selection of health assessment tools, including ethical considerations; (3) specific applications of health assessments; and (4) information on both the historic and prospective views of health assessment.

Although this discussion has revolved around the use of HRAs as means of providing information for a needs assessment, they have also been used to help motivate people to act on their health, to increase awareness, to serve as cues to action, and to contribute to program evaluation. However, the reliability, validity, and effectiveness in predicting risk and prompting behavior change is questionable (Edington, Yen, & Braunstein, 1999).

The following conclusions relative to HRAs can be made:

1. The reliability of HRA risk scores can vary greatly from one instrument to another.

2. Reliability scores decrease when users calculate their own score, as opposed to computer scoring.

3. There is a great variance in the self-reporting of specific risk factors and clinical physiologic measurements.

4. Only those HRAs for which reliability can be demonstrated should be used for evaluating the effectiveness of health education.

Table 4.2 summarizes the advantages and disadvantages of the various methods of collecting primary data.

Table 4.2   Methods of collecting primary data

Method	Advantages	Disadvantages
Self-Report		
Written questionnaire via mail	Large outreach No interviewer bias Convenient Low cost Minimum staff time required Easy to administer Quick Standardized	Possible low response rate Possible problem of representation No clarification of questions Need homogenous group if response is low No assurance addressee was respondent
Telephone interview	Moderate cost Relatively easy to administer Permits unlimited callbacks Can cover wide geographic areas	Possible problem of representation Possible interviewer bias Requires trained interviewers
Face-to-face interview	High response rate Flexibility Gain in-depth data Develop rapport	Expensive Requires trained interviewers Possible interviewer bias Limits sample size Time-consuming
Electronic mail*	Low cost Ease and convenience Almost instantaneous	Must have email access Self-selection Lack anonymity Risk of being "purged" Lack of "cueing" Must be short Noninvasive items only

(Table 4.2 continues)

Table 4.2 *(continued)*

Method	Advantages	Disadvantages

Group interview	High response rate
	Efficient and economical
	Can stimulate productivity
	  of others
		May intimidate and suppress
		  individual differences
		Fosters conformity
		Group pressure may influence
		  responses

Delphi technique**	Pooled responses Spans time and distance Reduced influence of others Enhanced response quality and quantity Equal representation Consistent participant contact	High cost and time commitment Reduced clarification opportunities Reduced immediate reinforcement
Community Forum (Town Hall Meeting)**	Straightforward to conduct Relative inexpensive Hear view of all segments of priority population People participate on own terms Can identify most interested	Difficult to achieve good attendance Representation of special interest Could degenerate into gripe session Data analysis can be time-consuming
Meetings	Good for formative evaluation Low cost Flexible	Possible result bias Limited input from participants
Focus Groups**	Low cost Convenience Creative atmosphere Ease of clarification High flexibility potential	Just qualitative data Limited representativeness Dependence on moderator skill Preliminary insights Recruitment of participants may be difficult
Nominal Group Process**	Direct involvement of target groups Planned interactivity Diverse opinions Full participation Creative atmosphere Recognition of common ground	Time commitment Competing issues Participant bias Segmented planning involvement
Observation	Accurate behavioral data Can be obtrusive Moderate cost	Requires trained observers May bias behavior Possible observer bias May be time-consuming
Self-assessments	Convenient No interviewer bias Convenient Moderate cost Minimum staff time required Easy to administer Flexibility	Possible low response rate Possible problem of representation Self-selection

*From McDermott and Sarvela (1999).

**From Gilmore and Campbell (2005).

Sources of Secondary Data

Several sources of secondary needs assessment data are available to planners. The main sources include data collected by government agencies at multiple levels (federal, regional, state, or local), data available from nongovernment agencies and organizations, data from existing records, and data or other evidence that are presented in the literature (see **Table 4.3**).

Table 4.3 Sample sources of secondary data available from governmental and nongovernmental agencies and organizations

Type of Agency/ Organization	Type of Data	URL (Web Address)
Government Agencies		
U.S. Bureau of Census	Demographic	
	U.S. Census	http://www.census.gov/
	Statistical Abstract of the United States	http://www.census.gov/ compendia/statab/
Centers for Disease Control and Prevention (CDC)	Health and Vital Statistics	
	National Center for Health Statistics (NCHS)	http://www.cdc.gov/nchs/
	Morbidity Mortality Weekly Report (MMWR)	http://www.cdc.gov/mmwr/
	CDC WONDER	http://wonder.cdc.gov/ welcome.html
	Behavioral Risk Factors	
	Behavioral Risk Factor Surveillance System (BRFSS)	http://www.cdc.gov/brfss/
	Youth Risk Behavior Surveillance System (YRBSS)	http://www.cdc.gov/ healthyyouth/yrbs/
Food & Drug Administration (FDA)	Health and Vital Statistics from States	http://www.fda.gov/oca/ sthealth.htm
Environmental Protection Agency (EPA)	Environmental Data and Statistics	http://www.epa.gov/
Substance Abuse & Mental Health Services Administration (SAMSHA)	Substance & Mental Health Statistical Information	http://www.samhsa.gov/
National Cancer Institute	Cancer Statistics	http://www.cancer.gov/
Nongovernmental Agencies and Organizations		
American Cancer Society	Cancer Information and Statistics	http://www.cancer.org/
American Heart Association	Heart Disease and Stroke Information and Statistics	http://www.americanheart.org/
The Henry J. Kaiser Family Foundation	Health Care Statistics	http://www.kff.org/

Data Collected by Government Agencies   Certain government agencies collect data on a regular basis. Some of the data collection is mandated by law (i.e., census, births, deaths, notifiable diseases, etc.), whereas other data are collected voluntarily (i.e., usage rates for safety belts). Since the data are collected by the government, program planners can gain free access to them by contacting the agency that collects the data or by finding them on the Internet, or in a library that serves as a United States government depository. Many college and university libraries and large public libraries serve as such depositories.

Data Available from Nongovernment Agencies and Organizations   In addition to the data available from government agencies, planners should also consult with nongovernment agencies and groups for data. Included among these are health care systems, voluntary health agencies, and business, civic, and commerce groups. For example, most of the national voluntary health agencies produce yearly "facts and figures" booklets that include a variety of epidemiological data. In addition, local agencies and organizations often have data they have collected for their own use. For example, it is not unusual for a local United Way to have performed a needs assessment in the community before distributing funds.

Data from Existing Records   These are health data that are often "collected as a by-product of a service effort, such as managing a clinic, an immunization program, or a water pollution control program" (Pickett & Hanlon, 1990, p. 151). These data can also serve as useful secondary needs assessment data. Using such data may be an efficient way to obtain the necessary information for a needs assessment (or an evaluation) without the need for additional data collection. The advantages include low cost, minimum staff needed, and ease in randomization. The disadvantages include difficulty in gaining access to the necessary records and the possible lack of availability of all the information needed for a needs assessment or program evaluation.

Examples of the use of existing records include checking medical records to monitor blood pressure and cholesterol levels of participants in an exercise program, reviewing insurance usage of employees enrolled in an employee health promotion program, and comparing the academic records of students engaging in an after-school weight loss program with those who are not. In these situations, as with all needs assessments using existing records, the cooperation of the agencies that hold the records is essential. At times, agencies may be willing to collect additional information to aid in the needs assessment for (or an evaluation of) a health promotion program. Keepers of records are concerned about confidentiality and the release of private information. The importance of privacy for those planners working in health care settings was further emphasized in 2003 with the enactment of the *Standards for Privacy of Individually Identifiable Health Information* section (The Privacy Rule) of the Health Insurance Portability and Accountability Act of 1996 (officially known as Public Law 104-191 and referred to as **HIPAA,** pronounced "hip-a"). The Rule sets national standards that health plans, health care clearinghouses, and health care providers who conduct certain health care transactions electronically must implement to protect and guard against the misuse of individually identifiable health information. Failure to implement the standards can lead to civil and criminal penalties (USDHHS, OCR, 2006). Planners can deal with these privacy issues by getting permission from all participants to use their records or by using only anonymous data.

Data from the Literature   Planners might also be able to identify the needs of a priority population by reviewing any available current literature about that priority population. An example would be a planner who is developing a health promotion program for individuals infected by the human immunodeficiency virus (HIV). Because of the seriousness of this disease and the number of people who have studied and written about it, there is a good chance that present literature could reflect the need of a certain priority population.

The best means of accessing data from the literature is by using the available literature databases. Most literature databases today are available in several different forms, including computer databases and the Internet. Computer access depends upon the capacity of the library or unit housing the databases. Depending on the database used, planners can expect to find comprehensive listings of citations for journal articles, book chapters, and books, and, in some databases, abstracts of the literature. Within the listings, most databases cite sources by both author and subject/title. **Figure 4.3** provides an example of what planners might find when searching a database.

Many literature databases are available to planners. Next is a short discussion of those databases that have proven helpful to health promotion planners.

PsycINFO   PsycINFO is an abstract (not full-text) database produced by the American Psychological Association (APA) that includes journal articles, book chapters, and book citations on literature in psychology and related subjects. The database is divided into several major categories, but two of particular interest to planners are (1) behavioral science and (2) mental health.

Medline   Medline, the primary component of and accessed through PubMed (http://www.ncbi.nlm.nih.gov/entrez/query.fcgi), is the U.S. National Library of Medicine's® (NLM) premier bibliographic database that contains over 15 million references from more than 5,000 journals covering the fields of medicine, nursing, dentistry, veterinary medicine, the health care system, and the preclinical sciences. "A distinctive feature of MEDLINE is that the records are indexed with NLM's Medical Subject Headings (MeSH®)" (NLM, 2006, ¶ 1).

Author Citation

Authors   Article title
↓   ↓
Thackeray, R., & Neiger, B. L., Use of social marketing to develop culturally-innovative diabetes interventions. <u>Diabetes Spectrum</u>. 2003; 16(1), 15–20.
                                    ↑   ↓   ↓
                              Journal   Journal volume   Pages
                                         (number)

Subject/Title

Article title
↓
Use of social marketing to develop culturally-innovative diabetes interventions. Thackeray, R., & Neiger, B. L., <u>Diabetes Spectrum</u>. 2003; 16(1), 15–20.

Figure 4.3 Sample citations

Education Resource Information Center (ERIC)   ERIC is an internet-based digital library of education literature sponsored by the Institute of Education Sciences (IES) of the U.S. Department of Education. ERIC provides free access to more than 1.2 million bibliographic records of journal articles and other education-related materials that have been indexed from 1966 to the present (ERIC, 2007).

Cumulative Index to Nursing & Allied Health Literature (CINAHL)   The CINAHL grew out of the work of a hospital librarian in the 1940s who created an index for nursing journals. Demand for this work grew over the years until in 1961 the first volume of *Cumulative Index to Nursing Literature (CINL)* was published. In order to keep pace with the trend toward a multidisciplinary approach to health care, the scope of coverage was expanded in 1977 to include allied health journals. That is the year its name changed to CINAHL. This database went online in 1984.

ETHXWeb   ETHXWeb is a database that "covers ethical, legal, and public policy issues surrounding health care and biomedical research. Citations are derived from the literature of law, religion, ethics, social sciences, philosophy, the popular media, and the health sciences" (Cottrell et al., 2009, p. 292).

Steps for Conducting a Literature Search

General Search Procedures   The process of searching a database is not difficult, and with the exception of a few individual differences, most indexes are arranged in a similar format. As Figure 4.3 indicated, most indexes include both an author and a subject/title index. An item that is specific to each index is its thesaurus, a listing of the key words the indexes used to index the subject/titles. Planners can find the thesauri online or in a separate volume with or near a hard copy of the indexes.

Figure 4.4 provides planners with a literature search strategy in the form of a flowchart. The chart begins by identifying the need of the priority population or topic to be searched. At this point, planners can search either by subject/title or by author. If planners know of an author who has done work on their topic, they can search the database using the author's last name. If they do not have information on authors, they will need to match their topic with the key words presented in the thesaurus. Since there are times when a topic is not expressed in the same terms used in the thesaurus, planners will need to look for related terms. Once they have a list of key words, they need to search the database for possible matches. In conducting this search, they need to ensure that they are using the database that covers the years of literature in which they are interested. This search should identify possible sources and citations.

Once sources are identified, planners may review abstracts (or entire documents) online or locate a hard copy of the document. Then, planners must determine the quality and usefulness of the publication in the needs assessment process. One means by which planners can judge the quality of the literature is to examine the references at the end of the publications. First, this reference list may lead planners to other sources not identified in the original search. Second, if the sources found in the database include all those commonly cited in the literature, this can verify the exhaustiveness of the search.

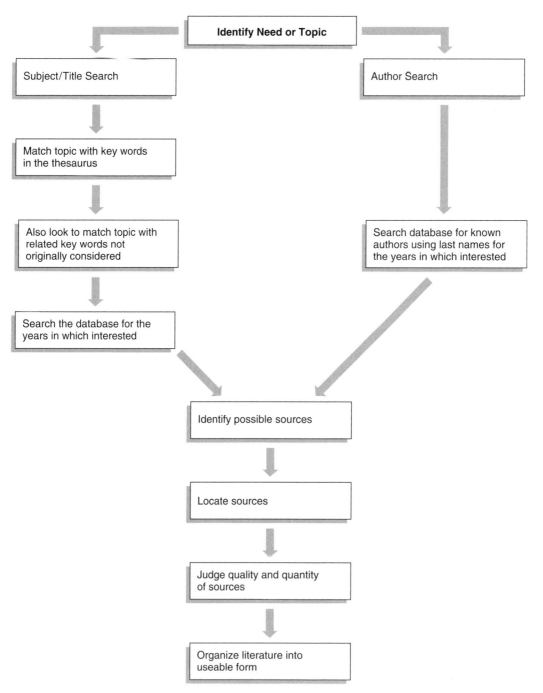

Figure 4.4 Literature search strategy flowchart

Source: Adapted from Deeds (1992) and Macarin (1995).

Searching via the World Wide Web   The continued development of the *World Wide Web* (WWW) has enhanced the opportunities for planners to obtain a variety of needs assessment data with the "touch of a button" from their home or office. Many of the government and nongovernment agencies and organizations, as well as the databases, discussed in this chapter have websites that planners can access if they have the web address, also known as the *Uniform Resource Locator* (URL). If the web address is unknown, planners can use a search engine to identify appropriate websites.

Popular search engines include Yahoo, Google, and WebCrawler. Planners can experiment with and select the sites that best fit their needs. If planners are using a term that has more than one word (i.e., *heart disease*), it is best to use quotation marks around the term when entering it on the search engine. "This will let the search engine know that the exact phrase, as contained in the quotation marks, is to be used when seeking sites that match. If the quotation marks are not used, the search engine will find sites that contain all the words in the query" (Cottrell et al., 2009, p. 296) and thus many of the sights found may not be of use.

As with any data source, planners need to be aware that not all data found via the WWW are valid and reliable. Thus planners need to scrutinize sources just as they would data found in hard copies. Several authors (Jadad & Gagliardi, 1998; Kotecki & Chamness, 1999; Pealer & Dorman, 1997; Silberg, Lundberg, & Musacchio, 1997; Tillman, 1997; Venditto, 1997) have published useful guides for evaluating information obtained via the Internet.

Using Technology to Collect Needs Assessment Data

As has already been mentioned in this chapter, more and more needs assessment data are being obtained through the use of technology (i.e., electronic interviews and computerized searchers of the World Wide Web and databases). In addition to these methods of data collection, program planners have used two other processes with increasing frequency. The first is the use of a commercial company to create an online data collection questionnaire with its own web address (URL). A number of different companies do such work (e.g., Zoomerang, SurveyMonkey, and Vovici). Most of these companies offer similar services. This is how they work. Customers sign up and pay a fee. For the most part, the fee is based upon the amount of service provided, and the length of time the service is used. Typical services offered include: design and preparation of the questionnaire, translation of the questionnaire into another language, customizing the questionnaire with organization logo/branding, personalized email cover letter introducing the questionnaire, personalized email "thank you" letters for those who complete the instrument, data tallying and analysis, various trainings, and customer support. The costs of the services vary depending on the type of customer, but most companies provide a discount for not-for-profit and educational organizations.

The second process that is being used more frequently is the use of geographic information systems (GIS) to help provide meaning to collected data. Being able to "map" the data provides this meaning. **Mapping** is the visual representation of data by geography or location, linking information to a place (Kirschenbaum & Russ, 2005). "Mapping is a powerful tool for two reasons: (1) it makes patterns based on place much easier to identify and analyze, and (2) it provides a visual way of communicating those patterns to a broad audience, quickly and dramatically" (Kirschenbaum & Russ, 2005, p. 450). The process of mapping involves (1) identifying the geographic area that the map will cover, (2) collecting the necessary data, (3) importing the data into GIS software so that the data can be placed on maps, and (4) analyzing what is found in the maps. In more technical terminology, "with GIS, digital maps and databases are stored with linked geo-referenced identifiers to facilitate rapid computer manipulation, analysis, and spatial display of information" (Riner, Cunningham, & Johnson, 2004, p. 57). The use of GIS in the needs assessment process will continue to grow as the development of such software becomes more widely available and easier to use. A helpful listing of existing GIS software is available at http://www.geoplan.ufl.edu/software.html.

Conducting a Needs Assessment

A number of different approaches can be used to determine the needs of the priority population. "Need assessments range from informal approaches, using educated and informed observations to formal, comprehensive research projects. However, the informal approaches are less reliable than a planned and scientifically developed research approach" (Timmreck, 2003, p. 89). Oftentimes, informal approaches are used because of limited time, personnel, and money. However, as noted in the beginning of this chapter, needs assessment may be the most critical step in the planning process and should not be taken lightly. Resources used on need assessments usually pay dividends many times over. Therefore the authors present a six-step process that is more formal in nature: (1) determining purpose and defining the scope of the needs assessment, (2) gathering data, (3) analyzing the data, (4) identifying the risk factors linked to the health problem, (5) identifying the program focus, and (6) validating the need before continuing on with the planning process (see **Figure 4.5**).

Step 1: Determining the Purpose and Scope of the Needs Assessment

The initial step in the needs assessment process is to determine the purpose and the scope of the needs assessment. In other words, what is the goal of the needs assessment? What does the planning committee hope to gain from the needs assessment? How extensive will the needs assessment be? What kind of resources will be available to conduct the needs assessment? In reality, the first challenge associated with conducting a needs assessment

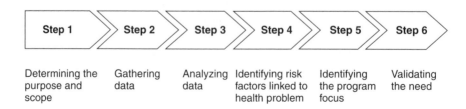

Figure 4.5 Steps in conducting a needs assessment

is determining whether an assessment should even be performed, and if so, what type of needs assessment is appropriate. For example, a great deal of health promotion today is driven by categorical funding. This means that the funding that supports programs is earmarked or dedicated to a specific health problem or determinant (i.e., risk factor). If this is the case, planners will not assess needs related to what health problem they should address since this is already predetermined by the funding agency. Likewise, if a planner works for the American Heart Association, he or she will not assess needs to determine a priority health problem—that has already been identified as heart disease.

Even if a health problem is already identified, it may be necessary to identify which determinants are most significant or which intervention strategies demonstrate the most promise in addressing the problem at hand. For example, heart disease may be the priority health problem, but it may be critical to assess the comparative importance of smoking, high blood pressure, and high blood cholesterol to identify appropriate interventions. The extent to which a needs assessment is necessary and appropriate should be determined by stakeholders, including key decision makers.

Some times, it is important to perform a needs assessment even if the health problem or determinant has been identified. For example, if the priority health problem is breast cancer, it is still necessary to collect current information on the degree to which women are either dying or suffering from the disease. It will be important to know how prevalent breast cancer is, where it is most prevalent in the population, high risk subpopulations, economic costs, and general trends over time. Stakeholders will want continual status reports on the extent of the problem.

In other cases, a planner may be found in a situation where a community needs assessment has not been performed for a long period of time or where categorical funding does not dictate what health problem(s) should be addressed. This will require planners and their partners to collect a wide range of data, compare the importance of multiple health problems, and set priorities. In a general sense, this is the process that is often referred to as community assessment. This implies that all significant health problems are examined to assess their relative significance. Stakeholders and planning groups will also usually determine how many health problems will be analyzed in the needs assessment. This will be influenced by how much time, and how many resources, can be directed to the needs assessment.

Another important decision that must be made is the extent to which actual consumers or clients will be involved in the needs assessment. The term **action** or **participatory research** has gained popularity in recent years, though it is often misunderstood or used inappropriately. In its truest sense, action research is characterized by at least four factors: (1) **community empowerment** (i.e., community members control decision making); (2) collaboration; (3) acquisition of knowledge through hands-on participation; and (4) a focus on social change. What often results is a scenario where planners invite a few community representatives to participate in assessing needs and setting priorities, but this is rarely representative of the population to be served.

Once the basic purpose and scope of the needs assessment is identified, planners may proceed to data collection. However, planners must not treat this first step too lightly. Although a natural tendency is to move forward quickly, an understanding of why a needs assessment is being performed will give proper direction to all other steps that follow.

Step 2: Gathering Data

The second step in the needs assessment process is gathering data. As noted earlier in this chapter, there are many different sources of needs assessment data. A part of the art of conducting a needs assessment is to be able to identify the most relevant data possible. By *relevant data,* we mean those data that are most applicable to the planning situation and that will do the best job of helping planners to identify the actual needs of the priority population. Because of the cost and availability, it is recommended that planners begin the data-gathering process by trying to locate relevant secondary data. For example, if a national program is being planned, then national secondary data should be sought from appropriate national government and nongovernment agencies. If a local program is being planned, then appropriate local data should be sought. When planning a local program, it is not unusual to find that local data do not exist. If that is the case, planners may need to use state, regional or national data (in that order) and apply them to the local area. For example, let's assume diabetes mellitus mortality data are needed for local planning and the only data available are national level data. Planners could use national data (e.g., 25.3 per 100,000 people died of diabetes in 2003) to estimate the number of deaths in a local community. If the population of a local city is 250,000, planners could infer that the number of deaths due to diabetes in the city during 2003 totaled 63 (i.e., 25.3 × 2.5). If the city's population were older, 63 deaths could be viewed as a low estimate since diabetes deaths are more prevalent in older populations. Conversely, if the population were younger, 63 deaths could be viewed as a high estimate. Obviously, as noted at the beginning of this chapter, there are disadvantages of using secondary data, but good planners use and interpret them in light of their limitations (McDermott & Sarvela, 1999).

Once relevant secondary data have been identified, planners need to turn their attention to gathering the appropriate primary data in order to fill in the "data gaps" to better understand the needs of the priority population. For example, if secondary data show that there is a need for cancer education programming, but does not specifically identify the type of cancer or segment the priority population by useful demographic characteristics (i.e., age or sex), then efforts should be made to collect such data. Or, it may be that all the secondary data are *quantitative data* such as how frequently a service is used, and thus it might be very useful to collect primary data that are *qualitative* in nature such as detailed explanations of why a service was not used. It should be noted that primary data collection could have a dual purpose. Not only do primary data collections provide valuable information about the specific planning situation that cannot be obtained from secondary data, they also provide an opportunity to get those in the priority population actively involved and contributing to the program planning process. Thus, planners need to decide what primary data are needed, from whom should they be collected (e.g., All? Some? Just certain demographic groups?), and what methods (e.g., Interviews? Questionnaires? Focus groups?) would be best for not only collecting the needed information but also in getting active participation from the priority population.

As planners conclude the second step in the needs assessment process, they must remember that each planning situation is different. It is desirable to have both primary and secondary needs assessment data in order to gain a clear picture of needs; however, depending on the resources and circumstances, planners may have access to only one or the other. In addition, there is usually a trade-off between quality and quantity of data. Planners must use the best data available under the challenges and constraints facing them.

Step 3: Analyzing the Data

At this point in the needs assessment process, the planners must analyze all the data collected, with the goal of identifying and prioritizing the health problems. The goal of data analysis is easily stated, but this step may be the most difficult to complete. There are those rare occasions where the data analysis is not very complicated because the need is obvious. For example, the data may clearly show that breast cancer rates have continued to rise in the community, while the number of breast screenings have been dropping, and those in the priority population recognize the problem. Or, in another setting the data analysis shows a very clear correlation between the health status of the priority population and the lack of primary health care received. However, not all analyses of data yield such obvious needs. More often than not, planners are faced with trying to compare data that are not easily compared. The data may be mixed (i.e., apples and oranges) or confusing. For example, they may have mortality data for one health problem, morbidity data for another, and perhaps behavioral risk factor data for yet another. Or, if planners are working with a multicultural priority population, data analysis may even be more confusing, because health concepts held by one culture may be very different than the health concepts held by the planners. These cultural differences "often involve family, community, and/or supernatural agents in cause and effect, placation, and treatment rituals to prevent, control, or cure illness. A failure to understand and appreciate these 'differences' can have serious implications for success of any health promotion/disease prevention effort" (Kline & Huff, 1999, p. 106).

One systematic way to analyze the data is to use the first few phases of the PRECEDE-PROCEED model for guidance. Start by asking and answering the following questions:

1. What is the quality of life of those in the priority population?

2. What are social conditions and perceptions shared by those in the priority population?

3. What are the social indicators (e.g., absenteeism, crime, discrimination, performance, welfare, etc.) in the priority population that reflect the social conditions and perceptions?

4. Can the social conditions and perceptions be linked to health promotion? If so, how?

5. What are the health problems associated with the social problems?

6. Which health problem is most important to change?

The last question in this list is really asking the question, Which health problem/ need should get priority? The health problems/needs must be prioritized not because the lowest-priority problems/needs are not important, but because organizations have limited resources. Thus planners need to see how the health promotion dollars can best be used. Therefore, in setting priorities, the planners should seek answers to these questions:

1. What is the most pressing need?

2. Are there resources adequate to deal with the problem?

3. Can the problem best be solved by a health promotion intervention, or could it be handled better through another means?

4. Are effective intervention strategies available to address the problem?

5. Can the problem be solved in a reasonable amount of time?

After answering these questions, the planners should be able to prioritize the identified problems/needs.

The actual process of setting priorities can take many different forms and range from basic rank ordering by a group of stakeholders, to use of the nominal group process, to a more complex process called the **Basic Priority Rating (BPR)** process. The BPR process was first presented by Hanlon (1974) (it has been more recently presented in Pickett & Hanlon, 1990) and will be discussed here in greater detail because it can greatly help program planners quantify the subjective process of prioritizing. The process requires planners to rate four different components of the identified needs and insert the ratings into a formula in order to determine a rating between 0 and 100. The components and their possible scores (in parenthesis) are:

A. size of the problem (0 to 10)

B. seriousness of the problem (0 to 20)

C. effectiveness of the possible interventions (0 to 10)

D. propriety, economics, acceptability, resources, and legality (PEARL) (0 or 1)

The formula in which the scores are placed is:

$$\text{Basic Priority rating (BPR)} = \frac{(A + B)C}{3} \times D$$

Component A, size of the problem, can be scored by using epidemiological rates or determining the percentage of the priority population at risk. The higher the rate or percentage, the greater the score. Pickett and Hanlon (1997) offer the scale noted in **Table 4.4** for scoring the size of the problem when using incidence and prevalence rates.

Component B, seriousness of the problem, is examined using four factors: economic loss to community, family, or individuals; involvement of other people who were not initially affected by the problem, as with the spread of an infectious disease; the severity of the problem measured in mortality, morbidity, or disability; and the urgency of solving the problem because of additional harm. Because the maximum score for this component is 20, raters can use a 0 to 5 score for each of the four factors.

Component C, effectiveness of the interventions, is often the most difficult of the four components to measure. The efficacy of some intervention strategies is known, such as immunizations (close to 100%) and smoking cessation classes (around 30%), but for many, it is not. Planners will need to estimate this score based upon the work of others or their own expert opinions. In scoring this component, planners should

Table 4.4 Scoring the size of the problem

Incidence or Prevalence per 100,000 Population	Score
50,000 or more	10
5,000 to 49,999	8
500 to 4,999	6
50 to 499	4
5 to 49	2
0.5 to 4.9	0

Source: G. Pickett and J. J. Hanlon, *Public Health: Administration and Practice.* Copyright ©
1997. Reprinted by permission of McGraw-Hill Companies, Inc.

consider both the effectiveness of intervention strategies in terms of behavior change, as
well as the degree to which the priority population will demonstrate interest in the intervention strategy.

Component *D*, PEARL, consists of several factors that determine whether a particular intervention strategy can be carried out at all. The score is 0 or 1; any need that
receives a zero will automatically drop to the bottom of the priority list because a score of
zero (a multplier) for this component will yield a total score of zero in the formula. Examples of when a zero may result are if an intervention is economically impossible, unaccept-
able to the priority population or planners, or illegal. Ideally, some of these assessments
will be made before a health problem is considered in the priority setting process.

Once the score for the four components is determined, an overall priority rating for
each need can be calculated, and the prioritizing can take place.

Other means of quantifying the prioritization of the needs may include getting the
priority population or key people from the community, such as opinion leaders, to rank-
order the identified needs.

How will planners know when they have completed Step 3 (Analyzing the Data) of
the needs assessment process? Planners should be able to list in rank order the health
problems/needs of the priority population.

Step 4: Identifying the Risk Factors Linked to the Health Problem

Step 4 of the needs assessment process is parallel to the second part of Phase 2 of the
PRECEDE-PROCEED model: epidemiological assessment. In this step, planners need
to identify the determinants of the health problem identified in the previous step. That
is, what genetic, behavioral, and environmental risk factors are associated with the
health problem? Because most genetic determinants either cannot be changed or interact with the behavior and/or environment, the task in this step is to identify and prioritize the behavioral and environmental factors that, if changed, could lessen the health
problem in the priority population. In essence, modifying these factors or determinants is the real work of health promotion. Thus, if the health problem is lung cancer,
planners should analyze the health behaviors and environment of the priority population for known risk factors of lung cancer. For example, higher than expected smoking behavior may be present in the priority population, and the people may live in a

community where smokefree public environments are not valued. Once these risk factors are identified, they too need to be prioritized (see Figure 2.3 for a means of prioritizing these risk factors).

Step 5: Identifying the Program Focus

The fifth step of the needs assessment process is similar to the third phase of the PRECEDE-PROCEED model: educational and ecological assessment. With behavioral and environmental risk factors identified and prioritized, planners need to identify those predisposing, enabling, and reinforcing factors that seem to have a direct impact on the risk factors. In the lung cancer example, those in the priority population may not have (1) the skills necessary to stop smoking (predisposing factor), (2) access to a smoking cessation program (enabling factor), or (3) people around them who support efforts to stop smoking (reinforcing factor). "Study of the predisposing, enabling, and reinforcing factors automatically helps the planner decide exactly which of the factors making up the three classes deserve the highest priority as the focus of the intervention. The decision is based on their importance and any evidence that change in the factor is possible and cost-effective" (Green & Kreuter, 1999, p. 42).

In addition, when prioritizing needs, planners also need to consider any existing health promotion programs to avoid duplication of efforts. Therefore, program planners should seek to determine the status of existing health promotion programs by trying to answer as many questions as possible from the following list:

1. What health promotion programs are presently available to the priority population?

2. Are the programs being utilized? If not, why not?

3. How effective are the programs? Are they meeting their stated goals and objectives?

4. How were the needs for these programs determined?

5. Are the programs accessible to the priority population? Where are they located? When are they offered? Are there any qualifying criteria that people must meet to enroll? Can the priority population get to the program? Can the priority population afford the programs?

6. Are the needs of the priority population being met? If not, why not?

There are several ways to seek answers to these questions. Probably the most common way is through **networking** with other people working in health promotion and the health care system—that is, communicating with others who may know about existing programs. (See Chapter 9 for a more detailed discussion of networking.) These people may be located in the local or state health department, in voluntary health agencies, or in health care facilities, such as hospitals, clinics, nursing homes, extended care facilities, or managed care organizations.

Planners might also find information about existing programs by checking with someone in an organization that serves as a clearinghouse for health promotion programs or by using a community resource guide. The local or state health department, a local chamber of commerce, a coalition, the local medical/dental societies, a community task force, or a community health center may serve as a clearinghouse or produce such a guide. Another avenue is to talk with people in the priority population. Although they may not know about all existing programs, they may be able to share information on the effectiveness and accessibility of some of the programs. Finally, some of the information could be collected in Step 2 through separate community forums, focus groups, or surveys.

Step 6: Validating the Prioritized Needs

The final step in the needs assessment process is to validate the identified need(s). *Validate* means to confirm that the need that was identified is the need that should be addressed. Obviously, if great care were taken in the needs assessment process, validation should be a perfunctory step. However, there have been times when a need was not properly validated; much energy and many resources have thereby been wasted on unnecessary programs.

Validation amounts to "double checking," or making sure that an identified need is the actual need. Any means available can be used, such as (1) rechecking the steps followed in the needs assessment to eliminate any bias, (2) conducting a focus group with some individuals from the priority population to determine their reaction to the identified need (if a focus group was not used earlier to gather the data), and (3) getting a "second opinion" from other health professionals.

SUMMARY

This chapter presented several definitions of needs assessment and a discussion of primary and secondary data. The sources of these data were discussed at length. Also, presented in this chapter was a six-step approach that planners can follow in conducting a needs assessment on a given group of people. It is by no means the only way of conducting an assessment, but it is one viable option.

No matter what procedure is used to conduct a needs assessment, the end result should be the same. Planners should finish with a clearly defined program focus.

REVIEW QUESTIONS

1. What is a need? What does *needs assessment* mean?

2. What should program planners expect from a needs assessment?

3. What is the difference between primary and secondary data?

4. Name several different sources of both primary and secondary data.

5. What advice might you give to someone who is interested in using previously collected data (secondary data) for a needs assessment?

6. What is the difference between a single-step (cross-sectional) and a multistep survey?

7. Explain the difference between a community forum and a focus group.

8. What is a health assessment (HA)?

9. What are the six steps in the needs assessment process, as identified in the chapter? What is the most difficult step to complete?

ACTIVITIES

1. Assume a local health department (LHD) that serves a rural population of about 100,000 people has hired you. After a few months on the job, your supervisor has given you the task of conducting a needs assessment. The last one completed by this LHD was 15 years ago. Based upon the annual reports of the LHD over the past 5 years, it has been determined that the needs assessment should focus on the needs of the elderly. For the purpose of this needs assessment, the LHD has defined elderly as those 65 years of age and older. Working with the six-step approach to needs assessment presented in this chapter, complete the first two steps. Complete Step 1 by writing a purpose and scope for the needs assessment. Complete the first part of Step 2 by identifying at least four sources of relevant secondary data. Also, describe what you think would be the best way to go about collecting primary data and defend your choice. Then complete this activity by creating a list of things you would like to find out by gathering primary data.

2. Visit the website of a commercial company (e.g., Zoomerang, SurveyMonkey, and Vovici) that is in the business of helping others collect primary data via the Internet. Once at the site, find out as much as you can about using the service. What specific services does the company offer? How much do the services cost? What group of program planners do you think would most benefit from using the services? Summarize the results of your "fact-finding" experience in a one-page paper.

3. Using secondary data provided by your instructor or obtained from the World Wide Web (such as data from a Behavioral Risk Factor Surveillance System, state or local secondary data, or data from the National Center for Health Statistics), analyze the data and determine the health problems of the priority population.

4. Administer an HHA/HRA to a group of 25 to 30 people. Using the data generated, identify and prioritize a collective list of health problems of the group.

5. Plan and conduct a focus group on an identified health problem on your campus. Develop a set of questions to be used, identify and invite people to participate in the group, facilitate the process, and then write up a summary of the results based on your written notes and/or an audiotape of the session.

6. Using the data (paper-and-pencil instruments, clinical tests, and health histories) generated from a local health fair, identify and prioritize a collective list of health problems of those who participated.

WEBLINKS

1. http://ctb.ku.edu/

   Community Tool Box

   This site provides excellent resources on community assessment, conducting surveys, identifying problems, and assessing community needs and resources. Topic sections include step-by-step instruction, examples, checklists, and related resources.

2. http://www.healthypeople.gov/state/toolkit/default.htm

   Healthy People 2010 Tool Kit: A Field Guide to Health Planning

   This tool kit provides valuable resources for identifying and securing resources, identifying and engaging community partners, and setting health priorities, all important components of conducting an effective needs assessment.

3. http://www.cdc.gov/nchs/express.htm

   National Center for Health Statistics

   This webpage of the National Center for Health Statistics (NCHS) provides an overview of all of the surveys and data collections systems of the NCHS. In addition, it provides the results of many of the surveys and examples of the questionnaires used to collect the data.

4. http://www.statehealthfacts.kff.org/cgi-bin/healthfacts.cgi

   Kaiser Family Foundation State Health Facts Online

   This site contains current state-level data on demographics, health, and health policy, including health coverage, access, financing, and state legislation. Planners can access information as tables, bar graphs, or color-coded maps.

5. http://wonder.cdc.gov/welcome.html

   CDC WONDER

   This is the home page for the Centers for Disease Control and Prevention's (CDC) Wide-ranging OnLine Data for Epidemiologic Research (WONDER). CDC WONDER is an easy-to-use, menu-driven system that provides access to a wide array of secondary public health information. It also has a link to the latest data to support the *Healthy People 2010* objectives.

5

Measurement, Measures, Measurement Instruments, and Sampling

After reading this chapter and answering the questions at the end, you should be able to:

- Define measurement.
- Explain the difference between quantitative and qualitative measures.
- Explain why measurement is such an important process when it comes to program planning and evaluation.
- Briefly describe the four levels of measurement.
- List the variables that are often measured by health educators.
- List the four desirable characteristics of data.
- Explain the various types of validity.
- Define *reliability* and explain why it is important.
- Define *bias* in data collection and discuss how it can be reduced.
- Explain why measurement instruments must be fair.
- Briefly describe the steps one can follow when identifying, obtaining, and evaluating existing measurement instruments.
- Briefly describe the process for creating a data collection instrument.
- Describe how a sample can be obtained from a population.
- Differentiate between probability and nonprobability samples.
- Describe how a pilot test is used.

census	content validity	culturally competent
cluster sampling	convergent validity	discriminant validity
concurrent validity	criterion-related validity	face validity
construct validity	culture	fairness

Key Terms, Continued

field study	population	sample
instrumentation	predictive validity	sampling
internal consistency	preliminary review	sampling frame
interrater reliability	prepilots	sampling unit
interval level measures	probability sample	sensitivity
intrarater reliability	proportional stratified	simple random sample (SRS)
levels of measurement	random sample	specificity
measurement instrument	psychometric qualities	strata
nominal level measures	public domain	stratified random sample
nonprobability samples	qualitative measures	survey population
nonproportional stratified	quantitative measures	systematic sample
random sample	random selection	test-retest reliability
ordinal level measures	rater reliability	universe
parallel forms reliability	ratio level measures	validity
pilot testing	reliability	

In Chapter 4, we discussed in detail the needs assessment process, emphasizing the importance of collecting and analyzing appropriate needs assessment data. Later, in Chapters 13 through 15, we will again be concerned about data, but then the discussion will revolve around data and its relationship to program evaluation. In this chapter, we will examine the concepts that are considered when trying to determine the quality of data, whether it is for a needs assessment or a program evaluation. Specifically, we will examine the (1) term *measurement,* (2) types of data generated from measurement, (3) importance of measurement, (4) levels of measurement, (5) types of measures, (6) desirable characteristics of measures, (7) measurement instruments, (8) sampling, and (9) the importance of pilot testing data collection processes.

Box 5.1 identifies the responsibilities and competencies for health educators that pertain to the material presented in this chapter.

Box 5.1 RESPONSIBILITIES AND COMPETENCIES FOR HEALTH EDUCATORS

Because of the importance of measurement to program planning and evaluation, the content of Chapter 5 cuts across a couple different areas of responsibility. Those responsibilities and related competencies include:

Responsibility I: Assess Individual and Community Needs for Health Education

                Competency B: Collect health-related data

Responsibility IV: Conduct Evaluation and Research Related to Health Education

                Competency B: Review research and evaluation procedures

                Competency C: Design data collection instruments

Source: NCHEC, SOPHE, & AAHE (2006).

Measurement

Measurement has been defined as the process of assigning numbers or labels to objects, events, or people according to a particular set of rules (Kerlinger, 1986). For example, planners/evaluators can measure the level of fitness of program participants by asking them a question. Using the numbers *1, 2,* and *3,* planners/evaluators can assign the number *1* to those with poor fitness, *2* to those with average fitness, and *3* to those with good fitness. Further, the planners/evaluators need to specify what constitutes poor, average, and good fitness. In other words, measurement means that the program planners/evaluators need to "clearly specify the objects to be measured, the numbers to use, and the rules by which the numbers are assigned to the objects" (Green & Lewis, 1986, p. 58).

The data generated by measurement can be classified into two different categories, depending on the method by which they are collected. **Quantitative measures** "rely on more standardized data collection and reduction techniques, using predetermined questions or observational indicators and established response items" (Green & Lewis, 1986, p. 151). Quantitative data can be transformed into numerical data. Examples of quantitative data would be the number of participants in a smoking cessation program, the ratings on a patient satisfaction survey, and the pretest and posttest scores on a HIV knowledge test. **Qualitative measures** "tend to produce data in the language of the subjects, rarely with numerical values attached to observations" (Green & Lewis, 1986, p. 151). Qualitative data are usually assigned labels or categories (Morreale, no date) and often take the form of narrative (Weiss, 1998). Examples include data generated from case studies, focus groups, in-depth interviews, and descriptions and explanations of observations. Both quantitative and qualitative measures have their individual strengths and weaknesses, yet their greatest strength may come when both are used in the measurement process. **Table 5.1** provides a comparison of many of the qualities and characteristics of quantitative and qualitative measures.

Table 5.1 Comparison of quantitative and qualitative measures

Quantitative Measures	Qualitative Measures
Use deductive reasoning	Use inductive reasoning
Produce numerical data such as counts	Produce narrative data such as explanations
Often collected via structured design*	Often collected via flexible design*
Provide level of occurrence**	Provide depth of understanding**
Are objective**	Are subjective**
Ask "what"? "how often"? and "how many"?**	Ask "why"?**
Describes**	Interprets**
Data collection often distant from participant*	Data collection often close to participant*
Often take shorter time to collect*	Often take longer time to collect*
Examples of methods to collect data:	Examples of methods to collect data:
Written questionnaires	Case studies
Telephone interviews	Focus groups
Tests	In-depth interviews

Source: Cottrell & McKenzie (2005).
**Source*: Debus (1988).

The Importance of Measurement in Program Planning and Evaluation

As noted earlier in the chapter (see Box 1.1), health educators are expected to have the knowledge and skills (NCHEC, SOPHE, & AAHE, 2006) to plan and carry out the processes associated with appropriate measurement. Health educators need to be both comfortable and competent with measurement because the measurement process is interwoven within the daily work of health educators. Here are several examples: (1) When reviewing literature in order to create a program rationale, health educators need to be able to understand the data generated by measurement in order to know if they have located strong evidence for a proposed program; (2) When conducting a needs assessment, health educators must understand the basic principles of measurement in order to select and use appropriate data collection instruments; (3) When health educators are planning an evaluation to measure whether or not the program participants have met the objectives of a program, they need to be skilled in order to measure the program outcomes; (4) When a funding agency wants some evidence that the program it is supporting is making a difference in a community, health educators must apply appropriate measurement techniques to generate the needed evidence; or (5) When health educators are asked to interpret the results of a program evaluation to a group of stakeholders, they need to be competent in communicating how the program outcome measures produced the program results. Each of these examples demonstrates the need for a good understanding of the processes associated with measurement. In other words, measurement is an integral part of program planning, implementation, and evaluation.

Levels of Measurement

A fundamental question of measurement is deciding how something should be measured (McDermott & Sarvela, 1999). What yardstick should be used to measure the object of interest? For example, consider planners/evaluators who need data on the income levels of their program participants. They could ask the participants' income level several different ways:

1. Are you on any type of welfare?

2. What income category best describes your family income? $0 to 10,000, $10,001 to 25,000, $25,001 to 40,000, $40,000+

3. What is your family income? _____

Each of these questions gets at one's income level, but each generates a different form of data. They not only generate certain types of data, but also use different wording that may be either acceptable or offensive to certain populations. Thus when planners/evaluators begin to think about data collection, they need to consider both the wording of the questions and the form(s) of data they want to use.

There are four **levels of measurement** used to determine how something is to be measured. They are hierarchical in nature, and the form of data collected determines what statistical test can be used to analyze them. The four levels of measurement are (Cottrell & McKenzie, 2005):

1. **Nominal level measures,** the lowest level in the measurement hierarchy, enable planners to put data into categories. "The two requirements for nominal measures are that the categories have to be mutually exclusive so that each case fits into one of the categories, and the categories have to be exhaustive so that there is a place for every case" (Weiss, 1998, p. 116). Nominal measures do not convey any value to what is measured but rather just identifies or names it (Dignan, 1995). An example question that would generate nominal data is, "What is your sex?" The possible answers include the categories of "female" and "male." These answers are exhaustive (contain all possible answers) and mutually exclusive (the respondent has to be one or the other, but not both). We can then assign numbers to these categories according to a particular rule we create (e.g., 1 = female, 2 = male).

2. **Ordinal level measures,** like nominal level measures, allow planners to put data into categories that are mutually exclusive and exhaustive, but also permits them to rank-order the categories. The different categories represent relatively more or less of something. However, the distance between categories cannot be measured. For example, the question "How would you describe your level of satisfaction with your health care? (select one) very satisfied – satisfied – not satisfied" creates categories (very satisfied – satisfied – not satisfied) that are mutually exclusive (the respondent cannot select two categories) and exhaustive (there is a category for all levels of satisfaction), and the categories represent more or less of something (amount of satisfaction, thus there is a rank order). We cannot, however, measure the distance (or difference) between the levels of satisfaction (e.g., what is the difference between very satisfied and satisfied?). Is the distance between very satisfied and satisfied the same distance between satisfied and not satisfied? Ordinal data categories are not necessarily equal distance apart.

3. **Interval level measures** enable planners to put data into categories that are mutually exclusive and exhaustive, and rank-orders the categories. Furthermore, the widths of the categories must all be the same (Hurlburt, 2003), which allows for the distance between the categories to be measured. There is, however, no absolute zero value. Thus, interval level measures assign numerical values to things according to a particular rule (Dignan, 1995). An example question that generates interval data is: "What was the high temperature today?" We know that a temperature of 70° F is different than a temperature of 80° F, that 80° is warmer than 70°, that there is 10° F difference between the two, and if the temperature drops to 0° F there is still some heat in the air (though not much) because 0° F is warmer than –10° F.

4. **Ratio level measures,** the highest level in the measurement hierarchy, enable planners to do everything with data that can be done with the other three levels of measures; however, they are done using a scale with an absolute zero. Example questions that generate interval data include: "What was your score on the test?" How tall are you in inches?" and "During an average week, how many minutes do you exercise aerobically?" An absolute zero "point means that the thing being measured actually vanishes when the scale reads zero" (Hurlburt, 2003, p. 17). For example, when a person has a blood pressure reading of zero over zero, there is in fact no blood pressure.

Because interval and ratio data are continuous and rank-ordered values with equal distance between them, and because most statistical procedures are the same for both types of data (Valente, 2002), some have combined them into a single level of measurement and refer to the resulting data as *numerical data*. However, if given the choice, planners should strive to collect ratio data because it still provides the greatest flexibility in data analysis.

Types of Measures

Many different types of measures are used to conduct needs assessments or evaluate programs. It is important to match the methods of measurement with the focus of the task, whether it be a needs assessment or program evaluation. Typically, health promotion programs focus on one or more of the following types of measures: demographic variables, awareness variables, cognitive variables, psychosocial variables, skill variables, behavioral variables, environmental variables, health variables, and quality of life variables. **Table 5.2**

Table 5.2   Types of measures, data generated, and methods of obtaining the data

Measure	Example Data	Commonly used methods of data collection
Demographic variables	Social characteristics of a population e.g., sex, age, race, income	Self-report questionnaires, existing records
Awareness variables	Conscious of, for example, location of services, identification of risk factors	Self-report questionnaires, proxy measures such as asking a significant other
Cognitive (knowledge) variables	Bloom's taxonomy* • knowledge (remembering) • comprehension (lowest level of understanding) • application (using learned material) • analysis (ability to analyze learned material) • synthesis (creating from learned material) • evaluation (ability to judge the value)	Written or oral tests
Pyschosocial variables	Attitudes, beliefs, motivation, and personality traits, for example, attitude about an issue, type-A personality	Self-report validated scales
Skill variables	Ability to perform a task, for example, CPR or give insulin shot	Observation (obtrusive and unobtrusive), skills test
Behavior variables	Performance, for example, stop smoking, exercise habits, stress management	Observation, proxy measure such as laboratory test
Environmental variables	Factors or conditions outside a person, for example, social support, access to care, clean air	Self-report questionnaires, checklists, laboratory tests
Health variables	Biological and clinical health, for example, level of health, number of risk factors, functional ability	Self-report questionnaires, health screenings, health risk appraisal (HRA)
Quality of life (QoL) variables	Satisfaction, happiness, and fulfillment, for example, goodness of life, health-related quality of life	Self-report validated scales

Source: Bloom (1956).

provides examples of how data can be generated for each of the different types of measures.

Desirable Characteristics of Data

The results of a needs assessment or program evaluation are only as good as the data that are used to gain the results. If a questionnaire was filled with ambiguous questions and the respondents were not sure how to answer, it is highly likely that the data collected would not reflect the true knowledge, attitudes, etc., of those responding. Therefore, it is of vital importance that planners and evaluators make sure that the data they collect are reliable, valid, fair, and unbiased. The collective term given to describe three of these characteristics—validity, reliability, and fairness—is **psychometric qualities** (Cottrell & McKenzie, 2005).

Reliability

Reliability refers to consistency in the measurement process. That is, **reliability** "is an empirical estimate of the extent to which an instrument produces the same result (measure or score), applied once or two or more times" (Windsor, Clark, Boyd, & Goodman, 2004, p. 93). However, no instrument will ever provide perfect accuracy in measurement. Green and Lewis (1986) illustrate the theory of reliability with an equation, where total score (obtained score) equals the true score (unobservable) plus an error score. The total score represents the individual's score obtained on the measuring instrument. The true score represents the score for the same individual if all conditions and the measuring instrument were perfect. The error score represents the portion of the total score that is generated from the "imprecision in measurement due to human error, uncontrollable environment occurrences, inappropriateness of measurement instruments, and other unanticipated things" (Dignan, 1995, p. 40). For example, suppose the total score of an individual on a knowledge test was 85 out of a possible 100 points. The question then becomes whether the 85% is a true indication of the person's knowledge. If the conditions under which the score was generated were perfect and the measurement instrument had perfect reliability, the error score would be zero and we could say, "yes the 85% is a true indication of the person's knowledge." However, if the conditions under which the score was generated were *not* perfect (e.g., the person did not have enough time to take the test) and the measurement instrument *did not* have perfect reliability (e.g., it included several poorly worded questions), the error score would *not* be zero and we say, "no the 85% is *not* a true indication of the person's knowledge. This person may really know more, or maybe less, than was indicated by the score." "Reliability coefficients are highest if no error exists ($r = 1.0$) and lowest when there is only error or no association ($r = 0.0$) between two measures" (Windsor et al., 2004, p. 95).

Planners need to strive to collect data under the best conditions with the most reliable measurement instruments possible (Cottrell & McKenzie, 2005). Several methods of determining reliability are available.

Internal Consistency   Internal consistency, is one of the most commonly used methods of estimating reliability (Windsor et al., 2004). It refers to the intercorrelations among the individual items on the instrument, that is, whether all items on the instrument are measuring part of the total area. This can be done by logically examining the instrument to ensure that the items reflect what is to be measured and that the level of difficulty of all items is the same. Statistical methods can also be used to determine internal consistency by correlating the items on the test with the total score.

Test-retest Reliability   Test-retest reliability, or stability reliability, "is used to generate evidence of stability over a period" (Torabi, 1994, p. 57) of time. To establish this type of reliability, the same instrument is used to measure the same group of people under similar, or the same, conditions at two different points in time, and the two sets of data generated by the measurement are used to calculate a correlation coefficient (Cottrell & McKenzie, 2005). The amount of time between the test and retest may vary from a few hours to a few weeks. A maximum amount of time should be allowed between the test and retest so that individuals are not responding on the basis of remembering responses they made the first time, but not be so long that other events could occur in the intervening time to influence their responses. To avoid the problems of retesting, parallel forms (equivalent forms) of the test can be administered to the participants and the results can be correlated.

Rater Reliability   Rater reliability focuses on the consistency between individuals who are observing or rating the same event or when one individual is observing or rating a series of events. If two or more raters are involved, it is referred to as **interrater reliability**. If only one individual is observing or rating a series of events, it is referred to as *intrarater reliability*. There are several different ways to calculate rater reliability. In a research study, most researchers would use Cohen's *K* or kappa (Cohen, 1960) to calculate rater reliability. However, a quicker and easier method (DiIorio, 2005) is to calculate it as a percentage of agreement between/among raters or within an individual rater. An example of interrater reliability would be the percent of agreement between two observers who are observing passing drivers in cars for safety belt use. If ten cars are observed by the raters and they agree eight out of ten times on whether the drivers are wearing their safety belts, the interrater reliability would be 80%. **Intrarater reliability** would be the degree to which one rater agrees with himself or herself on the characteristics of an observation over time. For example, when a rater is evaluating the CPR skills of participants in his or her program, the rater should be consistent while observing and evaluating the skills of the participants.

Parallel Forms Reliability   Parallel forms reliability, or equivalent forms or alternate-forms reliability, focuses on whether different forms of the same measurement instrument when measuring the same subjects will produce similar results (means, standard deviations, and item intercorrelations). The usefulness of having measurement instruments that possess parallel forms reliability is being able to test the same subjects on different occasions (e.g., using a pretest-posttest evaluation design) without worry that the subjects will score better on the second administration (posttest) because they remember questions from the first administration (pretest) of the instrument. A good example of parallel forms reliability is found in the different versions of the standardized college entrance examinations (Cottrell & McKenzie, 2005).

Validity

When designing a data collection instrument, planners/evaluators must ensure that it measures what it is intended to measure. This refers to the **validity** of the measurement—whether it is correctly measuring the concepts under investigation. Using a valid instrument increases the chance that planners/evaluators are measuring what they want to measure, thus ruling out other possible explanations for the results. We will discuss several types of validity.

Face Validity   The lowest level of validity is face validity. A measure is said to have **face validity** if, on the face, the measure appears to measure what it is supposed to measure (McDermott & Sarvela, 1999). It differs from the other forms of validity in that it lacks some form of systematic logical analysis of the content (Hopkins, Stanley, & Hopkins, 1990). An example of face validity might include a planner/evaluator asking a colleague to look over a series of questions to see whether the questions seem reasonable to include on a questionnaire about, for example, heart disease. Face validity is a good first step toward creating a valid measurement instrument, but is not a replacement for the other means of establishing validity (Cottrell & McKenzie, 2005).

Content Validity   Content validity refers to "the assessment of the correspondence between the items composing the instrument and the content domain from which the items were selected" (DiIorio, 2005, p. 213). For example, when planning a risk reduction program for cardiovascular disease, the program planner can conduct a review of the literature in the area of cardiovascular risk reduction in order to ensure that all major risk factors, such as smoking, exercise, and diet, are included on a questionnaire.

Content validity is usually established by using a group (jury or panel) of experts to review the instrument. After such a group is identified, they would be asked to review each element of the instrument for its appropriateness to be included. The collective opinion of the experts is then used to determine the content of the instrument. McKenzie and colleagues (1999) present a method of establishing content validity that includes both qualitative and quantitative steps.

Criterion-Related Validity   Criterion-related validity refers to "the extent to which data generated from a measurement instrument are correlated with data generated from a measure (criterion) of the phenomenon being studied, usually an individual's behavior or performance" (Cottrell & McKenzie, 2005, p. 307). Criterion-related validity can be divided into two subtypes: predictive and concurrent validity (DiIorio, 2005).

If the measurement used will be correlated with another measurement of the same phenomenon at another time, as with the use of standardized test scores to predict future college success, the criterion validity is known as **predictive validity. Concurrent validity** is established when a new instrument and an established valid instrument that measure the same characteristics are administered to the same subjects, and the results of the new instrument are compared to the results of the valid instrument. For example, if a planner/evaluator wanted to establish the validity of a new test for breast cancer, he or she administers both the new instrument and another already valid breast cancer instrument to the same subjects and then compares the results. The new instrument would be valid if the results compared favorably with the established instrument. In both subtypes of criterion-related validity, the aim is to legitimize the inferences that can be made by establishing their predictive ability for a related criterion.

Construct Validity   Though criterion-related validity is very useful in establishing validity, there are times when there is not an existing criterion from which to compare, or the phenomenon that planners want to measure is more abstract than concrete, like many of the psychosocial constructs, such as the constructs of locus of control, self-efficacy, or subjective norm. In such cases, validity can be established via construct validity (Cottrell & McKenzie, 2005). **Construct validity** "is the degree to which a measure correlates with other measures it is theoretically expected to correlate with. Construct validity tests the theoretical framework within which the instrument is expected to perform" (Valente, 2002, p. 161). An instrument that has construct validity will possess both convergent validity and discriminant validity. **Convergent validity** "is the extent to which two measures which purport to be measuring the same topic correlate (that is, converge)" (Bowling, 2005, p. 12). For example, an instrument that purports to measure a person's self-efficacy for regular exercise should positively correlate with that person's exercise behavior. That is, a person who is self-efficacious with regard to exercise would exercise regularly regardless of the circumstances (i.e., normal day, busy day, inclement weather, while on vacation). **Discriminant validity** "(also known as divergent validity) requires that the construct should not correlate with dissimilar (discriminant) variables" (Bowling, 2005, p. 12). Thus in the exercise example above, the self-efficacy instrument would not be expected to correlate positively with a person's inactivity.

Sensitivity and Specificity   When speaking about validity, because of the possibility of reading health care literature, planners should also be familiar with the terms *sensitivity* and *specificity*. These terms are used in the health care settings and epidemiology to express the validity of screening and diagnostic tests (Cottrell & McKenzie, 2005). **Sensitivity** is defined as the ability of the test to identify correctly those with a disease or condition (Mausner & Kramer, 1985). It is recorded as the proportion of true positive cases correctly identified as positive on the test (Timmreck, 1997). The better the sensitivity, the fewer the false positives. **Specificity** is defined as the ability of the test to identify correctly those who do not have a disease or condition (Mausner & Kramer, 1985). It is recorded as the proportion of true negative cases correctly identified as negative on the test (Timmreck, 1997). And the better the specificity, the fewer the number of false negatives. "An ideal screening test would be 100% sensitive and 100% specific. In practice this does not occur; sensitivity and specificity are usually inversely related" (Mausner & Kramer, 1985, p. 217).

One final thought before leaving our discussion of validity: The validity of an instrument is thought to be a more important issue than reliability. If an instrument does not measure what it is supposed to, then it does not matter if it is reliable (Windsor et al., 2004) (**Table 5.3**).

Fairness

Fairness deals with the question of whether a measure "is appropriate for the individuals of various ethnic groups with different backgrounds, gender, educational levels, etc." (Torabi, 1994, p. 56). Because planners/evaluators often work with members of priority

Table 5.3   Types of reliability and validity

Reliability—"an empirical estimate of the extent to which an instrument produces the same result (measure or score), applied once or two or more times" (Windsor et al., 2004, p. 93).

 Internal consistency—the intercorrelations among individual items on the instrument, that is, whether all items on the instrument are measuring part of the total area

 Test-retest (or stability)—"used to generate evidence of stability over time" (Torabi, 1994, p. 57)

 Rater (or observer)—associated with the consistent measurement (or rating) of an observed event by the same or different individuals (or judges or raters) (McDermott & Sarvela, 1999)

 Parallel (or equivalent or alternate) **forms**—focuses on whether different forms of the same instrument when measuring the same participants will produce similar results

Validity—whether an instrument correctly measures what it is intended to measure

 Face—if, on the face, the measure appears to measure what it is supposed to measure (McDermott & Sarvela, 1999)

 Content—"the assessment of the correspondence between the items composing the instrument and the content domain from which the items were selected" (Dilorio, 2005, p. 213).

 Criterion-related—"the extent to which data generated from a measurement instrument are correlated with the data generated from a measure (criterion) of the phenomenon being studied, usually an individual's behavior or performance" (Cottrell & McKenzie, 2005, p. 307); two types: concurrent and predictive

 Construct—"the degree to which a measure correlates with other measures it is theoretically expected to correlate with. Construct validity tests the theoretical framework within which the instrument is expected to perform" (Valente, 2002, p. 161); an instrument with construct validity posseses both convergent and discrininant validity.

---

populations who are different than them, they need to be concerned about fairness. Unlike the other psychometric qualities of validity and reliability, there are no quantitative procedures for determining the fairness of a measure (Cottrell & McKenzie, 2005). Instead it becomes the responsibility of the planners/evaluators to work to seek fairness. A foundation for fairness is the planners/evaluators having an understanding of the culture of those in the priority population. **Culture** is defined as "the patterned ways of thought and behavior that characterize a social group, which are learned through socialization processes and persist through time" (Coreil, Bryant, & Henderson, 2001, p. 29). Therefore, people from different cultures are likely to possess different values, beliefs, traditions, and perceptions. These cultural values, beliefs, traditions, and perceptions affect nearly all activities of individuals, including their health-related behavior (Kline & Huff, 1999) and responding to questions related to health. "As cultures vary, so do notions of what the human body symbolizes, how it should appear, how it functions most appropriately and why, and when and how it should be treated" (AAHE, 1994, p. 5). Thus, culture influences program participants' ability to understand, internalize, and exercise positive health practices that will enhance the quality of life. For example, if we examine the diet of individuals from different cultures (i.e., religion, race), it is easy to see the impact of culture on what people eat. Some cultures see some foods as an important part of their diet, while others see the same foods as dirty and not to be consumed. Thus, when collecting data from diverse populations, planners/evaluators need to respond appropriately to cultural differences. In other words, planners/evaluators need to work toward being culturally competent. **Culturally competent** means having the ability "to understand and respect values, attitudes, beliefs, and mores that differ across cultures, and to consider and respond appropriately to these differences in planning, implementing and evaluating health education and health promotion programs and interventions" (Joint Committee, 2001, p. 99).

Unbiased

Biased data are those data that have been distorted because of the way they have been collected. In order to effectively plan and evaluate health promotion programs, planners/evaluators must work to eliminate bias. Windsor and colleagues (2004) describe ways in which bias can occur in data collection—for example, when participants do not feel comfortable answering a sensitive question, when participants act differently because they know they are being watched, when certain characteristics of the interviewer influence a response, when participants answer questions in a particular way regardless of the questions being asked, or when a bias sample has been selected from the priority population (see information later in this chapter on sampling). There are a number of steps planners/evaluators can take to limit bias. For example, if data are being collected via observation, the observation should be as unobtrusive as possible. If sensitive questions are being asked of respondents, then those collecting such data need to ensure that the data are being collected in a confidential way (the identity of the respondent can be determined but not released), and consider collecting the data via an anonymous means (there is no way of identifying the respondent). No matter how data are collected, the reduction of bias techniques will increase the accuracy of the results.

Measurement Instruments

As presented in Chapter 4, many different methods can be used to collect both primary and secondary data. The focus here is not to repeat that information but rather to present information on measurement instruments. By **measurement instrument,** we mean the item used to measure the variables (i.e., demographic, psychosocial, behavioral) of interest. Measurement instruments are also sometimes referred to as tools or data collection instruments. The term **instrumentation** is "a collective term that describes all measurement instruments used" (Cottrell & McKenzie, 2005, p. 311).

Measurement instruments can take many different forms and sizes. They can range from the very simple, like a ruler or yardstick, to a questionnaire, to a very complicated piece of machinery like one that breaks down the various components of an unknown liquid. Although at times health educators may use machines as instruments (e.g., to check blood cholesterol), more commonly they employ a sequence of questions to measure variables of interest (Windsor et al., 2004). These sequences of questions most often take the form of *tests*, *questionnaires*, and *scales*. The term "test" is most often used in the context of educational measurement (DiIorio, 2005), such as an HIV/AIDS knowledge test. Questionnaires (sometimes called *survey instruments*) are instruments that gather information about a variety of factors (e.g., awareness, skills, behaviors, health status) related to one or more specific topics. For example, a questionnaire may be developed about sleep habits and include questions about the average number of hours slept per night, normal bedtime, use of sleep aids, and techniques used to fall asleep. Further, the questionnaires can be administered orally via an interview, or people can be asked to respond in writing either on paper or on a computer. Most often, the answers to a questionnaire vary depending on the questions asked. In contrast, a scale is used to measure only one concept (DiIorio, 2005), often dealing with a psychosocial variable like attitudes, beliefs, or opinions. For example, health educators may be interested in collecting data about the attitudes of those in the priority population about abortion. In scales, often the response choice for every question is the same (e.g., always, sometimes, never).

Depending on the nature of the test, questionnaire, or scale, the instrument can also vary in length. Some can be as short as a single question, rating, or item to measure the variable, while others may be multipage instruments. There are advantages and disadvantages to various instrument lengths. Obvious advantages of a shorter instrument are the time for the participants to complete it and for the planners/evaluators to tally and analyze the data. However, longer instruments may do a better job of measuring less stable (i.e., change over time) variables like attitudes (DiIorio, 2005), and longer instruments may be more suitable for statistical calculations (Bowling, 2005).

Using an Existing Measurement Instrument

Before planners/evaluators ever go about creating their own measurement instrument, they should search for an already existing instrument that meets their needs. As you will discover in the next section, it takes a great deal of time, effort, and resources to create a measurement instrument with good psychometric qualities. The main advantages of using an existing valid and reliable instrument include less planning time and thus lower costs. The major disadvantage—one that prevents the use of many existing instruments—is that the items on the existing instrument may not be relevant or appropriate for the program being planned or evaluated. Cottrell and McKenzie (2005) presented four steps for identifying, obtaining, and evaluating existing measurement instruments.

Step 1: Identifying measurement instruments. Start by searching the literature to see what others have used. You may not find an actual copy of the measurement instruments in the literature, but you may find a reference to the original source. As you are aware by now, the U.S. government has created many health-related data collection instruments. Conducting a search of applicable websites (e.g., National Center for Health Statistics, CDC WONDER) can be useful. Remember, government publications are in the **public domain** (available for anyone to use) and thus free of charge and need no permission to use. Also, be aware that a number of commercial companies sell measurement instruments (e.g., Psychological Assessment Resources, Inc. [PAR]). In addition, note you may not find a measurement instrument that you can use in whole, but you may find a certain section of an instrument that may work for you.

Step 2: Getting your hands on the instrument. Once you have identified potential measurement instruments, you then have to physically get them in your hands. Unless an instrument is copyrighted, or there are plans to do so in the future, most are more than happy to share their measurement instrument. A phone call, letter, or sometimes a "formal" e-mail requesting a copy of an instrument is all that it takes to get a copy. Once the source of the measurement instrument is known, be aware that you may have to pay for an instrument, and have to meet certain criteria (i.e., being a licensed psychologist) to be able to obtain and use certain measurement instruments.

Step 3: Is it the right instrument? Here are some questions to ask to determine whether the instrument is the right one for your purposes: "(1) Is there evidence of the psychometric qualities (validity, reliability, and fairness) of the instrument? (2) Has it been used with participants similar to yours? (3) Are standard or normative scores available for various participants? (4) Is it culturally appropriate for your participants? (5) Has the reading level for the instrument been determined? (6) Is there a cost to administer or have the instrument scored? Can you afford it?" (Cottrell & McKenzie, 2005, p. 156).

Step 4: Final steps before proceeding. If you think you have found the right instrument, before proceeding make sure you have done everything necessary to be able to use it. Remember, for instruments that are not in the public domain "you need the permission of the author for any use of the instrument, usually in writing, and particularly if you need to make any changes" (Dignan, 1995, p. 67). You also may need to fulfill other conditions placed on the use of the instrument by the owner before you use it.

Creating a Measurement Instrument

Only when planners/evaluators are unable to use or adapt another instrument for their use should they undertake the process of developing their own (Janz, Champion, & Strecher, 2002). **Box 5.2** provides a list of steps to follow in creating a measurement instrument. Though the list was created to develop a data collection instrument for research projects, it illustrates the complexity in creating an instrument with good psychometric qualities. Each step in the list will not be discussed here; that has been done elsewhere (Cottrell & McKenzie, 2005), but rather a general discussion will be presented about the presentation, wording, and sequencing of questions in a measurement instrument.

The measurement instrument should begin with an introduction that includes a brief statement of purpose and directions for completing the instrument (see **Box 5.3**). This introduction can be followed by general questions to put the respondent at ease in the case of a written or electronic self-report instrument, or to develop a rapport between the interviewer and the respondent when data are collected via a face-to-face or telephone interview.

After several general questions come the questions of interest. Any questions that deal with sensitive topics should be posed at the end of the questionnaire or interview. Answers to questions about drug use, sexuality, or even demographic information, such as income level, are more readily answered when the respondents understand the need for the information, are assured of confidentiality or anonymity, and feel comfortable with the interviewer or the questionnaire. If the respondent ends the interview or does not complete the instrument when asked sensitive questions, the other information collected can still be used; this is another advantage of putting these questions at the end.

The way in which questions are worded is extremely important in gaining the needed information. The result of a poorly worded question was evident to one health promotion planner who was planning a smoking cessation program for employees. When asked, "Do you feel we need a smoking cessation program?" most employees said yes. The planner realized later that he should have also asked the question, "If offered, would you attend a smoking cessation program?" since very few employees participated.

| **Box 5.2** | Steps for Creating a Measurement Instrument |

Step 0: Be familiar with the related literature.

Step 1: Determine the specific purpose (or goal) and the objectives of the proposed instrument.

Step 2: Who are the individuals who are to be measured?

Step 3: Identify the conceptual theory/model that will provide the foundation for the instrument.

Step 4: Create a table of specifications and specifications for the instrument.

Step 5: Identify items from other existing instruments that could be used.

Step 6: Create new instrument items.

Step 7: Create directions for completing the instrument, and directions and instructions for administering the instrument.

Step 8: Establish procedures for scoring the instrument.

Step 9: Assemble an initial draft of the instrument.

Step 10: Establish face validity for the instrument.

Step 11: Check the readability of the instrument.

Step 12: Establish content validity for the instrument.

Step 13: Pilot-test the instrument.

Step 14: Conduct item analysis, factor analysis, and checks of psychometric qualities.

Step 15: Review, revise, and reassess.

Step 16: Conduct a second pilot-test, if necessary.

Step 17: Determine a cut score.

Step 18: Refine as needed and create the final version.

Source: R. R. Cottrell & J. F. McKenzie, "Health Promotion and Education Research Methods: Using the Five-chapter thesis/dissertation model." Copyright © 2005 Jones & Bartlett Publishers, Sudbury, MA. Reprinted by permission.

The questions should also be clear and unbiased. It is important to avoid questions with a specific direction ("How have you enjoyed the class?") that would guide the respondent's answer. Two-part (double-barreled) questions should also be avoided ("Do you brush and floss your teeth?"). Another problem with question design occurs when the question assumes knowledge that individuals may not have or includes terminology that they may not understand ("What cardiovascular benefits do you feel you gain from aerobic exercise?").

Many different types of questions can be used to create measurement instruments. Consideration must be given to whether or not the type of question will generate the needed data. For example, say planners/evaluators were interested in getting the ages of those in the priority population. A question like "How old are you?" could generate the best data (i.e., ratio level data), but some may not want to share their actual age and thus planners/evaluators may not collect enough data to describe the priority population. In this case, a question that generates ordinal level data such as "I am: 15–24 years old; 25–44 years old; 45–64 years old; 65+ years old" may be a better choice.

| **Box 5.3** | APPLICATION—INTRODUCTION FOR A DATA COLLECTION INSTRUMENT |

Health Questionnaire

Purpose: The Health Department is conducting a survey of those living in Delaware County in order to find out more about their health. Obtaining this information is important because it will provide us with a better understanding of the needs of our citizens so that we may in turn provide the programs to improve the health of those in our county.

Directions for completing the questionnaire: You are not required to complete this questionnaire, but your voluntary participation is requested. This is an anonymous survey so do not write your name on this instrument. Please read each of the questions carefully and respond to them by circling the response that best represents your feelings. There are no right or wrong answers. We recognize that some of the questions, by necessity, are quite personal. Be assured that your individual responses will not be shared with anyone and that only summarized group information will be reported. When you have completed the questionnaire, place it in the postage-paid business reply envelope and drop it in the mail. Thank you for your help with this survey.

Another consideration in creating questions is to determine how much freedom you want respondents to have in answering questions. Those with the least freedom are structured or closed questions. Examples of these are "true-false" or "multiple-choice" questions and are most often used for knowledge questions. These types of responses are the easiest to tabulate but do not allow the individual to elaborate on the answers. They may also force a person into a choice because of the limited number of responses to each question. An "other" category, with space to list the exact nature of the "other" response, may serve to give the respondent another option. However, giving the respondents an opportunity to provide their own answers on multiple-choice questions makes it more difficult to categorize responses when the data are analyzed, thus reducing one of the main benefits of such questions. One way to ensure that the most common responses to questions are included in the multiple choices is to involve several individuals (especially those in the priority population) in the formation of the instrument.

Attitude questions generally use less structured forms. Scales, such as Likert or semantic differentials, are often used, with the respondent choosing a response along a continuum, generally ranging from a five- to a seven-point scale. For example, responses to the statement, "I feel that it is important to limit my use of salt," might be rated on a five-point scale ranging from "strongly agree" to "strongly disagree."

Unstructured or open-ended questions—such as essay questions, short-answer questions, journals, or logs—may be used to gain descriptive information, but are generally not used when collecting quantitative data. Such responses are often difficult to summarize or to code for analysis. **Box 5.4** provides examples of structured and unstructured types of questions.

Box 5.4 EXAMPLES OF SELF-REPORT QUESTIONS

Structured (Closed)

I. Dichotomous

1. What is your gender?
a. Female   b. Male

2. A risk factor for heart disease is sedentary lifestyle.
a. True   b. False

II. Multiple Choice

1. The leading cause of death in the United States for adults is
a. Cancer   b. Heart disease
c. Injuries   d. AIDS

2. What type of computer do you use?
a. IBM   b. Apple
c. Gateway   d. Other (please specify): _____

III. Matching

Vitamin deficiencies
1. Vitamin A   a. Frequent infection
2. Vitamin C   b. Slow blood clotting
3. Vitamin D   c. Night blindness
4. Vitamin K   d. Bone softening

Grams of saturated fats
1. Butter, 1 tbsp.   a. 9
2. Ice cream, 4 oz.   b. 7.1
3. Chicken, 3 oz.   c. 5
4. One hot dog   d. 1.2

Less Structured (But Still Closed)

I. Likert

1. Women should be able to have an abortion if they choose to do so.

     Strongly   *Strongly*
     agree   *Agree*   *Neutral*   *Disagree*   *disagree*

2. I feel I can exercise
regardless of   *Strongly*   *Strongly*
weather conditions.   *agree*   *Agree*   *Neutral*   *Disagree*   *disagree*

II. Semantic Differentials

1. Smokeless tobacco is   Good   ___   ___   ___   ___   ___   Bad
2. When taking a test, I feel   Nervous   ___   ___   ___   ___   ___   Calm

III. Rank Order

1. Put the following values in order, from most important in your life to least
important:
a. health   _____   d. emotional security   _____
b. love   _____   e. financial security   _____
c. friendship   _____

> **Box 5.4**   CONTINUED
>
> **2.** Rank-order the following servings of foods from highest to lowest sources of protein:
>
> | | | | |
> |---|---|---|---|
> | a. tuna | ____ | d. cottage cheese | ____ |
> | b. rice | ____ | e. bread | ____ |
> | c. sirloin steak | ____ | f. broccoli | ____ |
>
> **Unstructured (Open)**
>
> *I. Completions*
>
>   **1.** I like to exercise because _____
>
>   **2.** The types of foods I generally eat are _____
>
> *II. Short-answer*
>
>   **1.** List five advantages to conducting a worksite health promotion program.
>
>   **2.** Describe the correct way to lift a heavy object to avoid straining your back.
>
> *III. Essay*
>
>   **1.** Explain the difference between aerobic and anaerobic exercise. Include examples of each type of exercise, and discuss the importance of each in total fitness.
>
>   **2.** Discuss the incidence of tuberculosis in the world today, including who is at risk and the public health measures to reduce the problem.

Sampling

The need to select participants from whom data will be collected can occur at several times during the processes of program planning or evaluation. Depending on the size of the priority population, planners/evaluators may want to collect data from all participants (**census**) or from only some of the participants (**sample**). Each of the participants is referred to as a sampling unit. A **sampling unit** is the element or set of elements considered for selection as part of a sample (Babbie, 1992). A sampling unit "may be an individual, an organization, or a geographical area" (Bowling, 2002, p. 166).

Figure 5.1 illustrates the relationship between groups of individuals. All individuals, unspecified by time or place, constitute the **universe**—for example, all U.S. citizens, regardless of where they reside in the world. Within the universe is a **population** of individuals specified by time or place, such as all U.S. residents in the 50 United States on January 1, 2008. Within this population is a **survey population**, composed of all individuals who are accessible to the planners. The key term here is *accessible*. For example, all U.S. citizens who are accessible and can be reached by telephone would be a survey population. Obviously, this would not include those without telephones, such as those who chose not to own them, those institutionalized, and the homeless.

A survey population may still be too large to include in its entirety. For this reason, a sample is chosen from the survey population, a process called **sampling**. These are the individuals who will be included in the data collection process. Using a sample rather than an entire survey population helps contain costs. For example, using a sample

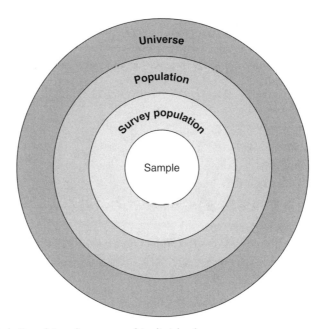

Figure 5.1 Relationship of groups of individuals

reduces the amount of staff time needed to conduct interviews, the cost of postage for written questionnaires, and the time and cost of travel to conduct observations.

How the sample is chosen is critical to the result of the needs assessment or evaluation: Does the information gained from the sample reflect the knowledge, attitudes, and behaviors of the survey population? According to Green and Lewis (1986), the sampling bias is the difference between the sampling estimate and the actual population value. The sampling bias can be controlled by controlling the sampling procedure—that is, how the sample is chosen. The ability to generalize the results to the survey population is greater when the sampling bias is reduced.

Probability Sample

Increasing the chance that the sample is representative of the survey population is achieved by **random selection**. "Randomness minimizes the likelihood that a systematic source of selection bias will occur among the sample, thereby influencing the degree of representativeness of the population" (Windsor et al., 2004, p. 110). When random selection is used, each person in the survey population has an equal chance or probability of being selected, thus creating a **probability sample**.

There are a number of different methods for selecting a probability sample. The most basic of the probability sampling methods is selecting a **simple random sample** **(SRS)**. In order to select a SRS, or for that matter any probability sample, the planner must have a list or "quasi-list" (Babbie, 1992) of all sampling units in the survey population. This list is referred to as the **sampling frame**. Often times sampling frames have the names and contact information for everyone in the survey population such as with membership lists, patients of a clinic, and parents of children enrolled in a certain school or program. Other times the frame may be just the title of an individual or organization, such as the Director of Environmental Services in the 94 local health departments in Indiana, or a list of all the voluntary health agencies in the county (Cottrell & McKenzie, 2005).

Once the sampling frame has been identified, the planner can proceed with the process of selecting a SRS. It begins with assigning a number with an equal number of digits to each sampling unit in the frame. Suppose, for example, we have a frame of 200 individuals. Thus the first person in the frame would be given the number 000. The rest of the individuals in the frame would be assigned consecutive numbers and the last person in the frame would be assigned the number 199. Once it is decided how large the sample should be, the sample can be selected. For the purpose of this example let's suppose a sample size of 20 is desired. To select these 20 individuals, a computer could be used to randomly select 20 numbers between 000 and 199, or it could be done manually by using a table of random numbers (see **Table 5.4**) (Cottrell & McKenzie, 2005).

In order to use a table of random numbers, the manner in which the table will be used needs to be set forth. Since these tables are generated randomly (by computer), it really does not matter which way one moves through the table as long as it is done in a consistent manner. For example, the process set forth could be to: (1) use the first three digits in the columns of numbers (because all individuals in the example frame have a three-digit number, that is, 000 to 199), (2) proceed down the columns (as opposed to up or across the rows), (3) at the bottom of the column proceed to the top of the next column to the right, and (4) proceed in this same manner until the 20 individuals are selected. To insure that this process is indeed random, the process must begin with a random start. That is, the planner cannot just pick the first number at the top of column one and proceed down through the column because every individual in the survey population would not have an equal chance of being selected. The planner can accomplish the random start by closing his/her eyes and pointing to a place on the table of random numbers then opening his/her eyes and proceeding through the table in the way that was set forth above (Cottrell & McKenzie, 2005).

Table 5.4 Abbreviated table of random numbers

Row/Column	A	B	C	D	E
1	75 51	02 17	71 04	33 93	36 60
2	42 75	76 22	23 87	56 54	84 68
3	00 47	37 59	08 56	23 81	22 42
4	74 01	23 19	55 59	79 09	69 82
5	66 22	42 40	15 96	74 90	75 89
6	09 24	34 42	00 68	72 10	71 37
7	89 22	10 23	62 65	78 77	47 33
8	51 27	23 02	13 92	44 13	96 51
9	17 18	01 34	10 98	37 48	93 86
10	02 28	54 60	01 11	28 35	54 32

A **systematic sample** also uses a frame and takes every Nth person (determined by dividing the survey population size by the sample size, N/n), beginning with a randomly selected individual. For example, suppose that we want to choose a sample of 10 people from a survey population of 100. We start by randomly choosing a number between 001 and 100, such as 026, using a table of random numbers. We then choose every tenth ($N/n = 100/10 = 10$) person (036, 046, 056, 076, 086, 096, 006, 016) until we have the 10 subjects for the sample. In this way, everyone in the survey population has an equal chance of being selected. A simple random sample or systematic sample can also be used to select "naturally occurring groups or clusters, such as schools, clinics, worksites, or census tracks" (Gilmore & Campbell, 2005, p. 59). When this occurs, it is called **cluster sampling**.

If it is important that certain groups should be represented in a sample, a **stratified random sample** can be selected. Such a method would be used if the planners felt that a certain variable (i.e., such as size, income, or age) might have an influence on the data collected from the participants. A stratified random sample might also be used if it is believed that because of the small numbers of a certain group in the survey population, representatives from that group may not be selected using a simple random sample. That is, you may have a survey population of 100 participants and in that 100 there are only eight of one group. If you were to select a sample of 10 from the 100, there is a good chance that none of the eight from the small group might be selected (Cottrell & McKenzie, 2005).

Here is an example of the use of a stratified random sample. To begin with, the planner first must divide the survey population into subgroups (or **strata**) then select a simple random sample from each strata. Suppose we were interested in collecting data from companies within a particular state concerning the number of health education programs offered for employees. Based upon past experience, we suspect the size of the business (i.e., number of employees) would affect the data we wanted to collect. That is, small companies might have fewer health education programs in general than large companies. Also, we know that only a couple of companies in the state have a large number of employees. We could then divide the companies into strata by size, say small (1–100 employees), medium (101–1,000), and large (1,001+). Once the planners decide how many to select from each strata, they have to decide whether to conduct a proportional stratified random sample or nonproportional stratified random sample. A **proportional stratified random sample** would be used if the planners wanted the sample to mirror, in proportion, the survey population. That is, draw out the companies in the same proportions that they are represented in the survey population. Say our example has 600 small companies, 350 medium companies, and 50 large companies, and the desired sample size is 100. Planners would then select simple random samples of 60 small, 35 medium, and 5 large companies (Cottrell & McKenzie, 2005).

A **nonproportional stratified random sample** may be used if the planners want equal representation from the different strata within the survey population. For example, suppose we wanted to collect information about the opinions of college students on a medium-size regional campus (the survey population) about a new alcohol use policy that was put in place by the administration and we wanted to hear equally from the different level of students (freshmen [$n = 4,000$], sophomores [$n = 3,000$], juniors [$n = 2,000$], and seniors [$n = 1,000$]) because it was thought that the policy would affect each class differently. If a sample size of 200 was desired, we would randomly select (using a simple random sample method) 50 students from each of the classes (Cottrell & McKenzie, 2005). (See **Table 5.5** for a summary of probability sampling procedures.)

Nonprobability Sample

There are times when a probability sample cannot be obtained or is not needed. In such cases, planners/evaluators can take **nonprobability samples,** samples in which all individuals in the survey population do not have an equal chance or probability of being selected to participate in the needs assessment or evaluation. Participants can be included on the basis of convenience (because they have volunteered, are available, or can be easily contacted) or because they have a certain characteristic.

Nonprobability samples have limitations in the extent to which the results can be generalized to the total survey population. Bias may also occur since those who are not included in the sample may differ in some way from those who are included. For example, including only the individuals who complete a health promotion program may bias the results; the findings might be different if all participants, including those who attended but did not complete the program, were surveyed.

Nonprobability samples can be used when planners/evaluators are unable to identify or contact all those in the survey population. These samples can also be used when resources are limited and a probability sample is too costly or time consuming. It is important that planners/evaluators understand the limitations of this type of sample when reporting the results. (See **Table 5.6** for a summary of nonprobability sampling procedures.)

Table 5.5 Summary of probability sampling procedures

Sample	Primary Descriptive Elements
Simple Random	Each subject has an equal chance of being selected if table of random numbers and random start are used.
"Fishbowl" (or "Out of a Hat")	Approximates simple random sampling, but not as precise. Can be done with or without replacement.
Systematic	Using a list (e.g., membership list or telephone book), subjects are selected at a constant interval (N/n) after a random start.
Nonproportional Stratified	The population is divided into subgroups based on key characteristics (strata), and subjects are selected from the subgroups at random to ensure representation of the characteristic.
Proportional Stratified	Like the nonproportional stratified random sample, but subjects are selected in proportion to the numerical strength of strata in the population.
Cluster or Area	Random sampling of groups (e.g., teachers' classes) or areas (e.g., city blocks) instead of individuals.
Matrix	The responses of several randomly selected subjects to different items are combined to form the response of one.

Source: Adapted from E. R. Babbie, *The Practice of Social Research,* 6th ed. (Belmont, CA: Wadsworth, 1992); P. C. Cozby, *Methods in Behavioral Research,* 3rd ed. (Palo Alto, CA: Mayfield, 1985); P. D. Leedy, *Practical Research: Planning and Design,* 5th ed. (New York: Macmillan, 1993); and R. J. McDermott and P. D. Sarvela, *Health Education Evaluation and Measurement: A Practitioner's Perspective,* 2nd ed. (New York: McGraw-Hill, 1999).

Table 5.6   Summary of nonprobability sampling procedures

Sample	Primary Descriptive Elements
Convenience	Includes any available subject meeting some minimum criterion usually being part of an accessible intact group.
Volunteer	Includes any subject motivated enough to self-select for a study.
Grab	Includes whomever investigators can access through direct contact, usually for interviews.
Homogeneous	Includes individuals chosen because of a unique trait or factor they possess.
Judgmental	Includes subjects whom the investigator judges to be "typical" of individuals possessing a given trait.
Snowball	Includes subjects identified by investigators, and any other persons referred by initial subjects.
Quota	Includes subjects chosen in approximate proportion to the population traits they are to "represent."

Source: R. J. McDermott & P. D. Sarveld, *Health Education Evaluation and Measurement: A Practitioner's Perspective, 2/e.* Copyright © 1999. Reprinted by permission of McGraw-Hill Companies, Inc.

Sample Size

An often-asked question associated with sampling is, how many individuals are needed for planners/evaluators to feel confident that sampling error is within an acceptable range so that reasonable conclusions can be drawn from the data analyzed? There is not an easy answer to this question. Appropriate sample size is determined by both practical and statistical considerations. From a practical standpoint, often the resources (i.e., personnel, financial) available to collect data are the determining factor on how large the sample will be. Asked another way, is the desired sample size affordable?

When analyzing sample size from a statistical standpoint, three major theoretical considerations are used: central limit theorem (CLT), precision and reliability, and power

Table 5.7   Sample sizes for studies describing population proportions when the population size is known

Population size	95% Confidence Interval Sample size for precision of		
	±1	±3	±5
500	*	*	222
1,000	*	*	286
5,000	*	909	370
10,000	5,000	1,000	385
100,000	9,091	1,099	398
S ∞	10,000	1,111	400

*=In these cases the assumption of normal approximation is poor, and the formula used to derive them does not apply.
Source: This table is derived from Yamane (1973).

Table 5.8   Sample sizes for the one-sample case for the mean

Directional ("one-tailed") test for numerical (interval or ratio) data				
	alpha = .05		alpha = .01	
Effect size/Power	.80	.90	.80	.90
.20	155	215	251	326
.50	27	37	43	55
.80	12	17	19	23

Nondirectional ("two-tailed") test for numerical (interval or ratio) data				
	alpha = .05		alpha = .01	
Effect size/Power	.80	.90	.80	.90
.20	197	263	292	372
.50	34	44	50	63
.80	15	19	22	27

Source: This table is derived from Hinkle, Oliver, & Hinkle (1985).

analysis (Norwood, 2000). The CLT can provide the quickest answer to the sample size question. Mathematically, it has been shown that when a sample size approaches 30 in number, characteristics of that group approach the normal distribution of the group from which it was drawn. Thus a general rule for comparison purposes is, no group should be smaller than 30.

Determining sample size using precision and reliability, or power analysis is much more complicated. There is not enough space in this chapter to provide for the detailed explanations needed. **Table 5.7** and **Table 5.8** are provided as examples of the application of these considerations. Detailed explanations of these concepts are presented in many statistics textbooks.

Pilot Testing

Pilot testing (sometimes referred to as *piloting* or a *pilot study*) is a set of procedures used by planners/evaluators to try out various processes during program development on a small group of participants prior to actual implementation. In other words, pilot testing can be thought of as a dress rehearsal for planners/evaluators (McDermott & Sarvela, 1999). The purpose of using pilot testing is to identify and, if necessary, correct any problems prior to implementation with the priority population. Thus pilot testing permits a thorough check of all planned processes to help increase the chances of having a successful program. Throughout the program planning process, planners/evaluators may use pilot testing to detect any problems with sampling, data collection instruments, data collection procedures, data analysis procedures, interventions, curricula, and program evaluation (McDermott & Sarvela, 1999). Because this chapter has focused on measurement and measures, the remaining portions of this discussion will focus on the pilot testing of data collection. Pilot testing will also be discussed in Chapter 12, as it relates to the implementation of a program.

Once the data collection method has been determined and the data collection instrument has been selected or created, a trial run of the instrument, data collection procedures, and analyses should be conducted. During the piloting process, it would not be uncommon for the planners/evaluators to find problems, such as ambiguous questions, difficulty with code sheets, and misunderstood directions. Further, the data collected during pilot testing should be statistically analyzed or compiled to make sure that there is no difficulty with this step in the data collection process. Revising the data collection process using the information gained from the pilot testing helps ensure that the actual data collection will proceed smoothly.

Several authors (Borg & Gall, 1989; McDermott & Sarvela, 1999; Parkinson and Associates, 1982; Stacy, 1987) have suggested processes for pilot testing. They have been combined here into a single process. Several of the preceding authors have presented hierarchies for pilot testing: preliminary review, prepilot, pilot tests, and field tests. The first, and lowest, level in the pilot testing hierarchy is a preliminary review. A **preliminary review** is conducted when those responsible for the data collection process ask colleagues, not people from the priority population, to review the data collection instrument. At a minimum, all data collection instruments should be subjected to this type of review. Specifically, in a preliminary review, colleagues would be asked to complete the instrument as if they were subjects in hopes of identifying problems, and also respond to several other questions about the instrument, such as the appropriateness of (1) the instrument's title, (2) the introductory statement explaining the purpose of the data collection, (3) the directions, (4) the order or grouping of the questions, (5) the questions (e.g. unclear or too personal), (6) the length of the instrument, and (7) the method of returning the instrument, to name a few. **Prepilots** (or mini-pilots) are used by planners/evaluators with five or six members of the priority population to assess the quality of materials, instruments, and data collection techniques. Methods used to collect this information include observations, interviews, and focus groups. The pilot test requires the actual implementation of the instrument. A representative sample of the priority population is used to determine the quality of the instrument. A **field study** is a final pilot test, combining all materials previously tested separately (e.g., instrument, curriculum materials) into a complete program. If enough subjects are used during the field study, it may be possible to check the validity and reliability of the instrument. If at all possible, the use of this sequence of pilot testing techniques is desirable, but planners/evaluators are often limited by time and resources, and so not all the steps can be completed.

Ethical Issues Associated with Measurement

Whenever people are being measured as part of a needs assessment or an evaluation, planners/evaluators need to be cognizant that many of their decisions made and actions taken throughout these processes could have ethical ramifications. Further, as noted in Chapter 4, planners/evaluators are obligated by law—via the *Health Insurance Portability and Accountability Act of 1996*—to guard against the misuse of individual identifiable health information.

Ethical issues associated with measurement begin with getting people to voluntarily participate in the process. Before people get involved they should be well informed about the nature of the process and what is expected when they do participate. Further, the potential participants should not be coerced or deceived to participate. And, once participation has begun, planners/evaluators should make it clear that participants have the right to discontinue participation at any time without penalty. A second issue is that of private and/or sensitive data. If planners/evaluators need to ask questions that reveal private and sensitive data, they need to ensure anonymity or confidentiality. During data collection, planners/evaluators may hear about illegal acts, such as drug use or other crimes, or the data collectors may be provided with access to confidential data. The planners/evaluators must consider the ethical issues and the legal ramifications of such issues. Weiss (1998) advises checking out state and national laws, and discussing these ethical situations with knowledgeable colleagues.

Once the data have been collected, several ethical issues could arise when the data are analyzed and reported. "Inappropriate data analyses can lead to, among other problems, harm to a person or property, implementation of inappropriate policies or procedures, and the waste of time, effort, and resources" (Cottrell & McKenzie, 2005 p. 107). Regardless of the purposes for which the analyzed data are used, planners/evaluators have an ethical obligation to ensure they do not mislead anyone who relies on them (Dane, 1990). Finally, when the results of a needs assessment or an evaluation are reported, planners/evaluators must ensure not to reveal the identity of those who participated, or individual results of participants, without their permission.

SUMMARY

This chapter focused on helping you understand the terms *measurement, measures, measurement instruments, sampling,* and *pilot testing.* A brief overview of measurement and measures was provided, along with the four levels of measurement: nominal, ordinal, interval, and ratio. Several different examples of questions used at each of the levels were also presented. Next, four desirable characteristics of data were discussed, including reliability, validity, fairness, and unbiased. Background information was provided to assist you with processes to identify existing measurement instruments and create new ones. Information was also presented on writing measurement instrument questions. This was followed by a discussion of techniques used to draw the various probability and nonprobability samples, and when the various sampling techniques might be most useful. The chapter concluded with short presentations on the importance of using pilot testing and the ethical issues associated with measurement.

REVIEW QUESTIONS

1. What is meant by *measurement,* and *qualitative* and *quantitative measures?*

2. Why is measurement such an important process when it comes to program planning and evaluation?

3. Name and give an example of each of the four levels of measurement.

4. What are the most common types of measures (variables) used in needs assessments and evaluations? Give an example of each type of variable.

5. What is validity? What is reliability? Why are they so important?

6. What is bias in data collection? Name three ways in which it can be reduced.

7. Why must measurement instruments be fair?

8. What are the steps one can follow when identifying, obtaining, and evaluating existing measurement instruments?

9. What are the advantages and disadvantages of using an existing measurement instrument?

10. What are the steps for creating a data collection instrument?

11. Define census, sample, sampling, and sampling frame.

12. Using a table of random numbers, explain how a simple random sample is selected.

13. Describe three types of probability samples.

14. When, if ever, should nonprobability samples be used?

15. What is the purpose of a preliminary review, a prepilot (or mini-pilot), a pilot test, and a field study? How is each conducted?

16. What ethical issues are associated with measurement?

ACTIVITIES

1. Construct a three-page written questionnaire on a health promotion topic of your choice that could be administered to a group of college students.

2. Conduct a prepilot test on your written questionnaire developed in activity number 1 on five or six of your friends, colleagues, or classmates. After pilot testing, identify any flaws you see in the questionnaire or data collection process.

3. Assume that your college or university has hired you to conduct a needs assessment on the student body for a new health promotion program. Because there are few secondary data on this group of people, other than national data on college students, you have decided to survey a random sample of students using a written instrument. Your task now is to develop the instrument. Create a draft of an instrument that includes questions that will collect data about the students' health behavior and demographic characteristics. Also, include some marketing questions that will provide data that help you know when and where the program should be offered. After completing the instrument, pilot test it on 10 students and then tally the data collected.

4. Assume that you are charged with the responsibility of collecting data from all the students on your campus who have enrolled in a fitness course. Assume also that

this group of students is too large to collect data from everyone. Explain how you would obtain a representative sample from this population.

5. Review a needs assessment or evaluation instrument. Identify the level of measurement for the questions, types of measurement, and types of questions.

6. Photocopy a page from a local telephone book. Let's assume that this page represents a sampling frame for your priority population. Go through the frame and divide it into groups of 10 by using the first 10 numbers as group 1, the second 10 as group 2, and so on, until all the numbers are used. Be sure you do not use fax or business numbers. If you have an odd number of telephone numbers (not an even 10), do not use that group. With this information, explain how you would select a simple random sample of 20 numbers, a systematic sample of 10 numbers, a proportional stratified sample of 40 numbers stratified on the first 3 numbers of the telephone numbers, and a cluster sample of 10 groups, assuming that the groups of 10s you formed are your clusters.

WEBLINKS

1. **http://ctb.ku.edu/tools/en/sub_section_main_1044.htm**

   Community Toolbox

   This is a page from the Community Toolbox website that was created and maintained by the Work Group on Health Promotion and Community Development at the University of Kansas in Lawrence, Kansas (U.S.A). This specific page defines and describes the process of developing baseline measures.

2. **http://www.welcoa.org/freeresources/pdf/data_dashboard.pdf**

   The Wellness Councils of America (WELCOA)

   This page of the WELCOA web site presents an article titled "Developing a Data Dashboard: The Art and Science of Making Sense." For those health educators interested in worksite wellness, this article presents a nice overview of the measures (metrics) with which those in the work setting are interested.

3. **http://www.cdc.gov/nchs/default.htm**

   National Center for Health Statistics (NCHS)

   This is the website for the NCHS. It is a rich source of measurement instruments used to collect the data about America's health.

4. **http://www.surveysystem.com/resource.htm**

   Creative Research Systems

   This is a page from the website for a commercial company called Creative Research Systems. This page includes a lot of information about survey instrument development data collection and includes a calculator for determining appropriate sample size.

6

Mission Statement, Goals, and Objectives

After reading this chapter and answering the questions at the end, you should be able to:

- Explain what is meant by the term *mission statement*.
- Define *goals* and *objectives*, and distinguish between the two.
- Identify the different levels of objectives as presented in the chapter.
- Describe a SMART objective.
- State the necessary elements of an objective as presented in the chapter.
- Specify an appropriate criterion for objectives.
- Write program goals and objectives.
- Describe the use for *Healthy People 2010*.
- Explain why a midcourse review is conducted for *Healthy People 2010*.

action or behavioral
   objectives
attitude objectives
awareness objectives
condition
criterion
environmental objectives

goal
impact objectives
knowledge objectives
learning objectives
mission statement
objectives
outcome

outcome or program
   objectives
process or administrative
   objectives
skill development/acquisition
   objectives
SMART

To plan, implement, and evaluate effective health promotion programs, planners must have a solid foundation in place to guide them through their work. The mission statement, goals, and objectives of a program can provide such a foundation. If prepared properly, a mission statement, goals, and objectives should not only give the necessary direction to a program but also provide the groundwork for the eventual program evaluation (**Box 6.1**). There are two old sayings that help express the need for a mission statement, goals, and objectives. The first is: If you do not know where you are going, then any road will do—and you may end up someplace where you do not want to be, or you may eventually end up where you want to be, but after wasted time and effort. The second is: If you do not know where you are going, how will you know when you have arrived? Without a mission statement, goals, and objectives, a program may lack direction, and at best it will be difficult to evaluate. **Figure 6.1** shows the relationship between a mission statement, goals, and objectives. The size of the rectangles presented in Figure 6.1 have special meaning. The rectangle that represents the mission statement is the largest, while the rectangle representing the objectives is the smallest, meaning that ideas presented go from broad to narrow in scope.

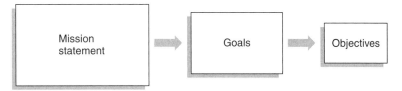

Figure 6.1 Relationship of mission statement, goals, and objectives

Mission Statement

Sometimes referred to as a program overview or program aim, a **mission statement** is a short narrative that describes the general focus or purpose of the program. The statement not only describes the current focus of a program but also may reflect the philosophy behind it. The mission statement also helps to guide planners in the development of

---

Box 6.1   RESPONSIBILITIES AND COMPETENCIES FOR HEALTH EDUCATORS

The content of Chapter 6 focuses on the mission, goals, and objectives of a program. Because the mission, goals, and objectives provide both the foundation on which programs are developed and the criteria used to evaluate the programs, the information presented in this chapter is applicable to two areas of responsibility:

Responsibility II: Plan Health Education Strategies, Interventions, and Programs
                      Competency C: Formulate appropriate and measurable program objectives

Responsibility IV: Conduct Evaluation and Research Related to Health Education
                      Competency D: Carry out evaluation and research plans

Source: NCHEC, SOPHE, & AAHE (2006).

| Box 6.2 | EXAMPLES OF MISSION STATEMENTS |

Setting	Mission Statement
Community Setting	The mission of the Walkup Health Promotion Program is to provide a wide variety of primary prevention activities for residents of the community.
Heath Care Setting	This program is aimed at helping patients and their families to understand and cope with physical and emotional changes associated with recovery following cancer surgery.
School Setting	School District #77 wants happy and healthy students. To that end, the district's personnel strives, through a coordinated school health program, to provide students with experiences that are designed to motivate and enable them to maintain and improve their health.
Worksite Setting	The purpose of the employee health promotion program is to develop high employee morale. This is to be accomplished by providing employees with a working environment that is conducive to good health and by providing an opportunity for employees and their families to engage in behavior that will improve and maintain good health.

program goals and objectives. **Box 6.2** presents examples of mission statements for several different settings.

Some people mistake the term vision statement for mission statement. They are different. While a mission statement provides a description of the current efforts of a program, a *vision statement* is more of an outline of where a program will be in the future. Vision statements are often a part of a strategic planning process in which organizations are defining a strategy or direction for their future. Most program plans do not include a vision statement.

Program Goals

Although some individuals use the terms *goals* and *objectives* synonymously, they are not the same: There are important differences between them. Ross and Mico (1980, p. 219) have stated that "a goal is a future event toward which a committed endeavor is directed; objectives are the steps to be taken in pursuit of a goal." Deeds (1992, p. 36) defined a goal as a "broad timeless statement of a long-range program purpose," whereas Neiger and Thackeray (1998) defined goals as general statements of intent. In comparison to objectives, a **goal** is an expectation that:

1. Is much more encompassing, or global

2. Is written to include all aspects or components of a program

3. Provides overall direction for a program

4. Is more general in nature

5. Usually takes longer to complete

6. Does not have a deadline (CDC, 2003)

7. Usually is not observed, but rather must be inferred because it includes words like *evaluate, know, improve,* and *understand* (Jacobsen, Eggen, & Kauchak, 1989)

8. Is often not measurable in exact terms

Program goals are not difficult to write and need not be written as complete sentences. They should, however, be simple and concise, and should include two basic components: who will be affected, and what will change as a result of the program. Goals typically include verbs such as *improve, increase, promote, protect, minimize, prevent,* and *reduce* (CDC, 2003). A program need not have a set number of stated goals. It is not uncommon for some programs to have a single goal while others have several. **Box 6.3** presents some examples of goals for health promotion programs.

Box 6.3 EXAMPLES OF PROGRAM GOALS

- To reduce the incidence of cardiovascular disease in the employees of the Smith Company.
- All cases of measles in the City of Kenzington will be eliminated.
- To prevent the spread of HIV in the youth of Indiana.
- To reduce the cases of lung cancer caused by exposure to secondhand smoke in Yorktown, IN.
- To reduce the incidence of influenza in the residents of the Delaware County Home.
- The survival rate of breast cancer patients will be increased through the optimal use of community resources.

Objectives

As Ross and Mico (1980) have indicated, **objectives** are more precise and represent smaller steps than program goals—steps that, if completed, will lead to reaching the program goal(s). Stated another way, objectives specify intermediate accomplishments or benchmarks that represent progress toward the goal (CDC, 2003). Objectives outline in measurable terms the specific changes that will occur in the priority population at a given point in time as a result of exposure to the program. "Objectives are crucial. They form a fulcrum, converting diagnostic data into program direction and resource allocation over time" (Green & Kreuter, 2005, p. 100). Objectives can be thought of as the bridge between needs assessment and a planned intervention. Knowing how to construct objectives for a program is a most important skill for planners.

Different Levels of Objectives

Several different levels of objectives are associated with program planning. The different levels are sequenced or placed in a hierarchical order to allow for more effective planning (Cleary & Neiger, 1998; Deeds, 1992; Parkinson & Associates, 1982). Objectives are created at each level in order to help attain the program goal. The "objectives should also be *coherent* across levels, with objectives becoming successively more refined and more explicit, and usually multiplied from one level to the next" (Green & Kreuter, 2005, p. 102). Achievement of the lower-level objectives will contribute to the achievement of the higher-level objectives and goals. **Table 6.1** presents the hierarchy of objectives and indicates their relationship to program outcomes and evaluation. Because the hierarchy of objectives was created from the work of several, the labels (names) given to the different levels of objectives have not been consistent. Thus, as we present the description of each type of objective, we identify the various labels that have been used.

Process or Administrative Objectives The **process or administrative objectives** are the daily tasks, activities, and work plans that lead to the accomplishment of all other levels of objectives (Deeds, 1992). They help shape or form the program and thus focus on all program inputs (all that are needed to carry out a program), implementation activities (actual presentation of the program), and stakeholder reactions. More specifically, these

Table 6.1 Hierarchy of objectives and their relation to evaluation

Type of Objective	Program Outcomes	Possible Evaluation Measures	Type of Evaluation
Process or Administrative Objectives	Activities presented and tasks completed	Number of sessions held, exposure, attendance, participation, staff performance, appropriate materials, adequacy of resources, tasks on schedule	Process (form of formative)
Learning Objectives			Impact (form of summative)
Awareness	Change in awareness	Increase in awareness	
Knowledge	Change in knowledge	Increase in knowledge	
Attitudes	Change in attitude	Improved attitude	
Skills	Change in skills	Skill development or acquisition	
Action or Behavioral Objectives	Change in behavior	Current behavior modified or discontinued, or new behavior adopted	Impact (form of summative)
Environmental Objectives	Change in the environment	Protection added to, or hazards or barriers removed from, the environment	Impact (form of summative)
Outcome or Program Objectives	Change in quality of life (QoL), health status, risk factors, and social benefits	(QoL) measures, morbidity data, mortality data, measures of risk (i.e., HRA), physiological measures, signs and symptoms	Outcome (form of summative)

Source: Adapted from Deeds (1992), Cleary and Neiger (1998), and Parkinson & Associates (1982).

objectives would focus on such things as program resources (materials, funds, space); appropriateness of intervention activities; priority population exposure, attendance, participation, and feedback; feedback from other stakeholders such as the funding and sponsoring agencies; and data collection techniques, to name a few.

Learning Objectives The second level of objectives in the hierarchy comprises **learning objectives**. They are the educational or learning tools needed in order to achieve the desired behavior change. They are based upon the analysis of educational and ecological assessment of the PRECEDE-PROCEED model.

Within this level of objectives, there is another hierarchy (Parkinson & Associates, 1982). This hierarchy includes four types of objectives, beginning with the least complex and moving toward the most complex. Complexity is defined in terms of the time, effort, and resources necessary to accomplish the objective. The learning objectives hierarchy begins with **awareness objectives** and moves through **knowledge, attitude,** and **skill development/acquisition objectives**. This hierarchy indicates that if those in the priority population are going to adopt and maintain a health-enhancing behavior to alleviate a health concern or problem, they must first be aware of the health concern. Second, they must expand their knowledge and understanding of the concern. Third, they must attain and maintain an attitude that enables them to deal with the concern. And fourth, they need to possess the necessary skills to engage in the health-enhancing behavior.

Action or Behavioral Objectives **Action or behavioral objectives** describe the behaviors or actions in which the priority population will engage that will resolve the health problem and move you toward achieving the program goal (Deeds, 1992). Action or behavioral objectives are commonly written about adherence (e.g., regular exercise), compliance (e.g., taking medication as prescribed), consumption patterns (e.g., diet), coping (e.g., stress-reduction activities), preventive actions (e.g., brushing and flossing teeth), self-care (e.g., first aid), and utilization (e.g, appropriate use of the emergency room).

Environmental Objectives **Environmental objectives** outline the nonbehavioral causes of a health problem that are present in the social, physical, and/or psychological environments. Environmental objectives are written about such things as the state of the physical environment (e.g., clean air or water), the social environment (e.g., access to health care), or the psychological environment (e.g., the emotional learning climate).

As we leave our discussion of environmental objectives, it should be noted that there are some who group the four types of learning objectives (i.e., awareness, knowledge, attitudes, and skills), action or behavioral objectives, and environmental objectives into a single category known as **impact objectives**. They get this label because they all form the groundwork for impact evaluation. (See the last column in Table 6.1. The term *impact objectives* is a parallel term with the terms *process objectives* and *outcome objectives*.)

Outcome or Program Objectives **Outcome or program objectives** are the ultimate objectives of a program and are aimed at changes in health status, social benefits, risk factors, or quality of life. "They are outcome or future oriented" (Deeds, 1992, p. 36). If these objectives are achieved, then the program goal will be achieved. These objectives are commonly written in terms of reduction of risk, physiologic indicators, signs and symptoms, morbidity, disability, mortality, or quality of life measures.

Developing Objectives

Does every program require objectives from each of the levels just described? The answer is no! However, too often, health promotion programs have too few objectives, all of which fall into one or two levels. Many planners have developed programs hoping solely to change the health behavior of a priority population. For example, a smoking cessation program may have an objective of getting 30% of the participants to stop smoking. Perhaps this program is offered, and only 10% of the participants quit smoking. Is the program a failure? If the program has a single objective of changing behavior, its sponsors would have a good case for saying that the program was not effective. However, it is quite possible that as a result of participating in the smoking cessation program, the participants increased their awareness of the dangers of smoking. They probably also increased their knowledge, maybe changed their attitudes, and developed skills for quitting or cutting back on the number of cigarettes they smoke each day. These are all very positive outcomes—and they could be overlooked when the program is evaluated, if the planner did not write objectives that cover a variety of levels.

Criteria for Developing Objectives

In addition to making sure that the objectives are written in an appropriate manner, planners also need to be realistic with regard to the other parameters of the program. These are some of the questions that planners should consider when writing objectives:

1. Can the objective be realized during the life of the program or within a reasonable time thereafter? It would be quite realistic to assume that a certain number of people will not be smoking one year after they have completed a smoking cessation program, but it would not be realistic to assume that a group of elementary school students could be followed for life to determine how many of them die prematurely due to inactivity.

2. Can the objective realistically be achieved? It is probably realistic to assume that 30% of any smoking cessation class will stop smoking within one year after the program has ended, but it is not realistic to assume that 100% of the employees of a company will participate in its fitness program.

3. Does the program have enough resources (personnel, money, and space) to obtain a specific objective? It would be ideal to be able to reach all individuals in the priority population, but generally there are not sufficient resources to do so.

4. Are the objectives consistent with the policies and procedures of the sponsoring agency? It would not be realistic to expect to incorporate a no-smoking policy in a tobacco company.

5. Do the objectives violate any of the rights of those who are involved (participants or planners)? Right-to-know laws make it illegal to withhold information that could cause harm to a priority population.

6. If a program is planned for a particular ethnic/cultural population, do the objectives reflect the relationship between the cultural characteristics of the priority group and the changes sought? It would not be realistic to have an objective that eliminates the use of tobacco in a priority population that is comprised of Native Americans because of the ceremonial pipe use in the Native American culture.

The CDCynergy planning model has created an acronym for the criteria for objectives presented above called SMART. **SMART** stands for specific, measurable, achievable, realistic, and time-phased (CDC, 2003). Every objective planners write for their programs should be SMART!

Elements of an Objective

For an objective to provide direction and be useful in the evaluation process, it must be written in such a way that it can be clearly understood, states what is to be accomplished, and is measurable. To ensure that an objective is indeed useful, it should include the following elements:

1. The *outcome* to be achieved, or what will change.

2. The *conditions* under which the outcome will be observed, or when the change will occur.

3. The *criterion* for deciding whether the outcome has been achieved, or how much change.

4. The *priority population,* or who will change.

The first element, the **outcome,** is defined as the action, behavior, or something else that will change as a result of the program. In a written objective, the outcome is usually identified as the verb of the sentence. Thus words such as *apply, argue, build, compare, demonstrate, evaluate, exhibit, judge, perform, reduce, spend, state,* and *test* would be considered outcomes (see **Box 6.4** for a more comprehensive listing of appropriate outcome words). It should be noted that not all verbs would be considered appropriate outcomes for an objective; the verb must refer to something measurable and observable. Words such as *appreciate, know, internalize, and understand* by themselves do not refer to something measurable and observable, and therefore are not good choices for outcomes. Some verbs work better than others for specific types of objectives. For example, the verb *list* is an appropriate verb for an awareness-level objective, but not for a knowledge-level objective. The verb *explain* would be much better suited for a knowledge-level objective.

The second element of an objective is the **condition** under which the outcome will be observed, or when it will be observed. "Typical" conditions found in objectives might be "upon completion of the exercise class," "as a result of participation," "by the year 2010," "after reading the pamphlets and brochures," "orally in class," "when asked to respond by the facilitator," "one year after the program," "by May 15th," or "during the class session."

The third element of an objective is the **criterion** for determining when the outcome has been achieved, or how much change will occur. The purpose of this element is to provide a standard by which the planners/evaluators can determine if an outcome has been

Box 6.4   OUTCOME VERBS FOR OBJECTIVES

abstract	copy	gather	offer	round
accept	count	(information)	order	score
adjust	create	generalize	organize	seek
adopt	criticize	generate	pair	select
advocate	deduce	group	participate	separate
analyze	defend	guess	partition	share
annotate	define	hypothesize	perform	show
apply	delay (response)	identify	persist	simplicity
approximate	demonstrate	illustrate	plan	simulate
argue	derive	imitate	practice	solve
(a position)	describe	improve	praise	sort
ask	design	infer	predict	spend
associate	determine	initiate	prepare	(money)
attempt	develop	inquire	preserve	state
balance	differentiate	integrate	produce	structure
build	discover	interpolate	propose	submit
calculate	discriminate	interpret	prove	subscribe
categorize	dispute	invent	qualify	substitute
cause	distinguish	investigate	query	suggest
challenge	effect	join	question	summarize
change	eliminate	judge	recall	supply
choose	enumerate	justify	recite	support
clarify	estimate	keep	recognize	symbolize
classify	evaluate	label	recommend	synthesize
collect	examine	list	record	tabulate
combine	exemplify	locate	reduce	tally
compare	exhibit	manipulate	regulate	test
complete	experiment	map	reject	theorize
compute	explain	match	relate	translate
conceptualize	express	measure	reorganize	try
connect	extend	name	repeat	unite
construct	extract	obey	replace	visit
consult	extrapolate	object	represent	volunteer
contrast	find	(to an idea)	reproduce	weigh
convert	form	observe	restructure	write

performed in an appropriate and/or successful manner. Examples might include "to no more than 105 per 1,000," "by 10% over the baseline," "300 pamphlets," "33% of the county residents," "75% of the motor vehicle occupants," "at least half of the participants," "according to CDC guidelines," or "all people who preregistered." One of the most difficult parts of creating appropriate objects for a program is to determine what would be the appropriate criterion for an objective. Should program planners expect a 10% increase over baseline? Should they anticipate half of the employees to participate? What should be expected? There is no hard and fast rule for determining the criterion, but remember SMART objectives should be realistic! Several different criterion-setting techniques were used in the writing of the *Healthy People 2010* objectives and for the *Healthy People 2010* Midcourse Review. **Box 6.5** provides a brief description of the target-setting methods used.

The last element that needs to be included in an objective is mention of the priority population, or who will change. Examples are "1,000 teachers," "25% of employees of the company," and "those residing in the Muncie and Provo areas." **Figure 6.2** summarizes the key elements in an objective. There is one exception to the priority population always being the *who* of an objective. That exception applies to process,

---

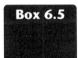

Box 6.5 TARGET (CRITERION) SETTING METHODS FOR *HEALTHY PEOPLE 2010* AND *HEALTHY PEOPLE 2010*'S MIDCOURSE REVIEW

Better than the best racial/ethnic group—when setting targets for disparities, when no baseline data were available, the criterion was set based upon a comparison to the racial/ethnic group with the best, or most favorable, rate [see *HP 2010 Midcourse Review: Appendix C: Technical Appendix* for full explanation (USDHHS, 2007b)].

- Percent improvement—target was set based upon a reasonable expected percent change in the priority population compared to previous improvement.
- Total coverage or elimination—target was set based upon the belief that a criterion of 100% could be achieved.
- Consistent with another program—target was set based upon the results of other already completed programs.
- Projection of a trend—target was set based upon available trend data.
- Retain year 2000 target—target was retained if, at the Midcourse Review, it was thought that the target set in 2000 when the objective was written was still appropriate. Thus, no change was made.
- Expert opinion—if no other data were available, the target was set based upon the opinion of experts.
- No increase from baseline—target was set based upon the belief there would be no change from the baseline.

Sources: Gurley (2007, April); USDHHS (2007b).

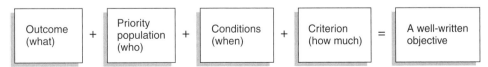

Figure 6.2 Elements of a well-written objective

formative, or administrative-level objectives. Because these objectives guide the work of the program planners and/or implementers, the *who* is the staff or group entrusted with instituting the program instead of the priority population (Cottrell & McKenzie, 2005). (See **Box 6.6** for examples of objectives that would include the four primary components.)

Box 6.6   EXAMPLES OF OBJECTIVES TO SUPPORT THE PROGRAM GOAL "TO REDUCE THE PREVALENCE OF HEART DISEASE IN THE RESIDENTS OF FRANKLIN COUNTY"

Process, Formative, or Administrative Objectives

A. During the next six months, the planning committee will increase participation in the programs by 50% over the baseline participation number.

Outcome (what): Will increase participation.
Priority Population (who): Planning committee.
Conditions (when): During the next six months.
Criterion (how much): By 50% over the baseline participation number.

B. By August 4, the volunteers will distribute the informational brochure to 33% of the county residents.

Outcome (what): Will distribute the informational brochure.
Priority Population (who): Volunteers.
Conditions (when): By August 4.
Criterion (how much): 33% of the county residents.

C. During the pilot testing, the program facilitators will receive a "good" rating from at least half of the participants.

Outcome (what): Will receive a "good" rating.
Priority Population (who): Program facilitators.
Conditions (when): During the pilot testing.
Criterion (how much): At least half of the participants.

D. Prior to the start of the program, the program staff will deliver the program notebooks to all people who preregistered for the program.

Outcome (what): Will deliver the program notebooks.
Priority Population (who): Program staff.
Conditions (when): Prior to the start of the program.
Criterion (how much): All people who preregistered.

Learning Objectives

A. Awareness level: After the American Heart Association's pamphlet on cardiovascular health risk factors has been placed in grocery bags, at least 20% of the shoppers will be able to identify two of their own risks.

Outcome (what): Identify their own risks.
Priority population (who): Shoppers.

Box 6.6 CONTINUED

Conditions (when): After distribution of the pamphlet.
Criterion (how much): 20%.

B. Knowledge level: When asked over the telephone, one out of three viewers of the heart special television show will be able to explain the four principles of cardiovascular conditioning.

Outcome (what): Able to explain the four principles of cardiovascular conditioning.
Priority population (who): Television viewers.
Conditions (when): When asked over the telephone.
Criterion (how much): One out of three.

C. Attitude level: During one of the class sessions, 50% of the participants will defend their reason for regular exercise.

Outcome (what): Defend their reason for regular exercise.
Priority population (who): Class participants.
Conditions (when): During one of the class sessions.
Criterion (how much): 50%.

D. Skill development/acquisition level: After viewing the video "How to Exercise," half of those participating will be able to locate their pulse and count it every time they are asked to do it.

Outcome (what): Locate their pulse and count it.
Priority population (who): Those participating.
Conditions (when): After viewing the video.
Criterion (how much): Half of those participating.

Action or Behavioral Objectives

A. One year after the formal exercise classes have been completed, 40% of those who completed a majority of the classes will still be involved in a regular aerobic exercise program.

Outcome (what): Will still be involved.
Priority population (who): Those who completed a majority of the classes.
Conditions (when): One year after the classes.
Criterion (how much): 40%.

B. During the telephone interview follow-up, 50% of the residents will report having had their blood pressure taken during the previous six months.

Outcome (what): Will report having their blood pressure taken.
Priority population (who): Residents.
Conditions (when): During the telephone interview follow-up.
Criterion (how much): 50%.

Environmental Objectives

A. By the year 2009, 10% of the clinic patients will have been able to schedule an appointment either after 5 p.m. or on a Saturday.

Outcome (what): Will have been able to schedule.
Priority Population (who): Clinic patients.
Conditions (when): By the year 2009.
Criterion (how much): 10%.

Box 6.6   CONTINUED

B. By the end of the year, all senior citizens will be provided transportation to the congregate meals.

Outcome (what): Provided transportation.
Priority population (who): Senior citizens.
Conditions (when): By end of year.
Criterion (how much): All.

Outcome or Program Objectives

A. By the year 2010, heart disease deaths will be reduced to no more than 100 per 100,000 in the residents of Franklin County.

Outcome (what): Reduce heart disease deaths.
Priority population (who): Residents of Franklin County.
Conditions (when): By the year 2010.
Criterion (how much): To no more than 100 per 100,000.

B. By 2010, increase to at least 25% the proportion of men in Franklin County with hypertension whose blood pressure is under control.

Outcome (what): Blood pressure under control.
Priority population (who): Men in Franklin County.
Conditions (when): By 2010.
Criterion (how much): To at least 25%.

C. Half of all those in the county who complete a regular, aerobic, 12-month exercise program will reduce their "risk age" on their follow-up health risk assessment by a minimum of two years compared to their preprogram results.

Outcome (what): Will reduce their "risk age."
Priority population (who): Those who complete an exercise program.
Conditions (when): After the 12-month exercise program.
Criterion (how much): Half.

D. Two-thirds of those who participate in a formal exercise program will use 10% fewer sick days during the life of the program than those who do not participate.

Outcome (what): Use fewer sick days.
Priority population (who): Those who participate.
Conditions (when): During the life of the program.
Criterion (how much): Two-thirds.

Although it is easy to describe the components of well-written objectives, it is not always easy to write them. **Box 6.7** provides a template to help program planners write objectives.

Goals and Objectives for the Nation

A chapter on goals and objectives would not be complete without at least a short discussion of the health goals and objectives of the nation. These goals and objectives have been most helpful to planners throughout the United States.

| **Box 6.7** | APPLICATION—TEMPLATE FOR WRITING OBJECTIVES FOR HEALTH PROMOTION PROGRAMS |

(insert one *when* from column A here), (insert one *how much* from column B here) of the (insert one *who* from column C here), will (insert one *what* from column D here).

Column A – *When?*

By December 2010

After the program

During a class session

One year after the classes

Column B – *How much?*

10%

half

a majority

at least 25

Column C – *Who?*

participants

people enrolled in the program

employees

university students

Column D – *What?*

be able to demonstrate how to prepare a low-fat meal

be able to explain the difference between exercise and physical activity

have stopped smoking

list the risk factors for skin cancer

The U.S. government is very interested in improving the health status of Americans. It is concerned about individuals and the population as a whole. The country is facing many problems and issues that revolve around health; the cost of ill health is the most obvious. Therefore, for at least some parts of the federal government, there is a goal to improve the health status of the public. Objectives have been developed to guide the work of reaching this goal. Some people have referred to these statements of objectives as the *health plan* or *agenda* or *blueprint of health* for the United States.

The first set of objectives was developed by many health professionals throughout the country; it was published in 1980 under the title *Promoting Health/Preventing Disease: Objectives for the Nation* (USDHHS, 1980). This volume was divided into three main areas: preventive services, health protection, and health promotion. Each of these contained five focus areas, or 15 in all. From these 15 areas came a total of 226 objectives. These objectives, which were based on the data collected for the U.S. Surgeon General's report *Healthy People* (1979), were the basis for health promotion and disease prevention planning during the 1980s.

Data for 1987 provided evidence that nearly half of those objectives had been achieved or were likely to be achieved by 1990, while about a quarter were unlikely to be achieved; the status of the remaining quarter was in doubt because tracking data were not available. Progress was slow for some of the 15 priorities identified in 1980, such as pregnancy and infant health, nutrition, physical fitness and exercise, family planning, sexually transmitted diseases, and occupational safety and health. Substantial progress was made, however, in high blood pressure control, immunization, unintentional injury prevention and control, control of infectious diseases, smoking, and alcohol and drugs (Mason & McGinnis, 1990, p. 442).

As the 1980s came to a close, it was obvious from the evaluation conducted on these national goals and objectives (USDHHS, 1986b) that there was a need to develop new goals and objectives to guide the country through the 1990s. Therefore a second set of goals and objectives called *Healthy People 2000: National Health Promotion and Disease Prevention Objectives* was developed (USDHHS, 1990a). That set was much more detailed than the first and was much more useful to all program planners. It included fewer goals and more objectives. In addition, subobjectives were established for people with low incomes, people who were members of some racial and ethnic minority groups, and people with disabilities to help meet their unique needs and health problems (USDHHS, 1994).

Just as the 1990 objectives were not all met, neither were the Healthy People 2000 objectives. In the mid–1990s, the U.S. government published *Healthy People 2000: Midcourse Review and 1995 Revisions* (USDHHS, 1995). That document served as a self-study of progress toward the year 2000 objectives and the beginning point for planning the year 2010 objectives. The context in which the *Healthy People 2010* was framed differed from the 2000 objectives in that planners were working with a broader scientific base, improved surveillance and data systems, and the knowledge that the public had a heightened awareness and demand for preventive services and quality health care (USDHHS, 1997). In January 2000, the latest version of the objectives for the nation, *Healthy People 2010*, was released.

Healthy People 2010 is the most sophisticated Healthy People planning document to date, which is reflective of the effort that went into creating it. The *Healthy People 2010* document is comprised of three parts. *Healthy People 2010: Understanding and Improving Health* is the first of three parts in the Healthy People 2010 series. In addition to providing a history of *Healthy People 2010* and the overall Healthy People initiative, this section presents the Determinants of Health model (see **Figure 6.3**) on which Healthy People is based, how to use Healthy People as a systematic approach to health improvement, and the Leading Health Indicators (LHIs). The LHIs are new to the Healthy People document and were created to provide a snapshot of the health of the nation. *Healthy People 2010* identifies 10 LHIs (physical activity, overweight and obesity, tobacco use, substance abuse, responsible sexual behavior, mental health, injury and violence, environmental quality, immunization, and access to health care). The LHIs highlight major health priorities for the nation and include the individual behaviors, physical and social environmental factors, and health system issues that affect the health of individuals and communities. Each of the 10 LHIs has one or more Healthy People measures associated with it and will be used to measure progress throughout the decade (USDHHS, 2000).

The second part of the document, *Healthy People 2010: Objectives for Improving Health*, contains the two overarching goals and detailed descriptions of 467 objectives to improve health. The two overarching goals for *Healthy People 2010* are:

- Increase quality and years of healthy life.
- Eliminate health disparities.

The first goal is to help individuals of all ages increase life expectancy and improve their quality of life, while the second goal is to eliminate health disparities among different segments of the population. These two goals are supported by specific objectives

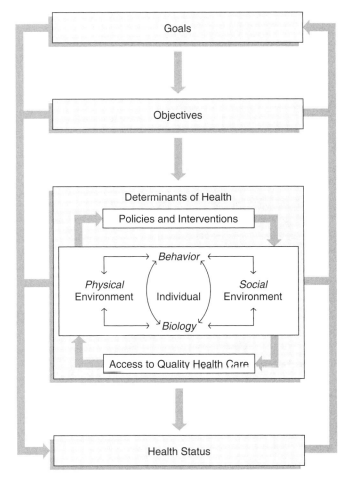

Healthy People in Healthy Communities
A Systematic Approach to Health Improvement

Figure 6.3 Determinants of health
Source: USDHHS (2000).

in 28 focus areas (see **Table 6.2**). In the document, each focus area is presented as a chapter. Each chapter contains a concise goal statement that frames the overall purpose of the area, an overview of the health issue that provides the context and background for the objectives, an interim progress report toward the year 2000 objectives, and the 2010 objectives. There are two types of objectives—measurable and developmental. The measurable objectives provide direction for action and include national baseline data from which the 2010 target was set. The developmental objectives provide a vision for a desired outcome or health status. The purpose of developmental objectives is to identify areas of emerging importance and to drive the development of data systems to measure them.

Table 6.2   *Healthy People 2010* focus areas

1. Access to Quality Health Services
2. Arthritis, Osteoporosis, and Chronic Back Conditions
3. Cancer
4. Chronic Kidney Disease
5. Diabetes
6. Disability and Secondary Conditions
7. Educational and Community-Based Programs
8. Environmental Health
9. Family Planning
10. Food Safety
11. Health Communication
12. Heart Disease and Stroke
13. HIV
14. Immunization and Infectious Diseases
15. Injury and Violence Prevention
16. Maternal, Infant, and Child Health
17. Medical Product Safety
18. Mental Health and Mental Disorders
19. Nutrition and Overweight
20. Occupational Safety and Health
21. Oral Health
22. Physical Activity and Fitness
23. Public Health Infrastructure
24. Respiratory Diseases
25. Sexually Transmitted Diseases
26. Substance Abuse
27. Tobacco Use
28. Vision and Hearing

Source: USDHHS (2000).

The third part of the document, *Tracking Healthy People 2010*, provides a comprehensive review of the statistical measures that will be used to evaluate progress. The purpose of this third part is to provide technical information so that others will be able to understand how the data are derived and the major statistical issues affecting the interpretation of the statistics. This is the first set of Healthy People objectives to have such a document (USDHHS, 2000).

Like the earlier versions of the Healthy People planning documents, *Healthy People 2010* had a midcourse review. The review assessed the status of the two overarching goals and the many national objectives. The purpose of such a review was to assess the data trends for the first half of the decade, consider new science and available data, and make changes to ensure that *Healthy People 2010* remained current, accurate, and relevant, while also assessing emerging public health priorities. The midcourse review was based upon available data and public comments on suggested changes for the objectives (USDHHS, 2006).

At the time of the midcourse review, some progress on the two overarching goals had been made, but the inability to measure the complex interactions of health, disease, disability, and early death make it difficult to quantify some of the progress. There were data to show that the first goal of increasing the quality and years of healthy life revealed that years of life—measured in terms of life expectancy—did improve. However, significant gender, racial, and ethnic differences remained. Women and whites continued to live longer than their comparison groups. While life expectancy continued to increase, the United States continued to have lower life expectancy than many other developed nations. Data for two measures of healthy life expectancy—expected years in good or better health and expected years free of activity limitations—showed slight improvements; however, a third measure of healthy life expectancy—expected years free of selected chronic diseases—declined slightly (USDHHS, 2006).

The midcourse review did show that there had been widespread improvements in rates for most of the populations associated with the social and demographic characteristics included in the second goal—eliminating disparities among segments of the population. However, there was little evidence of systematic reductions in disparity. Disparities—measured in terms of relative differences from the best racial/ethnic group rate—were generally not declining. That is, the health gap between certain racial and ethnic groups was getting wider. Unless greater reductions occur for the populations with the highest rates, disparities will not be eliminated any time soon (USDHHS, 2006).

The midcourse review not only provided an opportunity to measure the progress but also make changes to the objectives if necessary. Thus, the midcourse review yielded several changes. Of the 467 *Healthy People 2010* objectives, 28, or 6%, were dropped after the midcourse review because data were not available to track them or because of a change in science, and another 158, or 34%, of the objectives had no data on which to track their progress. However, of this 158 it was anticipated that data would be available by 2010 to assess 87 of these objectives. This left 281 objectives for which progress could be assessed at midcourse. As can be seen in **Figure 6.4**, a total of 59% of 281 objectives either moved toward the 2010 target or met or exceeded the target (USDHHS, 2006). However, it is clear that much work remains to be done before the end of the decade.

The importance of the Healthy People initiative serving as a blueprint for the nation's health agenda is evidenced by their widespread use. Since the publication of the first Healthy People goals and objectives in 1980, a number of other documents have been created that can help planners develop or adopt appropriate goals and objectives for their programs. A number of states and U.S. territories have taken the national objectives and created similar documents specific to their own residents (USDHHS, 1997). In addition, a number of agencies/organizations have taken similar steps to create documents that could be used by their members and clients in various planning efforts. Examples include the American College Health Association (2002) and the U.S. Department of Health and Human Services (2001a; 2001b).

The national goals and objectives have been important components in the process of health promotion planning since 1980. It is highly recommended that planners review these objectives before developing goals and objectives for programs. The national objectives may be helpful in providing a rationale for a program and in focusing program goals and objectives toward the areas of greatest need, as planners work toward the year 2010.

Finally, at the time this book went to press work had already begun on the *Healthy People, 2020* goal and objectives.

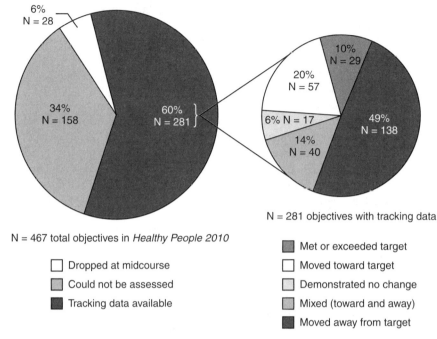

N = 281 objectives with tracking data

N = 467 total objectives in *Healthy People 2010*

☐ Dropped at midcourse
☐ Could not be assessed
■ Tracking data available

■ Met or exceeded target
☐ Moved toward target
☐ Demonstrated no change
■ Mixed (toward and away)
■ Moved away from target

Figure 6.4 *Healthy People 2010* objectives: status at the midcourse and summary of progress toward target attainment
Source: USDHHS (2006).

SUMMARY

The mission statement provides an overview of a program and is most useful in the development of goals and objectives. It should not be confused with a vision statement. The terms *goals* and *objectives* are sometimes used synonymously, but they are quite different. Together, the two provide a foundation for program planning and evaluation. Goals are more global in nature and often are not measurable in exact terms, whereas objectives are more specific and consist of the steps used to reach the program goals. Program objectives can and should be written for several different levels. For objectives to be useful, they should be written so as to be observable and measurable. At a minimum, an objective should include the following elements: a stated outcome (what), conditions under which the outcome will be observed (when), a criterion for considering that the outcome has been achieved (how much), and mention of the priority population (who). As planners develop their goals and objectives for their programs, they should find the *Healthy People 2010* document and data available at the Midcourse Review very useful.

REVIEW QUESTIONS

1. What is a mission statement? Why is it important? How is it different from a vision statement?

2. What is (are) the difference(s) between a goal and an objective?

3. What is the purpose of program goals and objectives?

4. What are the different levels of objectives?

5. What are the necessary elements of an objective?

6. What are the characteristics of a SMART objective?

7. What are the goals and objectives for the nation? How can they be used by program planners?

8. Briefly explain the Healthy People initiative.

9. How can planners use the *Healthy People 2010* goals and objectives in their program planning efforts?

10. What was the status of the *Healthy People 2010* goals and objectives at the time of the Midcourse Review?

ACTIVITIES

1. Write a mission statement, a goal, and supporting objectives (one at each level) for a program you are planning.

2. Identify which of the following objectives include all four elements necessary for a complete objective; revise those objectives that do not include all the elements:

    a. After the class on objective writing, the students will know the difference between a goal and an objective.

    b. The students know how a skinfold caliper works.

    c. After completing this chapter, the students will be able to write objectives for each of the levels based on the four elements outlined in the chapter.

    d. Given appropriate instruction, the employees will be able to accurately take blood pressure readings of fellow employees.

    e. Program participants will be able to list the reasons why people do not exercise.

3. Write a mission statement, a goal, and supporting objectives (one at each level) for a workshop on responsible use of alcohol by college students.

WEBLINKS

1. http://wonder.cdc.gov/data2010/

   CDC WONDER: DATA2010

   DATA 2010 is the data page from the CDC WONDER website. It is an interactive database system developed by staff of the Division of Health Promotion Statistics at the National Center for Health Statistics, and contains the most recent monitoring data for tracking *Healthy People 2010*.

2. http://www.cancer.org/docroot/AA/AA_0.asp

   American Cancer Society (ACS)

   This is a page from the ACS website. This page includes information about the ACS including its mission statement. If you click on the homepage of the ACS, you will find it to be a great source of cancer information and data.

3. http://www.americanheart.org/presenter.jhtml?identifier=10858

   American Heart Association (AHA)

   This is a page from the AHA website. This page includes information about the AHA including its mission statement. If you click on the homepage of the AHA, you will find it to be an excellent source of heart health information and data. It also includes links to other associations and organizations that have an interest in heart health.

4. http://www.acha.org/index.cfm

   American College Health Association (ACHA)

   This is the home page from the ACHA. From this page you can link to the page that describes the vision, mission, and goals of the ACHA. You can also find information about the Healthy Campus 2010—the health goals and objectives for institutions of higher learning.

Theories and Models Commonly Used for Health Promotion Interventions

After reading this chapter and answering the questions at the end, you should be able to:

- Define *theory*, *model*, *constructs*, *concepts*, and *variables*.
- Explain why health promotion interventions should be planned using theoretical frameworks.
- Describe how the concept of the ecological perspective applies to using theories.
- Explain the difference between a continuum theory and a stage theory.
- Briefly explain the theories and models presented in this chapter.
- Briefly describe some suggestions for applying theory to practice.

action stage
attitude toward
   the behavior
aversive stimulus
behavior change theories
behavioral capability
concepts
construct
contemplation stage
continuum theory
decisional balance
direct reinforcement
ecological perspective
efficacy expectations
elaboration

emotional-coping responses
expectancies
expectations
health belief model (HBM)
intention
lapse
likelihood of taking
   recommended preventive
   health action
locus of control
maintenance stage
model
negative punishment
negative reinforcement
outcome expectations

perceived barriers
perceived behavioral control
perceived benefits
perceived seriousness/
   severity
perceived susceptibility
perceived threat
planning models
positive punishment
positive reinforcement
precontemplation stage
preparation stage
processes of change
punishment
recidivism

Key Terms, continued

reciprocal determinism	self-efficacy	subjective norm
reinforcement	self-regulation	termination
relapse	self-reinforcement	theory
relapse prevention (RP)	stage	variable
self-control	stage theory	vicarious reinforcement

Whenever there is a discussion about the theoretical bases for health education and health promotion, we often find the terms *theory* and *model* used. We begin this chapter with a brief explanation of these terms, to establish a common understanding of their meaning.

One of the most frequently quoted definitions of **theory** is one in which Glanz, Lewis, and Rimer (2002b) modified an earlier definition written by Kerlinger (1986). It states, "A *theory* is a set of interrelated concepts, definitions, and propositions that presents a *systematic* view of events or situations by specifying relations among variables in order to *explain* and *predict* the events of the situations" (p. 25). Green and colleagues (1994, p. 398) have stated, "The role of theory is to untangle and simplify for human comprehension the complexities of nature." In other words, a theory is a systematic arrangement of fundamental principles that provide a basis for explaining certain happenings of life. Hochbaum, Sorenson, and Lorig (1992) defined theories in relationship to health education as "tools to help health educators better understand what influences health—relevant individuals, group, and institutional behaviors—and to thereupon plan effective interventions directed at health-beneficial results" (p. 298).

Nutbeam and Harris (1999) have stated that a fully developed theory would be characterized by three major elements: "It would explain:

- the major factors that influence the phenomena of interest, for example those factors which explain why some people are regularly active and others are not;

- the relationship between these factors, for example the relationship between knowledge, beliefs, social norms and behaviours [sic] such as physical activity; and

- the conditions under which these relationships do or do not occur: the how, when, and why of hypothesised [sic] relationships, for example, the time, place and circumstances which, predictably lead to a person being active or inactive" (p. 10).

In comparison, a **model** is a subclass of a theory. Models "are generalized, hypothetical descriptions, often based on an analogy, used to analyze or explain something" (Glanz & Rimer, 1995, p. 11). "Models draw on a number of theories to help understand a specific problem in a particular setting or content. They are not always as specific as theory" (Rimer & Glanz, 2005, p. 4). Unlike theories, models do "not attempt to explain the processes underlying learning, but only to represent them" (Chaplin & Krawiec, 1979, p. 68).

Though we just went to some effort to make a distinction between the words *theory* and *model*, when discussing the terms' theory-based endeavors (i.e., *theory-based health education/promotion practice* and *theory-based research*), it is commonly understood in our profession that the word theory is used in a general way to mean either a theory *or* model. Thus as we use the terms *theory* and *theory-based* through-out the remainder of this book, we use them to be inclusive of endeavors based on ei-ther a theory *or* a model.

Concepts are the primary elements or building blocks of a theory (Glanz et al., 2002b). When a concept has been developed, created, or adopted for use with a specific theory, it is referred to as a **construct** (Kerlinger, 1986). "The key concepts of a theory are its constructs" (Rimer & Glanz, 2005, p. 4). The operational (practical use) form of a construct is known as a **variable.** Variables "specify how a construct is to be measured in a specific situation" (Glanz et al., 2002b, p. 27). Thus, variables need to be matched "to constructs when identifying what needs to be assessed during evaluation of a theory-driven program" (Rimer & Glanz, 2005, p. 4).

> Now consider how these terms are used in practical application. A personal belief is a *concept* that has been shown to relate to various health behaviors. Using a *theory* that includes the concept of personal beliefs helps explain why people fear being trapped in a burning vehicle if they use their safety belts. This personal belief of fear acts as a per-ceived barrier to safety belt use. Perceived barrier is a part of a specific theory and is re-ferred to here as a *construct*. If a health educator develops a program around a theory to help people overcome this barrier and wear their safety belts, then safety belt use is the *variable* being studied. The health educator realizes that this theory, which empha-sizes personal beliefs, will not explain all the reasons why people do not wear safety belts. Thus other theories, which emphasize other concepts (i.e., knowledge, environ-ment, incentives, comfort, convenience, etc.) need to be considered.
>
> Eventually, all of these theories may be combined into a *model* that will explain, at least in part, why people wear safety belts. If a model were a perfect model, it would predict with 100 percent accuracy who would wear safety belts. Unfortunately, behav-ior is very complex and there are no perfect models in health education. It is therefore important for health educators to keep revising their models to improve their under-standing of health behavior. (Cottrell et al., 2009, p. 104).

Based on these descriptions, it seems logical to think of theories as the backbone of the processes used to plan, implement, and evaluate health promotion interventions. "A theory-based approach provides direction and justification for program activities and serves as a basis for processes that are to be incorporated into the health promotion pro-gram" (Cowdery et al., 1995, p. 248). For example, developmental theories can be used to ensure that the goals and objectives of programs are consistent with the participants' developmental stages and abilities. Theories also can guide program planners in select-ing the types of interventions that are needed to accomplish the stated goals and objec-tives. Appropriate use of learning and behavioral theories can help to ensure congruence between the planned interventions and expected outcomes. Stated a bit differently, "Theories can provide answers to program developers' questions regarding *why* people aren't already engaging in a desirable behavior of interest, *how* to go about changing their behaviors, and *what* factors to look at when evaluating a program's focus" (van Ryn & Heaney, 1992, p. 326). In addition, theoretical frameworks can alert planners to consider important influences outside the teaching-learning process, such as social and physical environments, that have an impact on targeted program outcomes (Parcel, 1983; Rimer & Glanz, 2005).

All health promotion interventions should be planned based upon proven theories. "Theory is not a substitute for professional judgment, but it can assist health educators in professional decision making. Insofar as the application of theory to practice strengthens program justification, promotes the effective and efficient use of resources, and improves accountability, it also assists in establishing professional credibility" (D'Onofrio, 1992, p. 394). However, this is not to say that a theory cannot be modified or expanded to include a logically valid idea or parts of other theories. "In fact, it is well understood that working with a theory has certain disadvantages; one of which is leaving out or ignoring factors that happen not to be theoretically relevant, even though they may be empirically significant" (Jessor & Jessor, 1977).

"Using theory as a foundation for program planning and development is consistent with the current emphasis on using evidence-based interventions in public health, behavioral medicine, and medicine" (Rimer & Glanz, 2005, p. 5). Getting people to engage in health behavior change is a complicated process that is very difficult under the best of conditions. Without the direction that theories provide, planners can easily waste valuable resources in trying to achieve the desired behavior change. Therefore, program planners should ground their planning process in the theories that have been the foundation of other successful health promotion efforts.

There are many theories that health educators could use to plan programs. "No single theory or conceptual framework dominates research or practice in health promotion and education today" (Glanz et al., 2002b, p. 30). Glanz, Lewis, and Rimer (1996) identified 66 theories and models that had been used in health promotion practice. We have no intention of introducing all of them. However, approximately 10 theories and models are used regularly to plan programs. The remaining sections of this chapter and Chapter 9 present an overview of the theories that are most often used in creating health promotion interventions. As you read about and study the various theories, you will find that some express the same general ideas, but employ "a unique vocabulary to articulate the specific factors considered to be important" (Glanz et al., 2002b, p. 26). Also, be aware that the presentation of theories that follows is by no means comprehensive in nature. For those readers who would like to examine these and other theories in more depth, we would recommend two books: *Health Behavior and Health Education: Theory, Research and Practice* (Glanz, Rimer, & Lewis, 2002a) and *Emerging Theories in Health Promotion Practice and Research: Strategies for Improving Public Health* (DiClemente, Crosby, & Kegler, 2002). **Box 7.1** identifies the responsibilities and competencies for health educators that pertain to the material presented in this chapter.

Types of Theories and Models

There are several ways of categorizing the theories and models associated with health education/promotion practice. One way of doing so is to divide them into two groups. The first group includes those theories and models used for planning, implementing, and evaluating health promotion programs. This group has been called **planning models** (or *theories/models of implementation*). The planning models were presented in Chapter 2. The second group is referred to as **behavior change theories** (or *change process theories*). Behavior change theories "specify the relationships among causal processes operating

> **Box 7.1** RESPONSIBILITIES AND COMPETENCIES FOR HEALTH EDUCATORS
>
> The content of Chapter 7 focuses on theories and models used in the practice of health promotion. Specifically, theories and models provide a "road map" for planners to use when creating interventions and evaluating the effectiveness of those interventions. The responsibilities and competencies related to these tasks include:
>
> Responsibility II: Plan Health Education Strategies, Interventions, and Programs
>
> Competency E: Design strategies, interventions, and programs consistent with specified objectives
>
> Responsibility IV: Conduct Evaluation and Research Related to Health Education
>
> Competency C: Design data collection instruments
>
> *Source*: NCHEC, SOPHE, & AAHE (2006).

both within and across levels of analysis" (McLeroy, Steckler, Goodman, & Burdine, 1992, p. 3). In other words, they help explain how change takes place.

Behavior Change Theories

As noted earlier, there are many behavior change theories that health educators could use to plan programs. Because of the peculiarities of the theories and multitude of factors that could impact a specific planning situation, some theories work better in some situations than others. Before we present the theories focusing on behavior change, it is important to introduce the concept of level of ecological perspective.

The **ecological perspective** is a multilevel, interactive approach to examining the influences on health-related behaviors and conditions (Cottrell et al., 2009). "The ecological perspective emphasizes the interaction between, and the interdependence of factors within and across all levels of a health problem" (Rimer & Glanz, 2005, p. 10). In other words, the ecological perspective recognizes that health-related behaviors and conditions are a part of a larger system and can be approached from multiple levels. McLeroy, Bibeau, Steckler, and Glanz (1988) identified five levels of influence: (1) intrapersonal or individual factors, (2) interpersonal factors, (3) institutional or organizational factors, (4) community factors, and (5) public policy factors. **Table 7.1** presents and defines each of the five levels, while **Box 7.2** provides an example of how the five levels can impact health behavior.

Because of the underlying concepts that are captured in the constructs of individual theories, certain theories are more useful in developing programs aimed at specific levels of influence. For example, some theories were developed to help explain behavior change in individuals, while others were developed to help explain change at the community level. Though there are five distinct levels of influence, for the purposes of program planning the five levels are often condensed to three—intrapersonal, interpersonal, and community (Glanz & Rimer, 1995; Rimer & Glanz, 2005). "In practice, addressing

Table 7.1   An ecological perspective: levels of prevention

Concept	Definition
Intrapersonal Level	Individual characteristics that influence behavior, such as knowledge, attitudes, beliefs, and personality traits
Interpersonal Level	Interpersonal processes and primary groups, including family, friends, and peers that provide social identity, support, and role definition
Community Level	
Institutional Factors	Rules, regulations, policies, and informal structures, which may constrain or promote recommended behaviors
Community Factors	Social networks and norms, or standards, that exist as formal or informal among individuals, groups, and organizations
Public Policy	Local, state, and federal policies and laws that regulate or support healthy actions and practices for disease prevention, early detection, control, and management

Source: Rimer and Glanz (2005, p. 11).

Box 7.2   APPLICATION OF THE ECOLOGICAL PERSPECTIVE

A good example of the use of the ecological perspective is the comprehensive approach used to reduce cigarette smoking in the United States. At the *intrapersonal* (or *individual*) *level*, a large majority of smokers know that smoking is bad for them and a slightly smaller majority have indicated they would like to quit. Many have tried—some have tried on many occasions. At the *interpersonal level*, many smokers are encouraged by their physician and/or family and friends to quit. Some smokers may attempt to quit on their own or join a formal smoking cessation group to try to quit. At the *institutional* (or *organizational*) *level*, a number of institutions (e.g., churches and worksites) have developed policies that prohibit smoking in and/or on institution property (i.e., buildings and grounds). At the *community level*, a number of towns, cities, and counties have passed ordinances that prohibit smoking in public places. And at the *public policy level*, a number of states have passed clean indoor air acts that limit smoking, and have passed laws increasing the tax on a package of cigarettes. Also at this level, the U.S. government has spent many dollars for public service announcements (PSAs) and other forms of media advertising the dangers of tobacco use. Attacking the smoking problem from all levels has contributed to the decrease in the percentage of smokers in the United States.

---

the community level requires taking into consideration institutional and public policy factors, as well as social networks and norms" (Rimer & Glanz, 2005, p. 11). To assist program planners with matching theories appropriate to level of influence, we have presented our discussion of the theories according to the level of influence at which they are most useful.

In addition to theories being placed into a level of influence at which they may be most useful, theories can also be categorized by the approach—continuum or stage theories—they use to explain behavior. The approach of a **continuum theory**

is to identify variables that influence action (such as perceptions of risk and precaution effectiveness) and to combine them in a prediction equation. When applied to a particular individual, the value generated by the equation indicates the probability that this person will act. Thus, each person is placed along a continuum of action of likelihood. Because each theory has only a single prediction equation, the way in which variables combine to influence action is expected to be the same for everyone (Weinstein, Rothman, & Sutton, 1998, p. 291).

A **stage theory** is one that is comprised of an ordered set of categories into which people can be classified, and which identifies factors that could induce movement from one category to the next (Weinstein & Sandman, 2002b). More specifically, stage theories have four principal elements (Weinstein & Sandman, 2002a): (1) a category system to define the stages, (2) an ordering of stages, (3) common barriers to change that people face in the same stage, and (4) different barriers to change that people face in different stages. **Table 7.2** lists the theories presented in this book by level of influence and theory approach.

Table 7.2   Theories by level of influence and category

Level of Influence	Chapter Where Found in This Book
• Intrapersonal Level	
Continuum Theory	
Stimulus Response Theory	Chapter 7
Theory of Reasoned Action	Chapter 7
Theory of Planned Behavior	Chapter 7
Theory of Freeing	Chapter 7
Health Belief Model	Chapter 7
Elaboration Likelihood Model of Persuasion	Chapter 7
Stage Theory	
Transtheoretical Model	Chapter 7
Precaution Adoption Process Model	Chapter 7
Health Action Process Approach	Chapter 7
• Interpersonal Level	
Continuum Theory	
Social Cognitive Theory	Chapter 7
• Community Level	
Continuum Theory	
Communication Theory	Chapters 8 & 11
Community Organizing	Chapter 9
Community Building	Chapter 9
Diffusion of Innovations	Chapter 11
Stage Theory	
Community Readiness Model	Chapter 7

Intrapersonal Level Theories

The intrapersonal or "individual level is the most basic one in health promotion practice, so planners must be able to explain and influence the behavior of individuals" (Rimer & Glanz, 2005, p. 12). Intrapersonal theories focus on factors within the individual such as knowledge, attitudes, beliefs, self-concept, mental history, past experiences, motivation, skills, and behavior (Glanz & Rimer, 1995). Because much of the work of health educators takes place at this level of influence, a number of theories could be used. They are discussed below.

Stimulus Response (SR) Theory   One of the theories used to explain and modify behavior is the stimulus response, or SR, theory (Thorndike, 1898; Watson, 1925; Hall, 1943). This theory reflects the combination of classical conditioning (Pavlov, 1927) and instrumental conditioning (Thorndike, 1898) theories. These early conditioning theories explain learning based on the associations among stimulus, response, and reinforcement (Parcel & Baranowski, 1981; Parcel, 1983). "In simplest terms, the SR theorists believe that learning results from events (termed 'reinforcements') which reduce physiological drives that activate behavior" (Rosenstock, Strecher, & Becker, 1988, p. 175). The behaviorist B. F. Skinner believed that the frequency of a behavior was determined by the reinforcements that followed that behavior.

In Skinner's view, the mere temporal association between a behavior and an immediately following reward is sufficient to increase the probability that the behavior will be repeated. Such behaviors are called *operants;* they operate on the environment to bring about changes resulting in reward or reinforcement (Rosenstock et al., 1988, p. 176). Stated another way, operant behaviors are behaviors that act on the environment to produce consequences. These consequences, in turn, either reinforce or do not reinforce the behavior that preceded.

There are two broad categories of environmental consequences: **reinforcement** or **punishment** (McDade-Montez, Cvengros, & Christensen, 2005): Individuals can learn from both. Reinforcement has been defined by Skinner (1953) as any event that follows a behavior, which in turn increases the probability that the same behavior will be repeated in the future. Stated differently, reinforcement has "a *strengthening effect* that occurs when operant behaviors have certain consequences" (Nye, 1992, p. 16). Behavior has a greater probability of occurring in the future (1) if reinforcement is frequent and (2) if reinforcement is provided soon after the desired behavior. This immediacy clarifies the relationship between the reinforcement and appropriate behavior (Skinner, 1953). If a behavior is complex in nature, smaller steps working toward the desired behavior with appropriate reinforcement will help to shape the desired behavior. This was found to be true in getting pigeons to play Ping-Pong, and it can be useful in trying to change a complex health behavior like smoking or exercise. While reinforcement will increase the frequency of a behavior, punishment will decrease the frequency of a behavior. However, both reinforcement and punishment can be either positive or negative. The terms *positive* and *negative* in this context do not mean good and bad; rather, *positive* means adding something (effects of the stimulus) to a situation, whereas *negative* means taking something away (removal or reduction of the effects of the stimulus) from the situation.

If individuals act in a certain way to produce a consequence that makes them feel good or that is enjoyable, it is labeled **positive reinforcement** (or *reward*). Examples of this would be an individual who is involved in an exercise program and "feels good" at the end of the workout, or one who participates in a weight loss program and receives verbal encouragement from the facilitator, again making that person "feel good." Stimulus response theorists would note that in both of these situations, the pleasant experiences (internal feelings and verbal encouragement, respectively) occur right after the behavior, which in turn increases the chances that the frequency of the behavior will increase.

While positive reinforcement helps individuals learn by shaping behavior, behavior that avoids punishment is also learned because it reduces the tension that precedes the punishment (Rosenstock et al., 1988). "When this happens, we are being conditioned by *negative reinforcement:* A response is strengthened by the *removal* of something from the situation. In such cases, the 'something' that is removed is referred to as a *negative reinforcer* or *aversive stimulus* (these two phrases are synonymous)" (Nye, 1979, p. 33). A good example of **negative reinforcement** is a weight loss program that requires weekly dues. When participants stop paying dues because they have met their goal weight, this removal of an obligation should increase the frequency of the desired behavior (weight maintenance). Or in the case of exercise, "negative reinforcements would include decreased poor self-image and decreased fatigue" (McDade-Montez et al., 2005, p. 64).

Some people think of negative reinforcement as a form of punishment, but it is not. While negative reinforcement increases the likelihood that a behavior will be repeated, punishment typically suppresses behavior. "Skinner suggests two ways in which a response can be punished: by *removing a positive reinforcer* or by *presenting a negative reinforcer* (aversive stimulus) as a consequence of the response" (Nye, 1979, p. 43). Punishment is usually linked to some uncomfortable (physical, mental, or otherwise) experience and decreases the frequency of a behavior. An aversive smoking cessation program that circulates cigarette smoke around those enrolled in the program as they smoke is an example of **positive punishment.** It decreases the frequency of smoking by presenting (adding) a negative reinforcer or **aversive stimulus** (smoke) as a consequence of the response. Examples of **negative punishment** (removing a positive reinforcer) would include not allowing employees to use the employees' lounge if they continue to smoke while using it, or reducing the health insurance benefits of employees who continue to participate in health-harming behavior such as not wearing a safety belt. Stimulus response theorists would note that taking away the privilege of using the employees' lounge or reducing health insurance benefits would decrease the frequency of smoking among the employees and increase the wearing of safety belts, respectively. **Figure 7.1** illustrates the relationship between reinforcement and punishment.

Finally, if reinforcement is withheld—or, stating it another way, if the behavior is ignored—the behavior will become less frequent and eventually will not be repeated. Skinner (1953) refers to this as extinction. Teachers frequently use this technique with disruptive children in the classroom. If a child is acting up in class, the teacher may choose to ignore the behavior in hopes that the nonreinforced behavior will go away.

Theory of Reasoned Action (TRA) Another theory that has received considerable attention in the literature of health behavior change is Fishbein's *theory of reasoned action (TRA)* (Fishbein 1967). This theory was developed to explain not just health behavior but all

		Consequences	
		Positive (adding to)	Negative (taking away)
Behavior	Increase in frequency	Positive reinforcement (reward)	Negative reinforcement
	Decrease in frequency	Positive punishment	Negative punishment

Figure 7.1 2 X 2 table of the stimulus response theory

volitional behaviors "that is, behaviors that can be performed at will" (Luszczynska & Sutton, 2005, p. 73). While the stimulus response theory discussed earlier in this chapter was concerned with behavior; however, this one provides a framework to study attitudes toward behaviors.

Fishbein and Ajzen (1975) distinguish among *attitude, belief, intention,* and *behavior,* and they present a conceptual framework for the study of the relationship among these four constructs. **Intention** "is an indication of a person's readiness to perform a given behavior, and it is considered to be an immediate antecedent of behavior" (Ajzen, 2006). According to this theory, individuals' intention to perform given behaviors are functions of their *attitudes* toward the behavior and their *subjective norms* associated with the behaviors. **Attitude toward the behavior** "is the degree to which performance of the behavior is positively or negatively valued. According to the expectancy-value model, attitude toward a behavior is determined by the total set of accessible behavioral beliefs linking the behavior to various outcomes and other attributes" (Ajzen, 2006). Thus a person who has strong beliefs about positive attributes or outcomes from performing the behavior will have a positive attitude toward behavior (Montano & Kasprzyk, 2002). For example, if a person feels strongly about exercise being able to help control weight, then that person will have a positive attitude toward exercise. The converse is true as well. Weak beliefs about the outcomes or attributes of exercise will produce a negative attitude toward it.

Subjective norm "is the perceived social pressure to engage or not engage in a behavior" (Ajzen, 2006). For many health behaviors, the social pressure comes from a person's peers, parents, partner, close friends, teachers, role models, boss, and co-workers, as well as experts or professionals like physicians or lawyers. Thus individuals who believe that certain people think they should perform a behavior and are motivated to meet the people's expectations will hold a positive subjective norm (Montano & Kasprzyk, 2002). Similar to behavioral beliefs, the converse is also true. An example of a positive subjective norm are employees who see their co-workers as important people in their lives and believe that these people approve of them participating in a company exercise program.

Theory of Planned Behavior (TPB)   The theory of reasoned action has proved to be most successful when dealing with purely volitional behaviors, but complications are encountered when the theory is applied to behaviors that are not fully under volitional control. A good example of this is a smoker who intends to quit but fails to do so. Even though intent is high, nonmotivational factors—such as lack of requisite opportunities, skills, and resources—could prevent success (Ajzen, 1988).

The *theory of planned behavior (TPB)* (see **Figure 7.2**) is an extension of the theory of reasoned action that addresses the problem of incomplete volitional control. The major difference between TPB and TRA is the addition of a third, conceptually independent determinant of intention. Like TRA, TPB includes attitude toward the behavior and subjective norm, but it has added the concept of perceived behavioral control. Perceived behavioral control is similar to the SCT's concept of self-efficacy. **Perceived behavioral control** "refers to people's perceptions of their ability to perform a given behavior" (Ajzen, 2006). Stated differently, perceived behavioral control refers to the perceived ease or difficulty of performing the behavior and is assumed to reflect past experience as well as anticipated impediments and obstacles. As a general rule, the more favorable the attitude and subjective norm with respect to a behavior, and the greater the perceived behavioral control, the stronger should be the individual's intentions to perform the behavior under consideration (Ajzen, 1988).

Figure 7.2 illustrates two important features of this theory. First, perceived behavioral control has motivational implications for intentions. That is, without perceived control, intentions could be minimal even if attitudes toward the behavior and subjective norm were strong. Second, there may be a direct link between perceived behavioral control and behavior. Behavior depends not only on motivation but also on actual control. *Actual behavioral control* "refers to the extent to which a person has the skills, resources, and other prerequisites needed to perform a given behavior. Successful performance of the behavior depends not only on a favorable intention but also on a sufficient level of behavioral control. To the extent that perceived behavioral control is accurate, it can serve as a proxy of actual control and can be used for the prediction of behavior" (Ajzen,

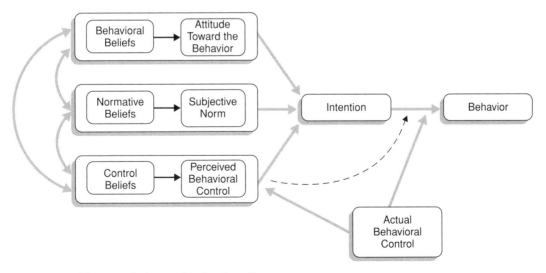

Figure 7.2 Theory of planned behavior diagram
Source: © 2007 Icek Aizen. Used with permission.

2006). To use the example of smoking once again as a behavior not fully under volitional control, TPB predicts that individuals will give up smoking if they:

1. Have a positive attitude toward quitting

2. Think others whom they value believe it would be good for them to quit

3. Perceive that they have control over whether they quit

Evidence to support the usefulness of the TPB to explain a variety of health behaviors seems to be mounting (Armitage & Conner, 1999; Godin & Kok, 1996; Montano, Kasprzyk, von Haeften, & Fishbein, 2001; Montano, Phillips, & Kasprzyk, 2000; and Montano, Thompson, Taylor, & Mahloch, 1997). Godin and Kok (1996) presented a review of 58 studies where the theory was applied to health-related behaviors. They found that the efficiency of the theory seemed "to be quite good for explaining intention, perceived behavioral control being as important as attitude across behavioral categories. The efficiency of the theory, however, varied between health-related behavior categories" (Godin & Kok, 1996, p. 87).

Theory of Freeing (TF)   A theory that takes a much different approach from the other theories presented is the theory of freeing (TF) (Freire, 1973, 1974). Like the others, it is not specific to health promotion, but does have application to health promotion. It is a theory aimed at empowering education. Wallerstein and Bernstein (1988, p. 380) define *empowerment* as "a social action process that promotes participation of people, organizations, and communities in gaining control over their lives in their community and larger society. With this perspective, empowerment is not characterized as achieving power to dominate others, but rather power to act with others to effect change."

The theory was first used in the late 1950s when the late Paulo Freire, a Brazilian educator, initiated a successful literacy and political consciousness program for shantytown dwellers and peasants in Brazil (Freire, 1973). Since that time, the theory has been applied to many other problems.

One of the first to apply this theory to health promotion was Greenberg. He stated (1978, p. 20) that the task of health education should be to "free people so they may make health-related decisions based upon their needs and interests as long as these needs and interests do not adversely affect others." In essence, Freire's concept of freeing contrasts "being free with being oppressed" (Walker & Bibeau, 1985/1986, p. 5). People become free by being critically conscious.

The underlying concept of this theory is that critical consciousness is determined by the interaction with culture. Consciousness is influenced by and influences the culture. Oppressed people are "of the world," and their consciousness is a product of the culture. Being "of the world" is defined by the lack of the person's ability to perceive, respond, and act with power to change concrete reality (Walker & Bibeau, 1985/1986). Free people are "in the world," and their consciousness is a producer of culture.

Education is the key to becoming critically conscious. However, the education that is meant here is not education in the traditional sense. Education occurs through dialogue, not through lecture. People who use dialogue are teachers, whereas those who just talk are lecturers. And in this type of education, participants replace pupils. All those involved in the educational process learn from one another.

A very useful summary of the applications of Freire's work to health promotion has been presented by Wallerstein and Bernstein (1988) and Wallerstein (1994). They state that Freire's theory includes three stages. Stage 1 is the listening stage, in which those in the priority population have the opportunity to share their thoughts, identify the problems, and set the priorities. Unlike in a more traditional planning process, the program planners do not collect data and determine the needs. Instead, the priority population is identifying the issues and prioritizing the needs.

Stage 2 is a dialogue process. The dialogue revolves around a *code*. "A 'code' is a concrete physical representation of an identified community issue in any form: role plays, stories, slides, photographs, songs, etc." (Wallerstein & Bernstein, 1988, p. 383). After experiencing a code, group facilitators lead the priority population through a discussion that helps the people move from a personal to a social analysis and action level. They do this by asking the priority population to respond to these five statements (Wallerstein & Bernstein, 1988):

1. Describe what you see and feel.

2. As a group, define the many levels of the problem.

3. Share similar experiences from your lives.

4. Question why this problem exists.

5. Develop action plans to address the problem.

Stage 3 of this theory is the action stage, in which those in the priority population try out the plans that came from the listening and dialogue stages. As the people put their plans into action, they reflect on their new experiences and create a thinking-acting cycle. "This recurrent spiral of action-reflection-action enables people to learn from their collective attempts at change and to become more deeply involved to surmount the cultural, social, or historic barriers" (Wallerstein & Bernstein, 1988, p. 383).

Health Belief Model (HBM)   The **health belief model (HBM)**, which is the one most frequently used in health behavior applications, is also a value-expectancy theory. It was developed in the 1950s by a group of psychologists to help explain why people would or would not use health services (Rosenstock, 1966). The HBM is based on Lewin's decision-making model (Lewin, 1935, 1936; Lewin et al., 1944). Since its creation, the HBM has been used to help explain a variety of health behaviors (Becker, 1974; Janz & Becker, 1984).

The HBM hypothesizes that health-related action depends on the simultaneous occurrence of three classes of factors:

1. The existence of sufficient motivation (or health concern) to make health issues salient or relevant.

2. The belief that one is susceptible (vulnerable) to a serious health problem or to the sequelae of that illness or condition. This is often termed **perceived threat**.

3. The belief that following a particular health recommendation would be beneficial in reducing the perceived threat, and at a subjectively acceptable cost. Cost refers to the **perceived barriers** that must be overcome in order to follow the health recommendation; it includes, but is not restricted to, financial outlays (Rosenstock et al., 1988, p. 177). In fact, the lack of self-efficacy is also seen as a perceived barrier to taking a recommended health action (Strecher & Rosenstock, 1997).

Figure 7.3 provides a diagram of the HBM as presented by Becker, Drachman, and Kirscht (1974).

In recent years, self-efficacy has become a more meaningful concept in the perceived barriers construct of the HBM. When the HBM was first conceived, self-efficacy was not explicitly a part of it. "The original focus of the model was on circumscribed preventive actions, usually one-shot in nature, such as accepting a screening test or an immunization, actions that generally were simple behaviors to perform" (Janz, Champion, &

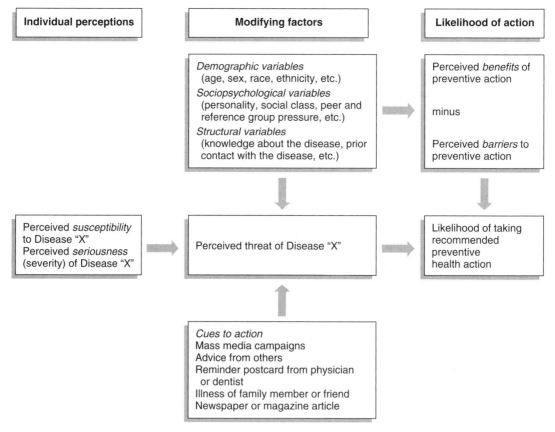

Figure 7.3 The HBM as a predictor of preventive health behavior

Source: M. H. Becker et al., "A New Approach to Explaining Sick-Role Behavior in Low Income Populations," *American Journal of Public Health, 64* (March 1974): 205–216. Copyright © 1974 by the American Public Health Association. Reprinted by permission.

Strecher, 2002, p. 50) and ones for which most people in the priority populations had adequate self-efficacy (Janz et al., 2002). However, when program planners want to use the HBM to plan health promotion interventions for priority populations in need of lifestyle behaviors requiring long-term changes, self-efficacy must be included in the model. "For behavior change to succeed, people must (as the original HBM theorizes) feel threatened by their current behavioral patterns (perceived susceptibility and severity) and believe that change of a specific kind will result in a valued outcome at acceptable cost. They must also feel themselves competent (self-efficacious) to overcome perceived barriers to taking action" (Janz et al., 2002, p. 51).

Here is an example of the HBM applied to exercise. Someone watching television sees an advertisement about exercise. This is a cue to action that starts her thinking about her own need to exercise. There may be some variables (demographic, sociopsychological, and structural) that cause her to think about it a bit more. She remembers her college health course that included information about heart disease and the importance of staying active. She knows she has a higher than normal risk for heart disease because of family history, poor diet, and slightly elevated blood pressure. Therefore, she comes to the conclusion that she is susceptible to heart disease (**perceived susceptibility**). She also knows that if she develops heart disease, it can be very serious (**perceived seriousness/severity**). Based on these factors, the individual thinks that there is reason to be concerned about heart disease (perceived threat). She knows that exercise can help delay the onset of heart disease and can increase the chances of surviving a heart attack if one should occur (**perceived benefits**). But exercise takes time from an already busy day, and it is not easy to exercise in the variety of settings in which she typically finds herself, especially during bad weather (perceived barriers). Her confidence in being able to exercise regularly will also be important. She must now weigh the threat of the disease against the difference between benefits and barriers. This decision will then result in a likelihood of exercising or not exercising (**likelihood of taking recommended preventive health action**).

The Elaboration Likelihood Model of Persuasion (ELM)   The Elaboration Likelihood Model of Persuasion, or Elaboration Likelihood Model (ELM) for short, was initially developed to help explain inconsistencies in the results from research dealing with the study of attitudes (Petty, Barden, & Wheeler, 2002). Specifically, the model was designed to help explain how persuasion messages (communications), aimed at changing attitudes, were received and processed by people. "Although the model has a rich history in the field of psychology, its application to health promotion is newly emerging" (Crosby, Kegler, & DiClemente, 2002, p. 9). Since its development, the framework has been found useful for interpreting and predicting the impact that health messages (communications) have on subsequent attitudes and behavior (Petty et al., 2002).

Before we continue with our explanation of this model, it is necessary to define what is meant by the term elaboration. **Elaboration** refers to the amount of effortful processing people put into receiving messages. By effortful processing, we mean careful cognitive consideration of the message, or stated another way "careful thinking about" the message. With that definition out of the way, let's examine the three major elements of this model (see **Figure 7.4**).

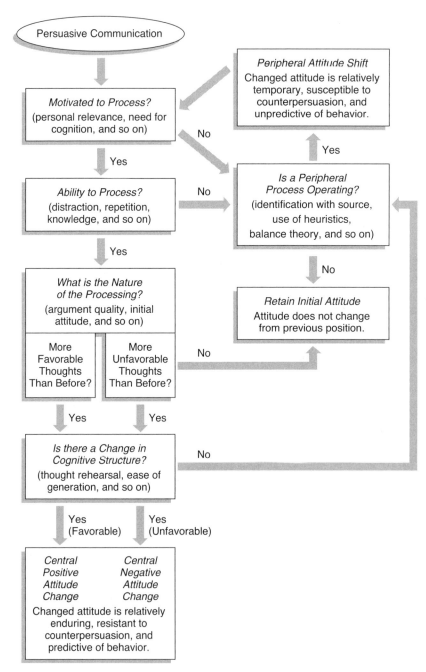

Figure 7.4 The elaboration likelihood model of persuasion

Source: From Petty et al., *Emerging Theories in Healthy Promotion Practice & Research*. Copyright © 2002 John Wiley & Sons. Used with permission.

First, the ELM organizes multiple persuasion processes into two routes of attitude change: *peripheral* and *central*. The peripheral processes are those that require little thought about issue-relevant information and instead rely on simple cues or mental shortcuts, called *heuristics,* as the primary means of attitude change (Petty et al., 2002). For example, a person may form an attitude after hearing a persuasive message simply because the person delivering the message is recognized as an expert in the field, such as when the Surgeon General makes a statement about a certain health behavior. Or, a person may form an attitude based solely on hearing the same message over and over. On the other hand, the central processes are those that require thoughtful consideration of issue-relevant information and its relationship to pertinent knowledge that one already has to form the primary bases for attitude change (Petty et al., 2002). "Two conditions are necessary for effortful processing to occur: the recipient of the message must be motivated and able to process it thoroughly" (Petty et al., 2002, p. 74). An example of central route processing would be a person's formation of an attitude about safety belt use based upon careful consideration of a message about the pros and cons of its use along with recalling the knowledge gained in drivers' education class and possibly the results of an automobile crash in which his/her cousin was involved.

It should be clear that the distinction between the peripheral and central routes is the amount of consideration given to the issue-relevant information and how the information is processed, not the type of information itself (Petty, Wheeler, & Bizer, 1999). Yet not all messages fall neatly into either peripheral or central categories of processing. People really receive messages along an *elaboration likelihood continuum*. The continuum stretches from one end anchored with processes requiring no thinking, like classical conditioning (see discussion of the Stimulus Response Theory earlier in this chapter), to processes requiring some effortful thinking such as making inferences based on one's experiences, to processes requiring careful consideration (Petty et al., 2002).

Second, when comparing the consequences of the two routes, research has shown that even though both routes "can sometimes result in attitudes with similar valence, the two processes typically lead to attitudes with different consequences" (Petty et al., 2002, p. 93). According to this model, the more effortful processing (or the more elaboration) people put into receiving messages, the more likely they are to form attitudes that are persistent over time, resistant to counterattack, and influential in guiding thought and behavior (Krosnick & Petty, 1995). Just the opposite is also true; the less elaboration, the less stable the attitude over time.

"Third, the model specifies how variables have an impact on persuasion" (Petty et al., 2002, p. 82). The variables can influence a person's motivation to think or ability to think, as well as the valence of one's thought or the confidence in the thoughts generated (Petty et al., 2002). Typical variables that have an influence on how persuasive messages are processed include the source of the message (i.e., Is the source credible? Is the source friendly? Is it coming from a friend, an authoritative figure, an expert?), the message itself (e.g., Is it understandable? Is it simple? Complex? Funny?), the context in which the message is presented (e.g., Is it delivered person-to-person? Where is the message received? Is the message coming by way of television or radio? Is the message being delivered to a group?), and the characteristics of the message recipient (e.g., How intelligent is the recipient? How attentive? In what mood is the recipient? How relevant is the topic to the recipient?) (Petty et al., 2002).

The ELM has been used to develop a variety of interventions for health promotion programs. The one area where the ELM has been most useful in health promotion has been with message tailoring. *Tailored messages* are those that are "crafted for and delivered to each individual based on individual needs, interests, and circumstances" (NCI, 2002, p. 251). In other words, tailored messages are matched to the needs, interests, and circumstances of the intended recipient. It has been found that the more tailored the persuasive communication, the more relevant it is to the recipient, and the more likely the message will be processed through the central route. And, if a message is processed through the central route the more likely it will impact attitude and behavior change.

For those readers who want more information on tailoring messages, please refer to the work of Kreuter, Farrell, Olevitch, & Brennan (2000).

The Transtheoretical Model (TTM)   "The Transtheoretical Model is an integrative framework for understanding how individuals and populations progress toward adopting and maintaining health behavior change for optimal health. The Transtheoretical Model uses stages of change to integrate processes and principles of change from across major theories of intervention, hence the name 'Transtheoretical'" (Prochaska, Johnson, & Lee, 1998, p. 59). The model has its roots in psychotherapy and was developed by Prochaska (1979) after he completed a comparative analysis of 18 therapy systems and a critical review of 300 therapy outcome studies. From the analysis and review, Prochaska found that some common processes were involved in change.

As this model has evolved, researchers have applied it to many different types of health behavior change, including but not limited to alcohol and substance abuse, anxiety and panic disorders, delinquency, eating disorders and obesity, exercise, high-fat diets, HIV/AIDS prevention, mammography screening, medication compliance, unplanned pregnancy prevention, pregnancy and smoking, sedentary lifestyles, sun exposure, and physicians practicing preventive medicine (Prochaska, Redding, & Evers, 2002; Spencer, Adams, Malone, Roy, & Yost, 2006).

The core constructs of the transtheoretical model include the stages of change, the processes of change, the pros and cons of changing, and self-efficacy (see **Table 7.3**). In addition, this model is "based on critical assumptions about the nature of behavior change and interventions that can best facilitate change" (Prochaska et al., 1998, p. 60). These constructs and assumptions will be discussed next.

Behavioral change does not occur overnight. A person does not go to bed at night as a nonexerciser and wake up the next morning as an exerciser. Behavior change occurs over a period of time. Thus the **stage** construct is an important part of the transtheoretical model because it represents the temporal dimension of change (Prochaska et al., 2002). The model suggests that "people move from *precontemplation*, not intending to change, to *contemplation*, intending to change within 6 months, to *preparation*, actively planning change, to *action*, overtly making changes, and into *maintenance*, taking steps to sustain change and resist temptation to relapse" (Prochaska, Redding, Harlow, Rossi, & Velicer, 1994). The **precontemplation stage** is defined as a time when "people are not intending to take action in the foreseeable future, usually measured as the next 6 months. People may be in this stage because they are uninformed or underinformed about the consequences of their behavior. Or they may have tried to change a number of times and become demoralized about their ability to change" (Prochaska,

Table 7.3 Transtheoretical model constructs

Constructs	Description
Stages of Change	
Precontemplation	No intention to take action within the next 6 months
Contemplation	Intends to take action within the next 6 months
Preparation	Intends to take action within the next 30 days and has taken some behavioral steps in this direction
Action	Has changed overt behavior for less than 6 months
Maintenance	Has changed overt behavior for more than 6 months
Decisional Balance	
Pros	The benefits of changing
Cons	The costs of changing
Self-Efficacy	
Confidence	Confidence that one can engage in the healthy behavior across different challenging situations
Temptation	Temptation to engage in the unhealthy behavior across different challenging situations
Processes of Change	
Consciousness Raising	Finding and learning new facts, ideas, and tips that support the healthy behavior change
Dramatic Relief	Experiencing the negative emotions (fear, anxiety, worry) that go with unhealthy behavioral risks
Self-Reevaluation	Realizing that the behavior change is an important part of one's identity as a person
Environmental Reevaluation	Realizing the negative impact of the unhealthy behavior, or the positive impact of the healthy behavior, on one's proximal social and/or physical environment
Self-Liberation	Making a firm commitment to change
Helping Relationships	Seeking and using social support for the healthy behavior change
Counterconditioning	Substitution of healthier alternative behaviors and/or cognitions for the unhealthy behavior
Reinforcement Management	Increasing the rewards for the positive behavior change and/or decreasing the rewards of the unhealthy behavior
Stimulus Control	Removing reminders or cues to engage in the unhealthy behavior and/or adding cues to reminders to engage in the healthy behavior
Social Liberation	Realizing that social norms are changing in the direction of supporting the healthy behavior change

Source: Redding et al., *SPM Handbook for Health Assessment Tools*. Copyright © 1999 The Society of Prospective Medicine. Used with permission.

2005, p. 111). People in this stage "tend to avoid reading, talking, or thinking about their high-risk behaviors" (Prochaska et al., 1998). The second stage, **contemplation** "is the stage in which people are intending to take action in the next six months" (Prochaska, 2005, p. 111). It occurs when people are aware that a problem exists and are seriously thinking about a behavior change but have not yet made a commitment to take action. They are more open to feedback and information about the problem behavior than those in the precontemplation stage (Redding et al., 1999). For example, most smokers know that smoking is bad for them and consider quitting, but are not quite ready to do so. The third stage is called **preparation** and combines intention and behavioral criteria. "Individuals in this stage are intending to take action in the next month and have unsuccessfully taken action in the past year" (Prochaska, DiClemente, & Norcross, 1992, p. 1104). In this stage, they may have taken some small steps toward action, such as buying the necessary clothes for exercising or cutting back on the fat grams they consume or the cigarettes they smoke, but they have not reached an effective criterion for effective action (Prochaska, Norcross, Fowler, Follick, & Abrams, 1992). "These are the people we should recruit for such action-oriented programs as smoking cessation, weight loss, or exercise" (Prochaska et al., 1998, p. 61).

People are in the fourth stage, the **action stage,** when they are overtly making changes in their behavior, experiences, or environment in order to overcome their problems. This stage of change reflects a consistent behavior pattern, is usually the most visible, and receives the greatest external recognition (Prochaska, DiClemente, & Norcross, 1992). Since the behavior change is very new in this stage and the chance of relapse is high, considerable attention still must be given to relapse prevention (Redding et al., 1999). Also, "not all modifications of behavior count as action in this model. People must attain a criterion that scientists and professionals agree is sufficient to reduce risks of disease" (Prochaska et al., 1998, p. 61). For example, in smoking, reduction in the number of cigarettes smoked does not count, only total abstinence (Prochaska et al., 1998). If those making changes continue with their new pattern of behavior, they will move into the fifth stage, maintenance.

Working to prevent relapse is the focus of the **maintenance stage.** People in this stage have changed their problem behavior for at least six months and are increasingly more confident that they can continue their changes (Prochaska et al., 1998; Redding et al., 1999). The person's change has become more of a habit and the chance of relapse is lower, but it still requires some attention (Redding et al., 1999).

The final stage is **termination.** This stage is defined as the time when individuals who have changed have zero temptation to return to their old behavior and they have 100% self-efficacy—that is, a lifetime of maintenance. No matter what their mood, they will not return to their old behavior (Prochaska et al., 1998). This is a stage that few people reach with certain behaviors (i.e., alcoholics). Since this may not be a practical goal for the majority of people, it has been given less attention in the research (Prochaska et al., 1998). **Figure 7.5** provides a summary of the stages of change.

The second major construct of the transtheoretical model is the **processes of change** (see Table 7.3 for an explanation of the 10 processes). "These are the covert and overt activities that people use to progress through the stages" (Prochaska et al., 1998, p. 62). Study over the years has indicated that some of the processes are more useful at specific stages of change. The experimental set of processes (consciousness raising, dramatic relief, self-reevaluation, environmental reevaluation, and social liberation) are most often emphasized in earlier stages (precontemplation, contemplation, and preparation) to increase intention and motivation, whereas the behavioral set of processes (helping relationships, counterconditioning, reinforcement management, stimulus control, and self-liberation) are most often utilized in the later stages (preparation, action, maintenance) as observable behavior change efforts get underway and need to be maintained (Redding et al., 1999) (see **Table 7.4**).

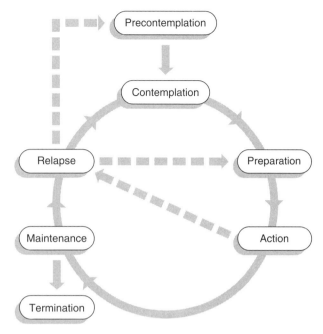

Figure 7.5 The stages of change

Source: M. G. Goldstein et al., "Models for Provider-Patient Interaction: Applications to Health Behavior Change," in S. A. Shumaker et al., *The Handbook of Health Behavior Change, 2/e.* Copyright © 1998.

Table 7.4   Stages of change in which processes are most emphasized

Stages of Changes				
Precontemplation	*Contemplation*	*Preparation*	*Action*	*Maintenance*
Consciousness raising				
Dramatic relief				
Environmental reevaluation				
	Self-reevaluation		Self-liberation	
			Contingency management	
			Helping relationships	
			Counterconditioning	
			Stimulus control	

Processes (row label to the left of the stages)

Source: M.G Goldstein et al., "Models for Provider-Patient Interaction: Applications to Health Behavior Change," in S.A. Shumaker et al., *The Handbook of Health Behavior Change, 2/e.* Copyright © 1998.

The construct of **decisional balance** refers to the pros and cons of the behavioral change. That is, individuals' decisions to move from one stage to the next is based on the relative importance (pro), or the lack thereof (con), of the behavior change for the individuals. "Characteristically, the pros of healthy behavior are low in the early stages and increase across the stages of change, and the cons of the healthy behavior are high in the early stages and decrease across the stages of change" (Redding et al., 1999, p. 90).

The final construct of the transtheoretical model is **self-efficacy.** The developers of this model see self-efficacy as it was defined by Bandura (1977b). As used in the TTM, Prochaska and colleagues (2002) break self-efficacy into two components: confidence and temptation. *Confidence* refers to the feelings of being able to engage in healthy behaviors across different challenging situations, while *temptation* refers to the situational temptation of those making change to engage in the unhealthy behavior. "Typically, three factors reflect the most common types of tempting situations: negative affect or emotional distress, positive social situations, and craving" (Prochaska et al., 2002, p. 103). As one might guess, temptation decreases as one moves through the stages; however, even in the maintenance stage temptation is still present.

As noted at the beginning of this discussion, the transtheoretical model not only includes the four core constructs but it is also based on five critical assumptions. The assumptions (Prochaska et al., 2002) include:

1. No single theory can account for all the complexities of behavior change. Therefore, a more comprehensive model will most likely emerge from an integration across major theories.

2. Behavior change is a process that unfolds over time through a sequence of stages.

3. Stages are both stable and open to change just as chronic behavioral risk factors are stable and open to change.

4. The majority of at-risk populations are not prepared for action and will not be served by traditional action-oriented prevention programs.

5. Specific processes and principles of change should be applied at specific stages if progress through the stages is to occur (p. 104).

Since its development, the transtheoretical model has been useful in several different ways. The first is that it makes program planners aware that not everyone is ready for change "right now," even though there is a program that can help them modify their behavior. People proceed through behavior change at different paces. Second, if individuals are not ready for action right now, then other programs can be developed to help them become ready for action. **Box 7.3** provides an example how to "stage" a person with a series of transtheoretical model type questions. With such information, planners can match a person's stage to a specific intervention, which in turn can increase the chances that the intervention will have an effect.

Precaution Adoption Process Model (PAPM)   The Precaution Adoption Process Model has been more recently developed than the transtheoretical model (TTM) (Weinstein, 1988; Weinstein & Sandman, 1992), and has been referred to as an *emerging theory* by DiClemente and colleagues (2002). Its goal "is to explain how a person comes to

---

Box 7.3 APPLICATION—AN EXAMPLE OF USING QUESTIONS BASED ON THE TRANSTHEORETICAL MODEL TO "STAGE" A PERSON

1. Do you eat at least five servings of fruits and vegetables each day?
Yes—Move to question #2
No—Skip to question #3

2. Have you been doing so for more than six months?
Yes—Maintenance stage
No—Action stage

3. Do you intend to in the next 30 days?
Yes—Preparation stage
No—Move to question #4

4. Do you intend to in the next six months?
Yes—Contemplation stage
No—Precontemplation stage

---

the decision to take action, and how he or she translates that decision into action" (Weinstein & Sandman, 2002a, p. 124). Though the TTM and PAPM are both stage models and appear similar, "it is mainly the names that have been given to the stages that are similar. The number of stages is not the same in the two theories, and those with similar names are defined quite differently" (Weinstein & Sandman, 2002a, p. 125). The PAPM is most applicable for use with the adoption of a new precaution, or the abandonment of a risky behavior that requires a deliberate action. It can also be used to explain why and how people make deliberate changes in habitual patterns. It is not applicable for actions that require the gradual development of habitual patterns of behavior such as exercise and diet (Weinstein & Sandman, 2002b). Weinstein and Sandman (2002a) report that PAPM has been successfully applied to osteoporosis prevention, mammography, hepatitis B vaccination, and home testing to detect radon gas.

The PAPM includes seven stages along the full path from ignorance to action (see **Figure 7.6**).

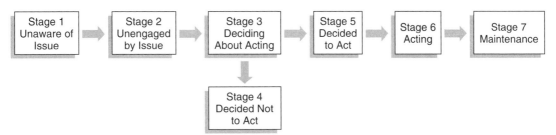

Figure 7.6 Stages of the precaution adoption process model

Source: From K. Glanz et al., *Health Behavior & Health Education, 3/e.* Copyright © 2002. Reprinted by permission of John Wiley & Sons, Inc.

At some initial point in time, people are unaware of the health issue (Stage 1) [Unaware]. When they first learn something about the issue, they are no longer unaware, but they are not necessarily engaged by it either (Stage 2) [Unengaged]. People who reach the decision-making stage (Stage 3) [Deciding about acting] have become engaged by the issue and are considering their response. This decision-making process can result in one of two outcomes. If the decision is to take no action, the precaution adoption process ends (Stage 4) [Decide not to act], at least for the time being. But if people decide to adopt the precaution (Stage 5) [Decide to act], the next step is to initiate the behavior (Stage 6) [Acting]. A seventh stage, if appropriate, indicates that the behavior has been maintained over time (Stage 7) [Maintenance] (Weinstein & Sandman, 2002b, p. 21. Note: names of the stages have been inserted by McKenzie, Neiger, & Thackeray).

Like with the TTM, the usefulness of this model is its ability to identify various stages of the behavior change process (see **Box 7.4**). Once it is known what stage the program participants are in, then the program planners can develop a stage-specific intervention to move the participants toward action. **Table 7.5** presents the important issues that need to be addressed to move participants from one stage to the next.

Health Action Process Approach (HAPA)   The Health Action Process Approach (HAPA) (Schwarzer, 2001) is a stage model that applies to all health-compromising and health-enhancing behaviors (Luszczynska & Sutton, 2005). Like the other stage theories discussed earlier in this chapter (i.e., Transtheoretical Model and the Precaution Adoption Process Model), this model provides a concise description of behavior change over time. The HAPA is divided into two distinct phases—motivation to change and self-regulatory processes—and five stages: intention, planning, initiative, maintenance, and recovery (see **Figure 7.7**).

The *motivation to change phase* includes the preintentional processes that lead to the development of behavioral intention (Luszczynska & Sutton, 2005). These processes revolve around the interaction of the variables of risk perception, outcome expectancies, and perceived self-efficacy. The motivation to change begins when people become aware that their actions are a threat to their health, that is *risk perception*. "People who are not aware at all of the risky nature of their actions will not develop the motivation to change them" (Schwazer, 2001, p. 48). Yet, perceiving a health threat is not enough

Box 7.4	Application—An example of using a question based on the Precaution Adoption Process Model to "stage" a person

What are your intentions for receiving the new vaccine for shingles?
a. I have already gotten it. (Stage 6)
b. I have decided to get it. (Stage 5)
c. I have thought about it and decided not to get it. (Stage 4)
d. I am not sure. I am still trying to decide whether to get it or not. (Stage 3)
e. I heard there was a vaccine, but I really haven't thought much about it. (Stage 2)
f. I was not aware there was a vaccine for shingles. (Stage 1)

Table 7.5   Issues likely to determine progress between stages of the PAPM

Stage Transition	Important Issues
Stage 1 to stage 2	• Media messages about the hazard and precaution
Stage 2 to stage 3	• Communication from significant other • Personal experience with hazard
Stage 3 to stage 4 or stage 5	• Beliefs about hazard likelihood and severity • Beliefs about personal susceptibility • Beliefs about precaution effectiveness and difficulty • Behaviors and recommendations of others • Perceived social norms • Fear and worry
Stage 5 to stage 6	• Time, effort, and resources needed to act • Detailed "how-to" information • Reminders and other cues to action • Assistance in carrying out action

Source: From K. Glanz et al., *Health Behavior & Health Education, 3/e.* Copyright © 2002. Reprinted by permission of John Wiley & Sons, Inc.

by itself to lead to intent to change. People "also need to understand the contingencies between their actions and subsequent outcomes. These *outcome expectations* are among the most influential beliefs in the motivation to change" (Schwarzer, 2001, p. 48). In addition to expecting certain results (outcomes) from a behavior change, people also

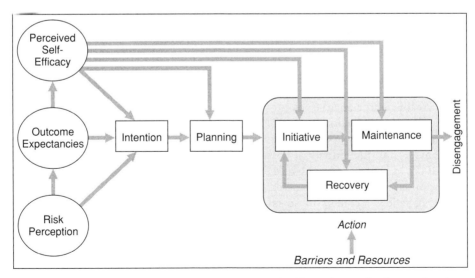

Figure 7.7 The health action process approach. The schematic shows the three predictors of behavioral change (in ovals) and the stages of change (in rectangles; the shaded rectangle highlights the action phase of behavioral change.

Source: R. Schwarzer, "Social Cognitive Factors in Changing Health-Related Behaviors" *Current Directions in Psychological Science*, 2001. Copyright © 2001. Used by permission of Blackwell Publishing.

have to possess beliefs that they are capable of engaging in the behavior change. Such beliefs are referred to as *perceived self-efficacy*. These beliefs are most important when "people approach novel or difficult situations or try to adopt strenuous self-regimes" (Schwarzer, 2001, p. 48). The stronger these beliefs, the greater the intention to change.

Though the motivation to change phase of HAPA is important, this model emphasizes the *self-regulatory phase* that leads to actual health behavior. "The pursuit of a goal of behavior change can be subdivided into a sequence of activities, such as planning, initiation, maintenance, relapse management, and disengagement" (Schwarzer, 2001, p. 48). Planning deals with determining the when, where, and how a behavior takes place. When that time takes place, people take the initiative to give the behavior a try. It is important at this stage that the people are self-efficacious with regard to the behavior. Trying behavior change is one thing, but maintaining it takes much work. Schwarzer (2001) states that:

> A health-related behavior is adopted and then maintained not through an act of will, but rather through the development of self-regulatory skills and strategies. In other words, individuals embrace a variety of means to influence their own motivation and behaviors. For example, they set attainable sub-goals, create incentives for themselves, draw from an array of options for coping with difficulties, and mobilize support from other people (p. 49).

Maintaining a behavior is difficult and many people lapse or relapse back to their old health-compromising behavior. When this occurs people need competent *relapse management* to recover from the setbacks (Schwarzer, 2001). That is, they need additional skills and strategies to deal with these slips. It may mean scaling back on the original behavior change goal and trying again. If they do not have the skills and strategies needed to deal with the relapse, they may not recover and thus disengage from the change all together. The real keys to the self-regulatory phase are successful completion of the previous stage and the optimistic sense of control over the next one (Schwarzer, 2001).

Interpersonal Level Theories

"At the interpersonal level, theories of health behavior assume individuals exist within, and are influenced by, a social environment. The opinions, thoughts, behavior, advice, and support of the people surrounding an individual influence his or her feelings and behavior, and the individual has a reciprocal effect on those people" (Rimer & Glanz, 2005, p. 19). Those individuals who have the greatest influence on others include spouse/partner, other family members, friends, peers (i.e., fellow students and coworkers), fellow members of social groups, health care providers, religious leaders, and others (Rimer & Glanz, 2005). There are a number of different interpersonal theories including those dealing with social learning, social power, interpersonal communication, social support, and social networks. This section presents a detailed description of the one interpersonal theory that has dominated health education practice for a number of years—the social cognitive theory.

Social Cognitive Theory (SCT)   The social learning theories (SLT) of Rotter (1954) and Bandura (1977b)—or, as Bandura (1986) relabeled them, the *social cognitive theory*

(SCT)—combine SR theory and cognitive theories. Stimulus response theorists emphasize the role of reinforcement in shaping behavior and believe that no "thinking" or "reasoning" is needed to explain behavior. However, Bandura (2001) stated "If actions were performed only on behalf of anticipated external rewards and punishments, people would behave like weather vanes, constantly shifting directions to conform to whatever influence happened to impinge upon them at the moment" (p. 7). Cognitive theorists believe that reinforcement is an integral part of learning, but emphasize the role of subjective hypotheses or expectations held by the individual (Rosenstock et al., 1988). In other words, reinforcement contributes to learning, but reinforcement along with an individual's expectations of the consequences of behavior determine the behavior. "Behavior, in this perspective, is a function of the subjective value of an outcome and the subjective probability (or 'expectation') that a particular action will achieve that outcome. Such formulations are generally termed 'value-expectancy' theories" (Rosenstock et al., 1988, p. 176). In brief, SCT explains human functioning in terms of triadic reciprocal causation (Bandura, 1986). "In this model of reciprocal causality, internal personal factors in the form of cognitive, affective, and biological events, behavioral patterns, and environmental influences all operate as interacting determinants that influence one another bidirectionally" (Bandura, 2001, pp. 14–15). The constructs of the SCT that have been most often used in designing health promotion interventions will be presented here.

As already noted, reinforcement is an important component of SCT. According to SCT, reinforcement can be accomplished in one of three ways: directly, vicariously, or through self-reinforcement (Baranowski, Perry, & Parcel, 2002). An example of **direct reinforcement** is a group facilitator who provides verbal feedback to participants for a job well done. **Vicarious reinforcement** is having the participants observe someone else being reinforced for behaving in an appropriate manner. This has been referred to as *observational learning* (Baranowski et al., 2002) or *social modeling*. In a system of reinforcement by **self-reinforcement,** the participants would keep records of their own behavior, and when the behavior was performed in an appropriate manner, they would reinforce or reward themselves.

If individuals are to perform specific behaviors, they must know first what the behaviors are and then how to perform them. This is referred to as **behavioral capability.** For example, if people are to exercise aerobically, first they must know that aerobic exercise exists, and second they need to know how to do it properly. Many people begin exercise programs, only to quit within the first six months (Dishman, Sallis, & Orenstein, 1985), and some of those people quit because they do not know how to exercise properly. They know they should exercise, so they decide to run a few miles, have sore muscles the next day, and quit. Skill mastery is very important. The construct of **expectations** refers to the ability of human beings to think, and thus to anticipate certain things to happen in certain situations. For example, if people are enrolled in a weight loss program and follow the directions of the group facilitator, they will expect to lose weight. **Expectancies,** not to be confused with expectations, are the values that individuals place on an expected outcome. "Expectancies influence behavior according to the hedonic principle: if all other things are equal, a person will choose to perform an activity that maximizes a positive outcome or minimizes a negative outcome" (Baranowski et al., 2002, p. 173). Someone who enjoys the feeling of not smoking more than that of smoking is more likely to try to do the things necessary to stop. The construct of **self-control** or **self-regulation** states that individuals may gain control of their own behavior through monitoring and adjusting it (Clark et al., 1992). When helping individuals to change their behavior, it is a common practice to have them monitor their behavior over a period of time, through 24-hour diet or smoking records or exercise diaries, and then to have them reward (reinforce) themselves based upon their monitored performance.

One construct of SCT that has received special attention in health promotion programs is self-efficacy (Strecher et al., 1986), which refers to the internal state that individuals experience as "competence" to perform certain desired tasks or behavior, "including confidence in overcoming the barriers to performing that behavior" (Baranowski et al., 2002, p. 173). "Unless people believe they can produce desired results and forestall detrimental ones by their actions, they have little incentive to act or to persevere in the face of difficulties" (Bandura, 2001, p. 10). Self-efficacy is situation specific; that is, individuals may be self-efficacious when it comes to aerobic exercise but not so when faced with reducing the amount of fat in their diet. People's competency feelings have been referred to as **efficacy expectations.** Thus, people who think they can exercise on a regular basis no matter what the circumstances have efficacy expectations. Even though people have efficacy expectations, they still may not want to engage in a behavior because they may not think the outcomes of that behavior would be beneficial to them. Stated another way, they may not feel that the reward (reinforcement) of performing the behavior is great enough for them. These beliefs are called **outcome expectations.** For example, in order for individuals to quit smoking for health reasons (behavior), they must believe both that they are capable of quitting (efficacy expectation) and that cessation will benefit their health (outcome expectation) (I. M. Rosenstock, personal communication, April 1986). **Figure 7.8** (Bandura, 1977b) illustrates efficacy and outcome expectations.

Individuals become self-efficacious in four main ways:

1. Through performance attainments (personal mastery of a task)

2. Through vicarious experience (observing the performance of others)

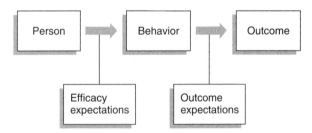

Figure 7.8 Diagrammatic representation of the difference between efficacy and outcome expectations

Source: Albert Bandura, *Social Learning Theory*. Copyright © 1977. Reprinted by permission of Pearson Education, Inc. Upper Saddle River, NJ.

3. As a result of verbal persuasion (receiving suggestions from others)

4. Through emotional arousal (interpreting one's emotional state)

The construct of **emotional-coping responses** states that for people to learn, they must be able to deal with the sources of anxiety that may surround a behavior. For example, fear is an emotion that can be involved in learning; according to this construct, participants would have to deal with the fear before they could learn the behavior.

The construct of **reciprocal determinism** states, unlike SR theory, that there is an interaction among the person, the behavior, and the environment, and that the person can shape the environment as well as the environment shape the person. All these relationships are dynamic. Glanz and Rimer (1995, p. 15) provide a good example of this construct:

> A man with high cholesterol might have a hard time following his prescribed low-fat diet because his company cafeteria doesn't offer low-fat food choices that he likes. He can try to change the environment by talking with the cafeteria manager or the company medical or health department staff, and asking that healthy food choices be added to the menu. Or, if employees start to dine elsewhere in order to eat low-fat lunches, the cafeteria may change its menu to maintain its lunch business.

Finally, there is one other construct that grew out of the social learning theory of Rotter (1954) that needs to be mentioned because of its association with health behavior. "Rotter posited that a person's history of positive or negative reinforcement across a variety of situations shapes a belief as to whether or not a person's own actions lead to those reinforcements" (Wallston, 1994, p. 187). Rotter referred to this construct as **locus of control**. Thus he felt that people with internal locus of control perceived that reinforcement was under their control, whereas those with external locus of control perceived reinforcement to be under the control of some external force. In the 1970s, Wallston and his colleagues at Vanderbilt University began testing the usefulness of this construct in predicting health behavior (Wallston, 1994). They explored the concept of whether individuals with internal locus of control were more likely to participate in health-enhancing behavior than those with external locus of control. They began their work by examining locus of control as a two-dimensional construct (internal vs. external), then moved to a multidimensional construct when they split the external dimension into "powerful others" and "chance" (Wallston, Wallston, & DeVellis, 1978). After a number of years of work by many different researchers, Wallston has come to the conclusion that locus of control accounts for only a small amount of the variability in health behavior (Wallston, 1992). The internal locus of control belief about one's own health status is a necessary but not sufficient determinate of health-enhancing behavior (Wallston, 1994). Since the rise of the construct of self-efficacy, Wallston (1994) feels that self-efficacy is a better predictor of health-promoting behavior than locus of control. This is not to say that locus of control is not a useful construct in developing health promotion programs. Knowing the locus of control orientation of those in the priority population can provide planners with valuable information when considering social support as part of a planned intervention. **Table 7.6** provides a summary of the constructs of the SCT and an example of how each construct might be operationalized.

Community Level Theories

As noted earlier in this chapter, the community level theories include any theory that would apply to the last three levels of the ecological perspective—institutional, community, or public policy. Community level theories "explore how social systems function and change and how to mobilize community members and organizations. They offer strategies that work in a variety of settings such as health care institutions, schools, worksites,

Table 7.6   Often-used constructs of the social cognitive theory and examples of their application

Construct	Definition	Example
Behavioral Capability	Knowledge and skills necessary to perform a behavior	If people are going to exercise aerobically, they need to know what it is and how to do it.
Expectations	Beliefs about the likely outcomes of certain behaviors	If people enroll in a weight-loss program, they expect to lose weight.
Expectancies	Values people place on expected outcomes	How important is it to people that they become physically fit?
Locus of Control	Perception of the center of control over reinforcement	Those who feel they have control over reinforcement are said to have internal locus of control. Those who perceive reinforcement under the control of some external force are said to have external locus of control.
Reciprocal Determinism	Behavior changes result from an interaction between the person and the environment; change is bidirectional (Glanz & Rimer, 1995)	Lack of use of vending machines could be a result of the choices within the machine. Notes about the selections from the nonusing consumers to the machine's owners could change the selections and change the behavior of the consumers to that of users.
Reinforcement (directly, vicariously, self)	Responses to behaviors that increase the chances of recurrence	Giving verbal encouragement to those who have acted in a healthy manner.
Self-Control or Self-Regulation	Gaining control over own behavior through monitoring and adjusting it	If clients want to change their eating habits, have them monitor their current eating habits for seven days.
Self-Efficacy	People's confidence in their ability to perform a certain desired task or function	If people are going to engage in a regular exercise program, they must feel they can do it.
Emotional-Coping Response	For people to learn, they must be able to deal with the sources of anxiety that surround a behavior	Fear is an emotion that can be involved in learning, and people would have to deal with it before they could learn a behavior.

community groups, and government agencies" (Rimer & Glanz, 2005, p. 22). Like the other levels already discussed in this chapter, a number of different community-level theories are available for health planners. Chapter 9 presents several of these theories in detail, specifically community organizing and developing. The following section presents a discussion of a stage model for communities—Community Readiness Model.

Community Readiness Model (CRM).   The Community Readiness Model is a stage theory for communities. The concept of community readiness got its beginnings back in the early-1990s and grew out of the need to understand the problems associated with developing and maintaining community programs. (See Edwards, Jumper-Thurman, Plested, Oetting, & Swanson, 2000, for a description of the origin of the CRM). What was evident from the beginning is that few communities were alike. They may have had similar problems, but the dynamics in each community did not mean that the starting point for dealing with the problem could be the same. "Communities are fluid—always changing, adapting, growing" (Edwards et al., 2000, p. 291), and like individuals, communities are in various stages of readiness for change. Yet, the stages of change for communities are not the same as for individuals. "The stages of readiness in a community have to deal with group processes and group organization, characteristics that are not relevant to personal readiness" Edwards et al., 2000, p. 296–297). Though the model was developed initially to deal with alcohol and drug abuse, it has been useful in helping with a variety of health and nutrition topics (e.g., AIDS awareness, elimination of heart disease, depression awareness, reduction of sexually transmitted diseases), environmentally centered programs (e.g., air quality and recycling), and social programs (e.g., intimate partner violence programs) (Edwards et al., 2000).

The Community Readiness Model defines nine stages: (1) *No Awareness* (The problem is not generally recognized by the community or leaders); (2) *Denial* (There is little or no recognition in the community that there is a problem; if so, the feeling is nothing can be done about it); (3) *Vague Awareness* (Feeling among some in the community there is a problem and something should be done, but no motivation or leadership to do so); (4) *Preplanning* (The clear recognition by some that there is a problem and something should be done. There are leaders, but no focused or detailed planning); (5) *Preparation* (There is planning going on but not based on collected data. There is leadership, resources are being sought, and there is modest support for efforts); (6) *Initiation* (Information is available to justify and begin efforts. Staff is in, or just completed, training. Leaders are enthusiastic and there is usually little resistance and involvement from the community members); (7) *Stabilization* (Program is running, staffed, and supported by community and decision makers. Program perceived as stable with no need for change. May include routine tracking, but no in-depth evaluation); (8) *Confirmation/Expansion* (Standard efforts are in place and supported by the community and decision makers. Program has been evaluated and modified, and efforts are in place to seek resources for new efforts. Data are collected on an ongoing basis to link risk factors and problems); and (9) *Professionalism* (Much is known about prevalence, risk factors, and cause of problems. Highly trained staff runs effective programs, aimed at general population and appropriate subgroups. Programs have been evaluated and modified. Community is supportive but should hold programs accountable.) (Edwards et al., 2000).

Table 7.7   Community readiness stages and goals

Stage	Goal
1. *No Awareness*	Raise awareness of the issue
2. *Denial*	Raise awareness that the problem or issue exists in the community
3. *Vague Awareness*	Raise awareness that the community can do something
4. *Preplanning*	Raise awareness with the concrete ideas to combat condition
5. *Preparation*	Gather existing information to help plan strategies
6. *Initiation*	Provide community-specific information
7. *Stabilization*	Stabilize efforts/programs
8. *Confirmation/Expansion*	Expand and enhance service
9. *Professionalism*	Maintain momentum and continue growth

Source: R. W. Edwards et al., "Community Readiness: Research to Practice," *Journal of Community Psychology,* 28(3), pp. 291–307, 2000. Copyright © 2000. Reprinted by permission of Wiley-Blackwell.

A community's readiness can be assessed through interviews with key informants. Once the stage of readiness is known, like the other stage theories, there are suggested processes for moving a community from one stage to the next. **Table 7.7** presents the nine stages and the goal for each stage.

Cognitive-Behavioral Model of the Relapse Process

For most people, relapse is a part of change. **Relapse** "refers to the breakdown or failure in a person's attempt to change or modify a particular habit pattern, such as stopping 'bad habits' or developing new, optimal health behaviors" (Marlatt & George, 1998, p. 33). Marlatt and George (1998) differentiate between relapse (an indication of total failure) and a **lapse** (a single slip or mistake). The first drink or cigarette following a period of abstinence would be considered a lapse. It has been said that getting people to change behavior is hard, but having them maintain the behavior is much harder. This is nicely illustrated by the old saying "Giving up smoking is easy; I've done it a hundred times." At one time, it was enough for program planners just to get people to change their behavior; now they need to do more. Because of the difficulty of maintaining a new behavior, program planners need to give special attention to helping those in the priority population avoid slipping back to their previous behaviors.

Although much of the early research dealing with this concept of slipping back was conducted using addictive behaviors, such as substance abuse and gambling, the concept applies to all behavior change, including preventive health behaviors. Marlatt (1982) indicates that a high percentage of individuals who enter programs for health behavior change relapse to their former behaviors within one year. More specifically, researchers have warned program planners of **recidivism** problems with participants in exercise (Dishman, Sallis, & Orenstein, 1985; Horne, 1975; Simkin & Gross, 1994), oral health care treatment (McCaul et al., 1990), weight loss (Stunkard & Braunwell, 1980), and smoking cessation (Leventhal & Cleary, 1980) programs. Therefore, planners need to make sure that program interventions include the skills necessary for dealing with those difficult times during behavior change.

Marlatt (1982) refers to the process of trying to prevent slipping back as relapse prevention. Relapse prevention, which is based on the social cognitive theory, combines behavioral skill-training procedures, cognitive therapy, and lifestyle rebalancing (Marlatt & George, 1998). **Relapse prevention (RP)** is "a self-control program designed to help individuals to anticipate and cope with the problem of relapse in the habit-changing process" (Marlatt & George, 1998, p. 33). Relapse is triggered by *high-risk situations*. "A high-risk situation is defined broadly as any situation (including emotional reactions to the situation) that poses a threat to the individual's sense of control and increases the risk of potential relapse" (Marlatt & George, 1998, p. 38). Cummings, Gordon, and Marlatt (1980), in a study of clients with a variety of problem behaviors (drinking, smoking, heroin addiction, gambling, and overeating), found high-risk situations to fall into two major categories: intrapersonal and interpersonal determinants. They found that 56% of the relapse situations were caused by intrapersonal determinants, such as negative emotional states (35%), negative physical states (3%), positive emotional states (4%), testing personal control (5%), and urges and temptations (9%). The 44% of the situations represented by interpersonal determinants included interpersonal conflicts (16%), social pressure (20%), and positive emotional states (8%). These determinants can be referred to as the *covert antecedents* of relapse. That is to say, these high-risk situations do not just happen; instead, they are created by what Marlatt (1982) calls *lifestyle imbalances.*

People who have the coping skills to deal with a high-risk situation have a much greater chance of preventing relapse than those who do not. **Figure 7.9** illustrates the possible paths one may take in a high-risk situation (Marlatt, 1982).

Marlatt has developed both global (see **Figure 7.10**) and specific (see **Figure 7.11**) self-control strategies for relapse intervention. Specific intervention procedures are designed to help participants anticipate and cope with the relapse episode itself, whereas

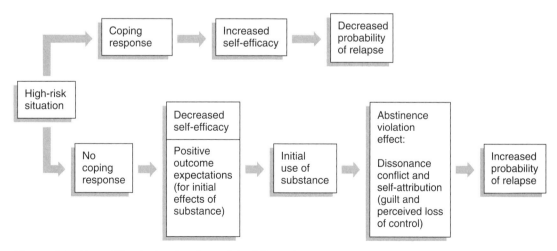

Figure 7.9 Cognitive-behavioral model of the relapse process

Source: G. A. Marlatt and J. R. Gordon, *Relapse Prevention,* p. 38. Copyright © 1985 The Guilford Press. Reprinted by permission.

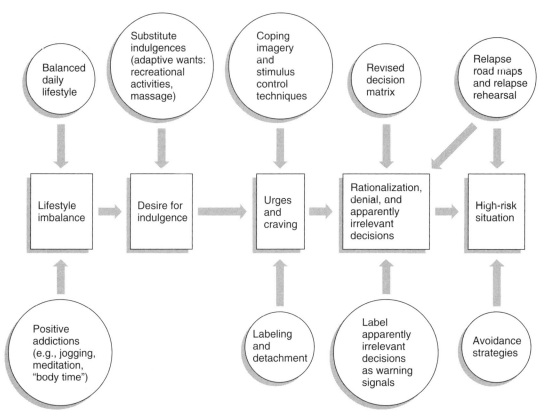

Figure 7.10 Relapse prevention: global self-control strategies

Source: G. A. Marlatt and J. R. Gordon, *Relapse Prevention,* p. 61. Copyright © 1985 The Guilford Press. Reprinted by permission.

the global intervention procedures are designed to modify the early antecedents of relapse, including restructuring of the participant's general style of life. A complete application of the relapse prevention model would include both specific and global interventions (Marlatt, 1982).

Applying Theory to Practice

Learning and understanding the theories presented in this chapter are manageable tasks. However, learning "how to apply given theories to 'real life' projects where theories usually have to be bent and twisted and adapted to uncontrollable conditions" (Hochbaum et al., 1992, p. 311) is a much more difficult task. Several authors (Burdine & McLeroy, 1992; Crosby et al., 2002; D'Onofrio, 1992; Glanz et al., 2002b; Hochbaum et al., 1992; McLeroy, 1993; van Ryn and Heaney, 1992) have reported the difficulties practitioners have had in applying theory. In the sections below, we will discuss the reported

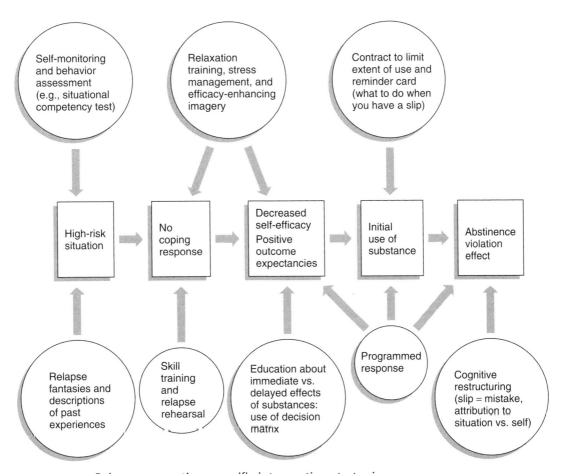

Figure 7.11 Relapse prevention: specific intervention strategies

Source: G. A. Marlatt and J. R. Gordon, *Relapse Prevention*, p. 54. Copyright © 1985 The Guilford Press. Reprinted by permission.

barriers to applying theory in the field and provide suggestions for choosing and applying theory.

Barriers to Applying Theory

Burdine and McLeroy (1992) have reported on semistructured interviews with health professionals on the use of theory in practice. Though the group was not randomly selected—it was part of a workgroup in eastern Pennsylvania—it was thought to be broadly representative of "practicing health educators." From these interviews came three primary reasons why practitioners were not using theory learned in their professional preparation courses in college. They included "(1) the failure of theory to adequately guide practice in specific settings or contexts; (2) the lack of appropriate theories to guide community-oriented interventions; and (3) difficulties in transferring theories from the academic training context to the practice environment" (Burdine & McLeroy, 1992, p. 336).

The concern about the failure of theory to adequately guide practice in specific settings or contexts stems from the fact that the theory on which the health promotion profession was built is borrowed from the social and behavioral sciences. It primarily revolves around individual behavior change. Even though behavior change is an important part of the work of health educators, the theories, except those aimed at the community level, do not match well with the expanded role of health educators when they address problems such as controlling environmental health hazards, increasing access to and utilization of health care facilities, limiting the commercial promotion of alcohol and tobacco (D'Onofrio, 1992), and organizing committees to deal with these problems (Burdine & McLeroy, 1992).

The third reason shared by Burdine and McLeroy (1992) for practitioners not using theory in practice is the means by which theory is taught by academicians. Instead of presenting the theories and asking how they apply to a problem, it is suggested (Burdine & McLeroy, 1992; D'Onofrio, 1992) that academicians should be teaching theory by starting with a specific health problem and asking how each of the theories helps one understand the problem.

Now that you know a bit about what appears to be some of the reasons for not using theory in practice, let's look at how it can be implemented.

Suggestions for Applying Theory to Practice

"Behavioral and social science theory provides a platform for understanding why people engage in health-risk or health-compromising behavior and why (as well as how) they adopt health-protective behavior" (Crosby et al., 2002, p. 1). Using the most appropriate theory and practice strategies for a given situation greatly enhances the chances for effective health promotion practice (Glanz et al., 2002b).

Several authors (D'Onofrio, 1992; Hochbaum et al., 1992; McGuire, 1983; van Ryn & Heaney, 1992) have suggested ideas for applying theory to practice. Following is a summary compilation of their ideas.

The first step is to have a basic grasp of the theories—old and new (D'Onofrio, 1992). Practitioners should take the time to review the theories and not depend on memory. Theories, like most other knowledge, are forgotten over time if they are not used. Also, the very nature of theory suggests that it can change and be updated. The theory of reasoned action and the theory of planned behavior are good examples. Practitioners also need to become familiar with new theories and models.

Once practitioners feel comfortable with the theories and models, they should examine their applicability to the problem they are addressing (D'Onofrio, 1992; van Ryn & Heaney, 1992). This can be done by taking the goals of a proposed program and matching them with the most applicable theories. For example, are the goals and objectives of the program to produce a lasting lifestyle change, or is the program designed to make a one-time decision and take action like having a child immunized for HPV? Also, at what level of influence (i.e., intrapersonal, interpersonal, or community) should the

Table 7.8   Major components of the theories that underlie health promotion interventions

Stimulus Response Theory	Social Cognitive Theory	Theory of Reasoned Action	Theory of Planned Behavior	Theory of Freeing
Operant behavior	Reinforcement 1. Direct 2. Vicarious 3. Self-management	Attitude toward behavior	Attitude toward behavior	Free
Consequences	Behavioral capability	Subjective norm	Subjective norm	Oppressed
Positive reinforcement	Expectations	Intentions	Perceived behavioral control	Critical consciousness
Negative reinforcement	Expectancies	Behavior	Intentions	Education
Positive punishment	Self-control		Behavior	
Negative punishment	Self-efficacy			
	Emotional-coping response			
	Reciprocal determinism			

Health Belief Model	Transtheoretical Model	Cognitive-Behavior Model of the Relapse Process	Elaboration Likelihood Model of Persuasion	Precaution Adoption Process Model	Health Action Process Approach	Community Readiness Model
Perceived susceptibility	Stages of change	High-risk situation	Central route	Stages	Motivation to change phase	Key informant interviews
Perceived seriousness	Decisional balance	Global self-control strategies	Peripheral route	Issues	Self-regulatory phase	Stages and goals
Perceived benefits	Processes of change	Specific intervention strategies	Elaboration likelihood continuum		Stages	Stategies
Perceived barriers	Self-efficacy		Variables			
Motivation (cues to action)						
Self-efficacy						

program be aimed to get the desired change in program participants? (See Table 7.2 for a refresher on what theories work best at what levels.) If planners feel that several theories could be applicable to the problem they are addressing, they should look for evidence that the theories or models will work in their particular situation. Have others used theories with success with the same or a similar problem or priority population (McGuire, 1983; van Ryn & Heaney, 1992)? Some theories may have to be adjusted or modified to be applicable to certain priority populations. For example, can the same theory apply to people from different cultural backgrounds within the United States? Or, what is the applicability of behavioral theories based on Western thought to people from non-Western cultures (D'Onofrio, 1992)?

It is also important to remember that seldom does a single theory address all the complexities of a problem. Planners will more than likely have to use more than one theory to adequately address all the components of the problem. To do so, planners will need to synthesize and integrate the theories to fit their particular situation (D'Onofrio, 1992). In bringing theories together, planners are warned against using only selected parts of a theory. Theories are based on the interaction of several variables. When some of those variables are removed, the theory is not the same. For example, if cues to action or motivation are removed from the health belief model, planners will not know the true effectiveness of the model. Thus the most effective use of a theory is to use it in total (Hochbaum et al., 1992).

In the final step in choosing a theory, planners need to select "a theory that makes sense to them, given their experience and what they know and believe about the world" (van Ryn & Heaney, 1992, p. 320). This is not to say that planners should not consider theories that may be different from their own views, but it "does not make sense to base a program on theoretical ideas that are at odds with one's own philosophy or belief system" (van Ryn & Heaney, 1992, p. 320).

SUMMARY

Many theories are available to program planners. One group of researchers identified no fewer than 66 theories that had been used to guide health promotion programs. This chapter presents an overview of the theories that are used most often in health promotion programs. These theories are important for planners because they provide information about: why people are, or are not, engaging in health-enhancing behaviors; how to create interventions; and what factors to look for when evaluating a program. Theories can be categorized in a number of ways. This chapter presents two categories. The first categorizes theories by the level of influence at which it is most effective; the second classifies theories as either the continuum or stage theories. The chapter also discusses some of the roadblocks to using theory and suggestions for applying theory to practice. **Table 7.8** summarizes the theories presented in the chapter and the major components of each.

Finally, the chapter provides a discussion of some of the roadblocks to using theory and suggestions for applying theory to practice.

REVIEW QUESTIONS

1. Define *theory*, using your own words.

2. How is a theory different from a model?

3. How do concepts, constructs, and variables relate to theories?

4. Why is it important to use theories when planning and evaluating health promotion programs?

5. How can the ecological perspective be used to select a theory for use?

6. What makes stage theories different from continuum theories?

7. What is the underlying concept for each of the following continuum theories?
   a. Stimulus response theory
   b. Social cognitive theory
   c. Theory of reasoned action
   d. Theory of planned behavior
   e. Health belief model
   f. Theory of freeing
   g. Elaboration likelihood model of persuasion

8. What are the major components of the following stage theories?
   a. Transtheoretical model
   b. Precaution adoption process model
   c. Health action process approach
   d. Community readiness model

9. What is the major difference between the transtheoretical model and the precaution adoption process model?

10. How is the community readiness model different from the other stage models?

11. How can program planners help to prepare those in the priority population for relapse prevention?

12. What are the major barriers to using a theory in practice?

ACTIVITIES

1. Assume that you have identified a need (health problem) for a given priority population. In a two-page paper:
   a. State who the priority population is and what the need is.
   b. Select a theory to use as a guide in developing an intervention to address the problem.

    c. Explain why you chose the theory that you did.

    d. Defend why you think this is the best theory to use.

    e. Show how the problem "fits into" the theory.

2. In a two-page paper, identify a theory that you plan to use in developing the intervention for the program you are planning. Explain why you chose the theory, and why you think it is a good fit for the problem you are addressing.

3. Write a paragraph on each of the following:

    a. Using the stimulus response theory, explain why a person might smoke.

    b. Using the social cognitive theory, explain how you could help people change their diets.

    c. Explain how the SCT construct of behavioral capability applies to managing stress.

    d. Explain the differences between, and the relationship of, the SCT constructs of expectations and expectancies.

    e. Explain what would have to take place for individuals to be self-efficacious with regard to taking their insulin.

    f. According to the theory of reasoned action, what would increase intent to exercise?

    g. Use the theory of planned behavior to explain how a smoker stops smoking.

    h. Using the theory of freeing, describe an ideal teacher.

    i. Apply the health belief model to getting a person to take a "flu shot."

    j. Apply the transtheoretical model to get a person to change any health behavior.

    k. Using the precaution adoption process model, explain how a person decides to get screened for blood cholesterol.

    l. Use the health action process approach to explain how planners could design an exercise program for sedentary adults.

    m. Explain how the community readiness model could be used by planners who are interested in getting a citywide smoking ordinance passed.

WEBLINKS

1. http://www.uri.edu/research/cprc/index-old.htm

   Cancer Prevention Resource Center (CPRC), University of Rhode Island

   This is the website for the CPRC which is the home of the Transtheoretical Model. Information about the model, as well as measures that can be used to "stage" a person, can be found at this site.

2. http://www.cdc.gov/std/program/community/9-PGcommunity.htm

   National Center for HIV, STD, and TB Prevention, Division of Sexually Transmitted Diseases

This website provides an overview of the following behavior change theories: Health Belief Model, Theory of Reasoned Action, Social (Cognitive) Learning Theory, Transtheoretical Model (stages of change), Diffusion of Innovations, and Empowerment Theory/Empowerment.

3. http://www.nci.nih.gov/PDF/481f5d53-63df-41bc-bfaf-5aa48ee1da4d/TAAG3.pdf

National Cancer Institute (NCI)

This is a file found at the NCI website. It presents *Theory at a Glance: A Guide for Health Promotion Practice*. This volume presents a single, concise summary of health behavior theories that is both easy to read and practical.

4. http://www.people.umass.edu/aizen/tpb.html

Theory of Planned Behavior

This is part of the website of Dr. Icek Ajzen, creator of the theory of planned behavior. The site provides great detail about the theory, as well as sample questionnaires to show how data can be collected using this theory.

8

Interventions

After reading this chapter and answering the questions at the end, you should be able to:

- Define the word *intervention* and apply it to a health promotion setting.
- Provide a rationale for selecting an intervention strategy.
- Explain the advantages of using a combination of several intervention strategies rather than a single intervention strategy.
- List and explain the different categories of intervention strategies.
- Explain the terms *curriculum*, *scope*, *sequence*, *units of study*, *lessons*, *lesson plans*, and *health advocacy*.
- Briefly explain the modified framework for instructional design.
- List some of the documents that provide guidelines or criteria for developing health promotion interventions.
- Discuss the ethical concerns related to intervention development.
- Create an intervention for a health promotion program.

best experience	disincentives	scope
best practices	dose	segmenting
best processes	health advocacy	sequence
codes of practice	incentive	strategy
communication channel	intervention	tailored
community advocacy	lessons	treatment
community building	lesson plan	units of study
community organization	multiplicity	
curriculum	penetration rate	

Once the goals and objectives have been developed, planners need to decide on the most appropriate means of reaching or attaining the goals and objectives. The planners must design an activity or set of activities that would permit the most *effective* (leads to desired outcome) and *efficient* (uses resources in a responsible manner) achievement of the outcomes stated in the goals and objectives. These planned activities make up the intervention, or what some refer to as **treatment**. The **intervention** is the theory-based strategy or experience to which those in the priority population will be exposed or in which they will take part. In the strictest sense, intervention means "to come or occur between two things, events, or points in time; to come in or between so as to hinder or alter an action" (Anderson, Fortson, Kleindler, & Schonthal, 2002, p. 447). When applied to the planning of health promotion programs, it is usually thought of as something that occurs between the beginning and the end of a program or between pre- and post-program measurements. For example, let's say that you want the employees of Company S to increase their use of safety belts while riding in company-owned vehicles. You can measure their safety belt use before doing anything else, by observing them driving out of the motor pool. This would be a pre-program measure. Then you can intervene in a variety of ways. For example, you could provide an incentive by stating that all employees seen wearing their safety belts would receive a $10 bonus in their next paycheck. Or you could put in each employee's pay envelope a pamphlet on the importance of wearing safety belts. You could institute a company policy requiring all employees to wear safety belts while driving company-owned vehicles. Each of these activities for getting employees to increase their use of safety belts would be considered part of an intervention. After the intervention, you would complete a post-program measurement of safety belt use to determine the success of the program.

The term *intervention* is used to describe all the activities that occur between the two measurement points. Thus an intervention may use a single activity, or it may be a combination of two or more activities. In the case of the example just given, you could use an incentive by itself and call it an intervention, or you could use an incentive, pamphlets, and a company policy all at the same time to increase safety belt use and refer to the combination as an intervention.

The above discussion about the number of activities that make up an intervention in part speaks to the *size* of an intervention. Two terms that relate to the size of an intervention are *multiplicity* and *dose*. **Multiplicity** refers to the number of components or activities that make up the intervention. We have known for a number of years (Erfurt et al., 1990; Kline & Huff, 1999; Shea & Basch, 1990) that interventions that include several activities are more likely to have an effect on the priority population than are those that consist of a single activity. Few people change their behavior based on a single exposure; instead, multiple exposures are generally needed to change most behaviors. It stands to reason that "hitting" the priority population from several angles or through multiple channels should increase the chances of making an impact. Although research has shown that using several activities is better than one, it has not identified an exact number of activities or a specific combination of activities that will ensure the most effective results (Kline & Huff, 1999). The right combination of activities will depend on the needs of those in the priority population and the specific planning situation.

When speaking about the **dose** of an intervention, we are referring to the number of program units delivered. For example, say that it was decided that the intervention for a skin cancer program would consist of multiple activities (*multiplicity*) and those activities would include an educational class for the public, distribution of brochures to those at high risk, and radio and television public service announcements (PSAs). The dose questions related to these activities would be: How many times would the class be offered? How many brochures would be distributed? And, how many times would the PSAs run? Again, like multiplicity, we know that the greater the dose of an intervention, the greater the chance for change. Chapter 14 includes additional information about multiplicity and dose as they relate to process evaluation.

Box 8.1 identifies the responsibilities and competencies for health educators that pertain to the material presented in this chapter.

Box 8.1 RESPONSIBILITIES AND COMPETENCIES FOR HEALTH EDUCATORS

The content of Chapter 8 focuses on the creation of the intervention that will be used in the program that is being planned. The intervention is really at the "heart" of a program. It is the component of the program that will cause the change in the priority population. The responsibility and competencies related to the tasks of creating an intervention include:

Responsibility II: Plan Health Education Strategies, Interventions, and Programs

Competency D: Develop a logical scope and sequence plan for health education practice

Competency E: Design strategies, interventions, and programs consistent with specified objectives

Competency F: Select appropriate strategies to meet objectives

Competency G: Assess factors that affect implementation

Source: NCHEC, SOPHE, & AAHE (2006).

Types of Intervention Strategies

As mentioned earlier, there are many different types of strategies that planners can use as part of an intervention. By **strategy,** we mean "a general plan of action for affecting a health problem. A strategy may encompass several activities" (CDC, 2003, glossary). Here, we present several categories of intervention strategies based on a modification of the Centers for Disease Control and Prevention's (2003) terminology for intervention strategies. These categories cover the more common strategies used by planners, but in actuality the variety of strategies is limited only by the planner's imagination. Note that the categories presented here are not always independent of each other—that is, some of the examples that we use to help explain the strategies could be used in more than one category. Even with this limitation, the strategies have been categorized into the following groups:

1. Health communication strategies
2. Health education strategies
3. Health policy/enforcement strategies
4. Environmental change strategies
5. Health-related community service strategies
6. Community mobilization strategies
7. Other strategies

Health Communication Strategies

Health communication strategies are designed to inform and influence individual and community decisions to enhance health (NCI, 2002). Of the various intervention strategies used in health promotion, we present health communication strategies first for several reasons. First, almost all health promotion interventions include some form of communication, whether it is as simple as speaking, reading, or writing, or more complex, such as the production of small media (i.e., handouts and brochures), or very complex in the development of mass media (i.e., radio, TV, or newspaper) campaigns. Second, communication strategies are useful in reaching many of the goals and objectives of health promotion programs. Specifically, they have been shown to be useful in: (1) increasing risk perceptions (Bartholomew et al., 2006); (2) providing cues and motivation to action; (3) reinforcing attitudes (e.g., regular exercise is important); (4) demonstrating simple skills (Bellicha & McGrath, 1990; Erickson, McKenna, & Romano, 1990); (5) increasing demand and support for health services (NCI, 2002); (6) increasing perceptions of one's ability to perform a behavior (NCI, 2002); (7) reinforcing behaviors (NCI, 2002); and (8) building social norms (NCI, 2002) (e.g., about not smoking in public places).

Third, communication strategies probably have the highest **penetration rate** (number in the priority population exposed or reached) of any of the intervention strategies. And fourth, they are also much more cost effective and less threatening than many other types of strategies.

The literally hundreds of communication activities can be subdivided by communication channels. A **communication channel** is the route through which a message is disseminated to the priority population. The four primary communication channels include intrapersonal (one-on-one communication), interpersonal (small group communication), organization and community, and mass media. These channels are hierarchical in nature with regards to the number of people they reach. The intrapersonal channel typically reaches the fewest number of people, while the mass media channel reaches the largest number of people. Note that the communication channels line up very closely to the levels in the ecological perspective.

Over the years, the *intrapersonal channel* has most often been used, but by no means exclusively, in health care settings when the health care provider and patient interact. This is a familiar channel for most people and one they trust. It is typically an effective communication channel, but it is also typically the most time and resource intensive channel for the number of people reached. In more recent years, this channel of communication has been greatly enhanced by the use of technology. For example, computers have been used to deliver tailored electronic mail messages (Kreuter, Farrell, Olevitch, & Brennan, 2000). Also, though most do not think of the telephone as "technology" it too is being used for health promotion interventions via the intrapersonal channel. Planners have used it for "gathering information, disseminating information, providing health education and counseling, promoting health education programs, offering cues to action and social support" (Soet & Basch, 1997, p. 760). Health education delivered by telephone "can be classified into two broad categories: *individual initiated,* where the individual must actively seek contact and assistance from a health information hotline; and *outreach,* where the individual is called by a health educator or counselor" (Soet & Basch, 1997, p. 760). Individual-initiated health information hotlines or help lines usually provide information, and sometimes education and counseling, whereas outreach activities range from brief, one-time preappointment reminders to long-term interactive professional health counseling (Soet & Basch, 1997) or coaching. Telephone-delivered intervention activities have been created for a variety of topics, including but not limited to cancer screening (Davis et al., 1997; Ludman et al., 1999; McDowell, Newell, & Rosser, 1989b), diabetes (Wilcox, 2006), medical appointments (Linkins et al., 1994), hypertension screening (McDowell, Newell, & Rosser, 1989a), smoking cessation (Koffman et al., 1998; Simmons, 1998), and weight loss (Hellerstedt & Jeffery, 1997). Soet and Basch (1997) present a generic process for developing a telephone intervention activity that includes three areas: "designing the intervention protocol, selection and training of the health educator/counselor(s), and developing the documentation and data collection protocol" (p. 763).

Examples of the *interpersonal channel* are support groups and small classes. This channel has many of the same characteristics of the intrapersonal channel, but reaches larger numbers of people with fewer resources.

Many people receive a lot of information through *organization* and *community channels.* Often health promotion programs have priority populations that are part of or entirely comprise already existing groups (i.e., workers of a particular company, social groups, or members of a religious organization), or who may participate in a community activity. As such, organizational and community channels provide excellent ways of reaching priority populations. Thus church bulletins, company or agency newsletters, organizations or community bulletin boards, and community activities are often used as a part of communication activities (e.g., the American Cancer Society's Great American Smokeout and health fairs).

Probably the most visible communication channel to most people is the *mass media channel.* This channel includes both print and electronic media formats such as: billboards; direct mail; daily papers with national or local circulation; local weekly newspapers; local, public, and network television, including cable television; public and commercial radio stations; and magazines with either a broad readership or a narrow focus. There are many ways to convey a message using the mass media. These include news coverage, public affairs coverage, talk shows, public service roundtables,

| Box 8.2 | PRODUCING MATERIALS FOR SPECIAL POPULATIONS |

Although planners should create/select materials that are applicable to each priority population, extra attention needs to be given to materials that are prepared for special populations. Consider the following:

A. For culturally diverse populations, remember:
   1. Interaction with the priority population and "intermediaries" familiar with the culture is especially important.
   2. Use of language may vary for different cultural groups (e.g., a word may have different meanings to different groups).
   3. Differences in priority populations extend beyond language to include diverse values and customs.
   4. Different channels of communication may be credible and more capable of reaching certain cultural groups.
   5. Don't assume that "conventional wisdom," published research studies, or "common knowledge" will hold true for different cultural groups. The degree of assimilation and mainstreaming is ever changing, so current information will be needed to choose the best channels and message strategies.
   6. Message appeals should be developed separately for each cultural group, since the perceived needs, values, and beliefs of one culture may differ from others.
   7. Print materials should be simply written, reinforced with graphics, and pretested. People perceive graphics and illustrations in different ways, just as their language skills differ.
   8. Bilingual materials assure that intermediaries and family members who are most comfortable with English can help the reader understand the content.
   9. Print materials should never be simply translated from English; concepts and appeals may differ by culture, just as the words do.
   10. Audiovisual materials or interpersonal communication may be more successful for some messages and audiences.

B. For patient populations, remember:
   1. Patients and their families facing a disorder or a disease may require different information in different formats at various points in the disease continuum.
   2. All patients are not alike, and may have nothing in common except their illness. Therefore, their interests in information and ability to understand the illness may vary.
   3. Few patients and family members can handle everything they need to know at once, and may find it particularly difficult to absorb information at the time of diagnosis.
   4. Patients' information needs may change as they emotionally adjust to their illness.

Source: Adapted from U.S. Department of Health and Human Services (1989).

entertainment, public service announcements (PSAs), paid advertisements, editorials, letters to the editor, comic strips, and columnists' commentaries (Arkin, 1990).

The cost of communication activities can range from almost nothing (e.g., elementary school children making posters for a health awareness campaign) to moderately priced (e.g., production of a brochure) to expensive (e.g., personal counseling) to very expensive (e.g., a prime-time television commercial). However, no matter what form the communication activities take or their cost, to be effective, they need to be carefully planned. See Chapter 2 for more information about health communication and the models commonly used to plan interventions using communication activities. Also, we recommend that health educators obtain a copy of the book *Making Health Communication Programs Work* (NCI, 2002), also fondly referred to as the "Pink Book" (see the *Weblinks* at the end of the chapter for the URL).

Before leaving our discussion on communication strategies, we would like to share some guidelines that we have found useful in preparing communication materials for priority populations with special needs. **Box 8.2** presents a list of items to consider when preparing materials for culturally diverse and patient populations. Planners also need to be concerned with creating written communication materials that are appropriate for the reading abilities of the priority population. Many health promotion materials are written at a reading level too difficult for many people in the general public to understand. That holds for both printed materials and those on the World Wide Web. Meyer and Rainey (1994) created a set of guidelines for health educators to follow when creating health promotion materials for low-literacy populations. We found their guidelines to be useful regardless of the priority population. Their eight guidelines have been modified and are summarized in **Table 8.1**. The only addition we would make to their list would be to check the reading level of the written materials. "For the general public, writing at the 6th grade reading level is usually safe. You can check if you're on target by using a readability test such as the SMOG, the Fog-Gunning Index, or the Fry Readability Formula" (USDHHS, 1991, p. 3). You can find such formulas in most reading methods books and on selected computer word-processing programs. **Box 8.3** presents the steps in the process of testing readability using the SMOG.

Health Education Strategies

As you may recall from Chapter 1, *health education* was defined as "any planned combination of learning experiences designed to predispose, enable, and reinforce voluntary behavior decisions conducive to health in individuals, groups, or communities" (Green & Kreuter, 205, p. G-4). You may be asking, "How is this definition different from the definition presented in the earlier section for health communication strategies?" There are some health communication strategies, because of the way they are designed, that could be classified as health education strategies. And, there are some health education strategies that could meet the definition of health communication strategies. There is no clear dividing line between these two categories of intervention strategies. That is, they are not mutually exclusive categories. In fact, it is for that reason that some authors have included health education strategies as part of the health communication strategies category or vice versa. Yet, we have decided to separate the two types of strategies. In general, we see health communication strategies as those that inform people (e.g., a brochure on skin cancer or a mass media campaign on preventing HIV), while health education strategies are those that are planned learning experiences that provide knowledge and skills to the learners in a

Table 8.1   Guidelines for preparing written materials

Guideline	Explanation
1. Needs and priority population identification	Identify the topic and the priority population (e.g., middle-aged women and mammography).
2. Plan the project	Develop a work plan and budget for your material.
3. Audience research	Segment your priority population using such factors as experience, attitude, culture, etc.
4. Material development	
a. Style	Use an active voice with familar terms that highlight key points. If possible, develop a behaviorally oriented interactive message.
b. Organization	Sequence or prioritize the message.
c. Content	Use words and terms that are understandable to lay people. Use short sentences and paragraphs.
d. Format	Make it appealing to the eye, making sure the reader can identify the main points.
5. Graphics and illustrations	Graphics and illustrations should be positive and easy to understand, and should summarize the message.
6. Pretesting	Make sure the materials work before you use them with the priority population. Also, make sure the reading level is appropriate.
7. Printing	Consider paper color, size, and cost.
8. Distribution and training	Develop a distribution system and instructions for use.

Source: Adapted from Meyer and Rainey (1994), pp. 372–374.

Box 8.3   THE SMOG READABILITY FORMULA

To calculate the SMOG reading grade level, begin with the entire written work that is being assessed, and follow these four steps:

1. Count off 10 consecutive sentences near the beginning, in the middle, and near the end of the text.

2. From this sample of 30 sentences, circle all of the words containing 3 or more syllables (polysyllabic), including repetitions of the same word, and total the number of words circled.

3. Estimate the square root of the total number of polysyllabic words counted. This is done by finding the nearest perfect square, and taking its square root.

4. Finally, add a constant of 3 to the square root. This number gives the SMOG grade, or the reading grade level that a person must have reached if he or she is to fully understand the text being assessed.

A few additional guidelines will help to clarify these directions:

• A sentence is defined as a string of words punctuated with a period (.), an exclamation point (!), or a question mark (?).

• Hyphenated words are considered as one word.

• Numbers that are written out should also be considered, and if in numeric form in the text, they should be pronounced to determine if they are polysyllabic.

Box 8.3	CONTINUED

- Proper nouns, if polysyllabic, should be counted, too.
- Abbreviations should be read as unabbreviated to determine if they are polysyllabic.

Not all pamphlets, fact sheets, or other printed materials contain 30 sentences. To test a text that has fewer than 30 sentences:

1. Count all of the polysyllabic words in the text.
2. Count the number of sentences.
3. Find the average number of polysyllabic words per sentence as follows:

$$\text{Average} = \frac{\text{Total \# of polysyllabic words}}{\text{Total \# of sentences}}$$

4. Multiply that average by the number of sentences *short of* 30.
5. Add that figure to the total number of polysyllabic words.
6. Find the square root and add the constant of 3.

Perhaps the quickest way to administer the SMOG grading test is by using the SMOG conversion table. Simply count the number of polysyllabic words in your chain of 30 sentences and look up the appropriate grade level on the chart.

SMOG Conversion Table*

Total Polysyllabic Word Counts	Aproximate Grade Level (±1.5 Grades)
0–2	4
3–6	5
7–12	6
13–20	7
21–30	8
31–42	9
43–56	10
57–72	11
73–90	12
91–110	13
111–132	14
133–156	15
157–182	16
183–210	17
211–240	18

*Developed by Harold C. McGraw, Office of Educational Research, Baltimore County Schools, Towson, Maryland.

Source: U.S. Department of Health and Human Services (1989).

more formal educational setting. We see health education strategies as those usually associated with settings such as classes, seminars, workshops, and courses. Some examples include prenatal classes for expectant parents, a workshop for parents on how to better communicate with their teenager, or a first aid and CPR course for potential babysitters.

While health communication strategies may be the most frequently used health promotion intervention strategy, health education strategies are the ones that provide the opportunity for the priority population to gain in-depth knowledge about a particular health topic. Well-designed health education strategies take an understanding of the educational process and take a great deal of effort to create. In order to better understand this process, several terms must be defined. The first is the word *curriculum*. **Curriculum** refers to a written plan outlining what those in the priority population will be taught (a course of study) (ASCD, 2007). Examples include the health education curriculum of a school district or the curriculum for a hospital's diabetes education program. To further define a curriculum it is important to understand the terms *scope* and *sequence*. **Scope** refers to the breadth and depth of the material covered in a curriculum, while **sequence** defines the order in which the material is presented. To further clarify these definitions, *scope* has been referred to as the horizontal organization of the substance of the curriculum (Goodlad & Su, 1992), while the *sequence* is the vertical relationship among the curricular areas (Ornstein & Hunkins, 1998). It is not unusual for the scope of a health education curriculum to be presented as **units of study**. These units are defined as "a segment of instruction focused on a particular topic" (ASCD, 2007, p. 3). Thus, a school health curriculum may have units on exercise, nutrition, chronic diseases, communicable diseases, and so forth, while the diabetes education curriculum might include units on self-management, working with a health care professional, and avoiding emergencies. And finally, units of study are further subdivided into **lessons**—the amount of material that can be presented during a single educational encounter, say for example the amount of material that can be presented in a one-hour class. The written outline of a lesson is referred to as a **lesson plan** and is typically comprised of three components—introduction, body, and conclusion. The introduction provides an overview of what will be covered; the body presents the health content, while the conclusion reviews what was presented. There is an old saying that summarizes these three parts that states *tell them what you are going to tell them* [introduction], *tell them it* [body], *and tell them what you told them* [conclusion]. (see **Figure 8.1** for an example lesson plan format).

The heart of any lesson is the body or the content portion of the lesson. Gagne (1985) has created a framework, called the *Nine Events of Instruction*, for designing educational experiences that provides a nice outline for creating the body of a lesson. More recently, Kinzie (2005) modified Gagne's framework for application to health promotion applications. The modified framework includes five stages instead of the original nine created by Gagne: (1) *gain attention* (convey health threats and benefits); (2) *present stimulus material* (tailor message to audience knowledge and values, demonstrate observable effectiveness, make behaviors easy to understand and do); (3) *provide guidance* (use trustworthy models to demonstrate); (4) *elicit performance and provide feedback* (to enhance *trailability*, and develop proficiency and self-efficacy); and (5) *enhance retention and transfer* (provide social support and deliver behavioral cues)

Title of Program: _____ Title of Lesson: _____ Page ___ of ___		
Unit: _____ Lesson No.: _____		
Priority Population: _____ Length of Lesson: _____		
Resources & References	Content	Teaching Method
	Introduction:	
	Body:	
	1.	
	2.	
	3.	
	Conclusion:	
Evaluation:		

Figure 8.1 Example lesson plan format

(Kinzie, 2005). **Table 8.2** provides an example of how these five stages can be applied to a health topic.

There are many different ways of presenting health education strategies such as lecture, discussion, group work, audiovisual materials, computerized instruction, laboratory exercises, and written materials (books and periodicals). **Box 8.4** provides a more complete listing of educational activities, and Gilbert and Sawyer (2000) have provided a detailed discussion of these activities.

Health Policy/Enforcement Strategies

Health policy/enforcement strategies include executive orders, laws, ordinances, policies, position statements, regulations, and formal and informal rules. These could be classified as mandated activities or regulated activities because they are activities that are required by an administrator, board, or legislative body to guide individual or collective behavior (Schmid, Pratt, & Howze, 1995). Examples include state laws requiring the use of safety belts and motorcycle helmets or raising the taxes on cigarettes, company policy stating that there will be no smoking in corporate offices and company-owned vehicles, and a board of education adopting a position statement that it will provide only well-balanced meals in its cafeterias. "An example of an executive order is a ban on tobacco advertising on city-owned buses" (Brownson et al., 1995, p. 479).

This type of intervention strategy may be controversial. It has been criticized by some because it mandates a particular response from an individual. It takes away individual freedoms and sometimes plays on a person's pride, "pocketbook," and

Table 8.2 Application of instructional design framework to lesson a on breast cancer

Stage	Content Covered	Method of Presentation
Gain attention	• Help participants identify personal risk to breast cancer • Share benefits of doing breast self-examinations (BSE), regular breast exams by physicians, and mammograms	• Use breast cancer risk appraisal or breast cancer pretest • Present a case study of women finding a lump in the breast early
Present stimulus material		
Tailor message to knowledge and values	• Using information from risk appraisal or pretest, tailor breast cancer information	• Lecture/discussion
Demonstrate observable effectiveness	• Explain importance of early diagnosis	• Use peer educators to role-play interaction with physician
Make desired behaviors easy to understand	• Present steps in BSE and making appointment with physician and for mammogram	• Use video showing correct steps for BSE or peer educators to demonstrate on models
Provide guidance	• Have others share experiences on how exams are conducted	• Use guest speakers who perform regular BSE and radiographers who do mammograms
Elicit performance and provide feedback	• Repeat steps in BSE and let participants practice BSE	• Use breast models for practice and provide critique
Enhance retention and transfer	• Encourage participants to share information learned with others and ways to remember to act	• Lecture/discussion • Brainstorm reminder ideas • Distribute BSE shower cards that explain importance of regular action for participants to place in their bathrooms

---

Box 8.4 COMMONLY USED EDUCATIONAL STRATEGIES

A. Audiovisual materials and equipment
   1. Audiotapes, records, and CDs
   2. Bulletin, chalk, cloth, flannel, magnetic, and peg boards
   3. Charts, pictures, and posters
   4. Films and filmstrips
   5. Instructional television
   6. Opaque projector or Elmo
   7. Slides and slide projectors
   8. Transparencies, Powerpoint ® Slides, and overhead projector
   9. Video (DVDs and tapes)

B. Computer based
   1. World Wide Web
   2. Desktop Publishing

Box 8.4 CONTINUED

    3. Presentation programs
    4. Individualized learning programs
    5. Video conferencing

C. Printed educational materials
    1. Instructor-made handouts and worksheets
    2. Pamphlets
    3. Study guides (commercial and instructor-made)
    4. Text and reference books
    5. Workbooks

D. Teaching strategies and techniques for the classroom
    1. Brainstorming
    2. Case studies
    3. Cooperative learning
    4. Debates
    5. Demonstrations and experiments
    6. Discovery or guided discovery
    7. Discussion
    8. Group discussion
    9. Guest speakers
    10. Lecture
    11. Lecture/discussion
    12. Newspaper and magazine articles
    13. Panel discussions
    14. Peer group teaching/coaching
    15. Poems, songs, and stories
    16. Problem solving
    17. Puppets
    18. Questioning
    19. Role playing and plays
    20. Simulation, games, and puzzles
    21. Tutoring
    22. Values clarification activities

E. Teaching strategies and techniques for outside of the classroom
    1. Community resources
    2. Field trips
    3. Health fairs
    4. Health museums
    5. Health education centers

psyche. This type of strategy must be sold on the basis of "common good." That is, the justification for this type of societal action is to protect the public's health. Health policy/enforcement strategies exist for the protection of the community and of individual rights.

Officials are willing to intercede into the private activities and lives of people in order to protect the larger population. When such intervention occurs it is usually very narrow and very specifically defined. There also tend to be sanctions attached if people do not comply. For example, in the case of inoculations, if a mother and father did not have their child inoculated that child cannot attend school. If parents do not send their child to school they are in violation of the law, and there are criminal and civil penalties that are involved (Rich & Sugrue, 1989, p. 33).

Some would say that health policy/enforcement strategies do not allow for the "voluntary behavior conducive to health" that are suggested by Green and Kreuter (2005, p. G-4) in their definition of health education. But, at the same time, this kind of activity can get people to change their behavior when other strategies have failed. For example, before the passage of safety belt laws, most states were reporting about a 14% use rate by drivers of automobiles and were trying to attack the problem through communication strategies using the mass media. Now that safety belt laws are in effect in states, usage rates in those states are closer to 75%; in some states where there is strict enforcement, usage rates approach 90%. Another example is the work of Sorensen and colleagues (1991), which showed a 21% reduction in the number of employees who smoked in a company that put a nonsmoking policy in effect. Both of these examples show that health policy/enforcement strategies are necessary to reinforce and support prevention messages.

Since health policy/enforcement strategies are often mandatory, it is particularly important to use good judgment and show respect for others when implementing them. In some instances, planners will be faced with ethical decisions. Also, if a program uses health policy/enforcement strategies, the planner should remember that, as in any political process, there are likely to be both pro and con feelings toward the "mandatory" action. Thus when developing and implementing any mandatory action, planners should bear in mind the following points:

1. Have top-level support for the mandated action (Emont & Cummings, 1989; Mikanowicz & Altman, 1995).

2. Have a representative group (committee) from the priority population help formulate the "mandatory" action.

3. Consider surveying those in the priority population to gain additional information regarding policy change (Mikanowicz & Altman, 1995).

4. Make sure expert advice on the subject of the mandated action is available to the group developing it.

5. Seek a legal opinion if necessary.

6. Examine the work of others and review the issues they faced when implementing "mandatory" actions.

7. Be sure that health policy/enforcement strategies are based on sound principles and, if possible, good research.

8. Seek input and debate/discussion concerning the mandated action from the priority population while it is being formulated.

9. Develop health policy/enforcement strategies that are written simply and include a rationale, a general policy statement, specific areas affected, and clearly defined complaint, grievance, and enforcement procedures (Mikanowicz & Altman, 1995).

10. Consider phasing in the new regulation a little bit at a time. For example, if a no-smoking policy is going to be implemented, the planner may want to begin by restricting smoking in certain areas before banning it altogether. This not only helps people change gradually but it also expresses concern for them.

11. Provide education and behavior change programs to assist those in the priority population with the implementation of the "mandatory" actions (Mikanowicz & Altman, 1995).

12. Ensure that, once formulated, the "mandatory" actions
    a. are actively communicated to those in the priority population.
    b. are reviewed on a regular basis for the purposes of evaluating and revising if necessary.
    c. apply to all in the priority population and not just to select groups.
    d. are consistently enforced. Be prepared to deal with the complaint and grievance processes (Mikanowicz & Altman, 1995).
    e. are enforced as a shared responsibility of all in the institution.

Environmental Change Strategies

Another group of strategies that have proved useful in reaching desired outcomes is the category of environmental change strategies. Environmental change strategies are those designed to change the structure or types of services, or systems of care, to improve the delivery of health promotion services (CDC, 2003). Examples of such strategies include equipping automobiles with safety belts, air bags, and child safety seats, placing speed bumps in parking lots by playgrounds to slow traffic where children are present, or installing fire and safety doors in apartment buildings to make them safer for the residents. These strategies are characterized by changes in those things "around" individuals that may influence their awareness, knowledge, attitudes, skills, or behavior. Often environmental change strategies do not necessarily require action on the part of the priority population (CDC, 2003) as noted in the examples above. Yet, some of these strategies provide a "forced choice" situation, as when the selection of foods and beverages in vending machines or cafeterias are changed to include only "healthy" foods. If people want to eat foods from these places, they are forced to eat certain types of foods. French and colleagues (1997) used a similar idea to the forced choice idea when they lowered the price by 50% on low-fat snacks in vending machines to try to influence food choices.

Other activities in this category may provide those in the priority population with health messages and environmental cues for certain types of behavior. Examples would be posting of no-smoking signs, eliminating ashtrays, providing lockers and showers, using role modeling by others, playing soft music in a work area, organizing a shuttle service or some other type of transportation system to get seniors to congregate for meals or to a health care provider, and providing point-of-purchase education, such as a sign on a vending machine or food labeling on the food options in the cafeteria.

Finally, like so many of the other intervention strategies, environmental change strategies often are more effective when combined (i.e., multiplicity) with intervention strategies from the other categories. For example, the inclusion of safety belts in automobiles is important but when combined with strict enforcement of safety belt laws (a health policy/enforcement strategy), it makes for a much more effective intervention.

Health-Related Community Service Strategies

Health-related community service strategies include things such as services, tests, or treatments to improve the health of those in the priority population (CDC, 2003). Examples of this type of intervention strategy include, but are not limited to, completing a health risk assessment (HRA) form (see Chapter 4 for a discussion of HRAs), offering low-cost flu shots or child immunizations, providing clinical screenings (sometimes called biometric screenings) for diabetes, blood pressure, or cholesterol, and providing professional health check-ups and examinations. Because a health-related community service strategy requires action on the part of those in the priority population, an important component of this type of strategy is to reduce the barriers to obtaining the service. Thus planners must be mindful of the affordability and accessibility of such services. Also, planners must weigh the consequences of including this type of strategy in an intervention. For example, if abnormal readings are found during a screening, those conducting the screening have an ethical obligation to follow up and make sure appropriate referrals for care are made. Chapman (2003a) has provided a nice review of many of the concerns associated with biometric screening.

Health-related community service strategies are often offered in settings such as grocery stores, shopping malls, health fairs, worksites, personal residencies, mobile units (e.g., vans equipped with mammography units), and easily accessible health care facilities. Such strategies usually have high credibility with priority populations because of their link with health care providers.

Community Mobilization Strategies

"Community mobilization strategies involve helping communities identify and take action on shared concerns using participatory decision making, and include such methods as empowerment" (Barnes, Neiger, & Thackeray, 2003, p. 60). In this book we present two subcategories of community mobilization strategies: (1) community organization and community building, and (2) community advocacy.

Community Organization and Community Building   Other than defining the terms *community organization* and *community building*, little will be presented here about these terms because all of Chapter 9 is dedicated to the discussion of these processes. **Community organization** has been defined as "the process by which community groups are helped to identify common problems or goals, mobilize resources, and in other ways develop and implement strategies for reaching the goals they have collectively set" (Minkler & Wallerstein, 2005, p. 26). **Community building** is not so much a process but rather "an orientation to community that is strength based rather than need based and stresses the identification, nurturing, and celebration of community assets" (Minkler, 2005a, p. 4).

Community Advocacy Community advocacy is a process in which the people of the community become involved in the institutions and decisions that will have an impact on their lives. It has the potential for creating more support, keeping people informed, influencing decisions, activating nonparticipants, improving service, and making people, plans, and programs more responsive (Checkoway, 1989). Community advocacy can have a big impact on social change issues, including those dealing with health. The community advocacy that deals with health issues is called **health advocacy**. This type of advocacy has been defined as "the processes by which the actions of individuals or groups attempt to bring about social and/or organizational change on behalf of a particular health goal, program, interest, or population" (Joint Committee on Terminology, 2001, p. 7). Galer-Unti, Tappe and Lachenmayr (2004) have identified several different ways of advocating for health and health education. They include: (1) voting behavior, (2) electioneering, (3) direct lobbying, (4) integrate grassroots lobbying into direct lobbying efforts, (5) use of the Internet, (6) media advocacy—newspaper letters to the editor and opinion-editorial (op-ed) articles, and (7) media advocacy—acting as a resource person. They have further presented these seven advocacy strategies in a three-tiered approach to show the varying levels of involvement in the advocacy process. These levels and examples of each are presented in **Table 8.3**.

Table 8.3 Advocacy strategies: good, better, best

Strategy	Good	Better	Best
Voting behavior	Register and vote	Encourage others to register and vote	Register others to vote
Electioneering	Contribute to the campaign of a candidate friendly to public health and health education	Campaign for a candidate friendly to public health and health education	Run for office or seek a political appointment
Direct lobbying	Contact a policy maker	Meet with your policy makers	Develop ongoing relationships with your policy makers and their staff
Integrate grassroots lobbying into direct lobbying activities	Start a petition drive to advocate a specific policy in your local community	Get on the agenda for a meeting of a policy-making body and provide testimony	Organize a community coalition to enact changes that influence health
Use the Internet	Use the Internet to access information related to health issues	Build a Web page that calls attention to a specific health issue, policy, or legislative proposal	Teach others to use the Internet for advocacy activities
Media advocacy: Newspaper letters to the editor and op-ed articles	Write a letter to the editor	Write an op-ed piece	Teach others to write letters and op-ed pieces for media advocacy
Media advocacy: Acting as a resource person	Respond to requests by members of the media for health-related information	Issue a news release	Develop and maintain ongoing relationships with the media personnel

Source: R. A. Galer-Unti et al., "Advocacy 100: Getting started in health education advocacy," *Health Promotion Practice,* 5(3), pp. 283–288, 2004. Copyright © 2004, Society for Public Health Education. Reprinted by permission of Sage Publications.

Auld (1997) offered a set of practical tips for influencing public policy. They are adapted here to apply to influencing public policy at the local as well as the state and federal levels.

1. *Opening doors.* Establish relationships that build trust and rapport with staff, legislative assistants, and, if possible, the elected officials themselves so that you can approach them for their support on an issue of concern. Know what committees your elected officials sit on and how they have voted on the issues.

2. *Identifying the players.* Identify who the stakeholders are on a particular issue and find out why they are.

3. *Making the link.* Find out how the issues you are interested in are linked to the health problems of the population/constituency of the elected officials. For example, if you are interested in chronic diseases, show how they are linked to the elderly in the population/constituency.

4. *Crafting your position.* Make sure your position on the issue(s) is (are) developed on the best available science and data.

5. *Organizing the troops.* Organize others who may be interested in your issue to show broad representation from the population/constituency (see Chapter 9 for organizing techniques).

6. *Visiting policymakers.* Schedule appointments with the elected official or staff to express your views on the issues. Take others with you who can help explain your views. Be on time, be brief, yet be prepared to educate by using practical examples.

7. *Demonstrating the power of press.* Demonstrate your link to the media and how you and your organization can get positive press for the elected official by activating (i.e., letters to the editor, etc.) your link.

8. *Reinforcing your message.* End your visit or follow up the visit with a packet that summarizes your position on the issues. Supporting scientific data should be included. Also, send a thank you letter. As the issue moves through the legislative process, let your elected official know your views on its direction.

9. *Serving as a resource.* Stay in contact with the staff and elected official and offer to be a resource person to help them as needed on the issue.

10. *Responding quickly.* Be prepared to respond quickly when asked to be a resource person or testify to a legislative group. Requests often come at the last minute.

11. *Reaching the finish line.* Follow up on a piece of legislation after it has been passed to help those who have to implement it and to advocate for funding to help the implementation.

To further assist planners with community advocacy activities, the Coalition of National Health Education Organizations (CNHEO) maintains a website for advocacy information. The website features advocacy alerts, how to take action, health legislation, links to other advocacy sites, and other policy tools for health education and health promotion (CNHEO, 2007). (See the *Weblinks* at the end of this chapter for more information about the site).

Other Strategies

The "Other Strategies" category includes a variety of intervention activities that do not fit neatly into one of the six categories noted above.

Behavior Modification Activities   Behavior modification activities, often used in intrapersonal-level interventions, include techniques intended to help those in the priority population experience a change in behavior. *Behavior modification* is usually thought of as a systematic procedure for changing a specific behavior. The process is based on the stimulus response and social cognitive theories. As applied to health behavior, emphasis is placed on a specific behavior that one might want either to increase (such as exercise or stress management techniques) or to decrease (such as smoking or consumption of fats). Particular attention is then given to changing the events that are antecedent or subsequent to the behavior that is to be modified.

In changing a health behavior, the behavior modification activity often begins by having those in the priority population keep records (diaries, logs, or journals) for a specific period of time (24 to 48 hours, one week, or one month) concerning the behavior (such as eating, smoking, or exercise) they want to alter. Using the information recorded, one can plan an activity to modify that behavior. For example, facilitators of smoking cessation programs often will ask participants to keep a record of all the cigarettes they smoke from one class session to the next (see **Figure 8.2** for an example of such a record). After keeping the record, participants are asked to analyze it to see what kind of smoking habit they have. They may be asked questions such as: "What three cigarettes seem to be the most important of the day to you?" "In what three places or activities do you find yourself smoking the most?" "With whom do you find yourself smoking most often?" "Is there a primary reason or mood for your smoking?" "When during the day do you find yourself smoking the most and the least?" Once the participant has answered these questions, appropriate interventions can be designed to deal with the problem behavior. For example, if participants say they smoke only when they are by themselves, then activities would be planned so that they do not spend a lot of time alone. If other participants seem to do most of their smoking while drinking coffee, an activity would be developed to provide some type of substitute. If participants seem to smoke the most while sitting at the table after meals, activities could be planned to get them away from the dinner table and doing something that would occupy their hands.

Another way of leading into a behavior modification activity is through a health status evaluation, or what is often referred to as a *health screening*. Such screenings could happen at home (e.g., BSE, TSE, hemocult), at a community health fair (e.g., blood pressure, cholesterol), or in the office of a health care professional (e.g., breast examination). Like record keeping via diaries, logs, or journals, health screenings can "grab the attention" (develop awareness) of those in the priority population to begin the behavior modification process.

Organizational Culture Activities   Closely aligned with environmental change strategies are activities that affect organizational culture. Culture is usually associated with norms and traditions that are generated by and linked to a "community" of people. Organizations,

Name _____

Date _____

Number of Cigarettes During the Day	Time of Day	Need Rating*	Place of Activity	With Whom	Mood or Reason
1.	_____	1 2 3	_____	_____	_____
2.	_____	1 2 3	_____	_____	_____
3.	_____	1 2 3	_____	_____	_____
4.	_____	1 2 3	_____	_____	_____
5.	_____	1 2 3	_____	_____	_____
6.	_____	1 2 3	_____	_____	_____
7.	_____	1 2 3	_____	_____	_____
8.	_____	1 2 3	_____	_____	_____
9.	_____	1 2 3	_____	_____	_____
10.	_____	1 2 3	_____	_____	_____
11.	_____	1 2 3	_____	_____	_____
12.	_____	1 2 3	_____	_____	_____
13.	_____	1 2 3	_____	_____	_____
14.	_____	1 2 3	_____	_____	_____
15.	_____	1 2 3	_____	_____	_____
16.	_____	1 2 3	_____	_____	_____
17.	_____	1 2 3	_____	_____	_____
18.	_____	1 2 3	_____	_____	_____
19.	_____	1 2 3	_____	_____	_____
20.	_____	1 2 3	_____	_____	_____
21.	_____	1 2 3	_____	_____	_____
22.	_____	1 2 3	_____	_____	_____
23.	_____	1 2 3	_____	_____	_____
24.	_____	1 2 3	_____	_____	_____
25.	_____	1 2 3	_____	_____	_____
26.	_____	1 2 3	_____	_____	_____
27.	_____	1 2 3	_____	_____	_____
28.	_____	1 2 3	_____	_____	_____
29.	_____	1 2 3	_____	_____	_____
30.	_____	1 2 3	_____	_____	_____

*Need rating: How important is the cigarette to you at this time?

    1 = Most important; I would miss it very much

    2 = Average

    3 = Least important; I would not miss it

Figure 8.2 Twenty-four-hour cigarette count

which are made up of people, also can have their own culture. The culture of an organization can be thought of as its personality. The culture expresses what is and what is not considered important to the organization. The nature of the culture depends on the type of organization—corporation, school, or nonprofit group.

Many people think that it takes a long time to establish norms and traditions, and it often does. Still, change can occur very quickly if the decision makers in an organization support it. For example, if organizational decision makers believe exercise is important, they may provide employees with an extra 20 minutes at lunchtime for exercise. Similarly, it is surprising to see how many young executives will use a corporation's exercise facility because the chief executive officer does. Other examples of organizational culture activities might include changing the types of foods found in vending machines, closing the "junk food" machines during lunch periods at school, offering discounts on the health foods found in the company cafeteria, and getting retailers to change the way they have done things in the past, such as moving their tobacco products from in front of a counter to behind a counter, so that an employee has to get them for the customer. Because these activities affect groups of people, they are usually used at the organizational or institutional level.

Incentives and Disincentives   The use of incentives and disincentives to influence health behaviors is a common type of activity, especially in worksite settings. An **incentive** is "an anticipated positive or desirable reward designed to influence the performance of an individual or group" (Chapman, 2005, p. 6). An incentive can increase the perceived value of an activity (Patton et al., 1986), motivate people to get involved, encourage health service use behavior (Chapman, 2005), encourage compliance with professional health advice (Chapman, 2005), and remind program participants of their commitment to and goals for behavior change (Wilbur, 1983). The key to motivating someone with an incentive is to know what will incite an individual to action. Thus for this type of activity to work, the planners need to match the incentives with the needs, wants, or desires of the priority population. However, this is not easy, for what is an incentive for one person may be a deterrent for another, and vice versa. If planners are not in touch with what program participants want, there is a chance of losing participant interest in the program (Hunnicutt, 2001). It has been suggested that incentives should even be tailored to the socioeconomic characteristics of the participants (Chenoweth, 1987) and, for that matter, the individual characteristics of each person.

For the planners, the task becomes one of matching the needs of the program participant or potential program participant with available incentives. Two approaches have been used to accomplish this. The first is to include questions about incentives as part of any needs assessment conducted in program planning. For example, a workforce needs survey might include a question on incentives, such as "What incentives would entice you to participate in the exercise program?" or "What would it take to get you to participate in this program?" or "What would it take to keep you involved in a health promotion program?" or "Would you continue to participate in an exercise program if you knew you were going to be given a nice tee shirt after logging 100 miles running or walking, or participating for 50 days in an aerobic dance or swimming program?" The responses to these questions should provide some indication of the type of incentives that would be most useful for this priority population. The second is the shotgun approach, based on previous experience or the experience reported by others. The shot-gun approach offers a variety of incentives to meet the needs of a large percentage of the program's priority population. However, the former approach is recommended as being more likely to meet the targeted needs and wants.

Based on the idea that incentives should meet the individual needs of the priority population, the number of different types of incentives is almost endless. Feldman (1983) suggests two major categories of incentives or reinforcers. The first group includes incentives that would be considered social reinforcers or intangible incentives; the second group includes incentives that are considered material reinforcers, or what may be referred to as tangible incentives (see **Figure 8.3**).

I. Social Reinforcers (Intangible Incentives)
  A. Special attention or recognition from instructors, peers, classmates, co-workers, or chief executive officers (Feldman, 1983; Shepard, 1985; Chapman, 2005)
  B. Praise/verbal reinforcement (Feldman, 1983; Shepard, 1985)
  C. Public and other recognition (i.e., name in newsletter, name on bulletin board) (Koffman et al., 1998)
  D. Encouragement (Feldman, 1983; Shepard, 1985)
  E. Friendship (Feldman, 1983; Shepard, 1985) and belonging (Chapman, 2005)
  F. Inclusion of family members in the program (Feldman, 1983; Shepard, 1985)
  G. Personal letter to those reaching goals (Bensley, 1991)
II. Material Reinforcers (Tangible Incentives)
  A. Inexpensive "token" incentives
    1. T-shirts, hats, caps, visors, warm-up jackets, calendars, key chains, flashlights, pens, windshield scrapers, wallets, tape measures, vacuum and water bottles, mugs, home fire extinguishers, smoke detectors, and auto safety kits (Cinelli, Rose-Colley, & Hayes, 1988; Kendall, 1984)
    2. Certificates
    3. Pins, buttons, patches, and decals that can be worn and plaques or markers that can be displayed in the work area
    4. Towels, lockers
    5. Preferred or free parking
  B. Program cost sharing between employer and employee
    1. Cost of registering for a program (Pollock et al., 1982)
    2. Membership at a fitness center/club (Chapman, 2005)
    3. Sliding-scale fee based on the ability to pay
    4. Refund of part or all of program fee based on participant's completion of an intervention
    5. Money to be used as an incentive (Koffman et al., 1998; Chapman, 2005)
  C. Health Insurance
    1. Sharing between employer and employee of money saved on health insurance from one year to the next (Toufexis, 1985)
    2. Employer picking up more of the insurance costs or reducing the deductible to reward good health practices or program participation (Harris, 2003; Chapman, 2005)
    3. Provision of a fund for each employee to pay for the person's health care costs during the year, with any unused money from this account given to the employee at the end of the year (Hosokawa, 1984; Toufexis, 1985)

Figure 8.3 Incentives: Social and material reinforcers

D. Monetary
  1. Tokens, Monopoly-style dollars, stamps, coupons, or points that are redeemable at a company store or a retail store, or for catalog shopping for prizes or merchandise (Kendall, 1984; Piniat, 1984; Toufexis, 1985)
  2. Drawings, lotteries, and raffles open to those who have participated or met a goal (Cinelli et al., 1988; Emont & Cummings, 1992; Health Insurance Association of America, 1983; Toufexis, 1985)
  3. Bonus, extra pay, rebates, or just plain pay for completion of contract, or participation (DiBlase, 1985; Pescatello et al., 2001; Poole, Kumpfer, & Pett, 2001; Toufexis, 1985)
  4. Financial rewards for both individuals and groups who have fewer and/or no work accidents during the year (DiBlase, 1985)
  5. "Well pay" for unused sick days (DiBlase, 1985)
  6. Gift certificates, from a small value, such as for a free ice cream cone, to something of greater value, such as a U.S. savings bond (Kendall, 1984)
  7. Registration fee refund for completing a program (Pescatello et al., 2001; Chapman, 2005)
  8. Retail store gift card for completing a health risk appraisal (B. Neilson Hahn, personal communication, October 17, 2003)
E. Work Hours
  1. Flex-time (flexible work hours) in order to participate
  2. Released time to participate
  3. Time off (Cinelli et al., 1988), well days (Chapman, 2005)
  4. Additional sick or vacation days (Chapman, 2005)
F. Contracts
  1. Contract (competition) with a buddy
  2. Contract with instructor to reach a specific goal, with a material incentive provided by instructor
  3. Forfeiture of money or time to charity for not fulfilling a contract (Bloomquist, 1981)
  4. Contract is entered into with the instructor in which money is withheld (via payroll deduction) while the person is enrolled in the program, so that if goal is met, the money is refunded; if not, it is forfeited (Bensley, 1991; Forster et al., 1985)
III. Miscellaneous
  A. Special medical examinations and screenings for those who participate
  B. Special events, such as contests or luncheons (Kendall, 1984; Patton et al., 1986)
  C. Providing special "space," such as a table in the lunchroom for those on a special diet (Bensley, 1991)
  D. Lottery opportunities for airplane tickets (Chapman, 2005)
  E. Special privilege or service (i.e., special parking spot)

Figure 8.3 (*continued*)

The following advice is offered to planners who choose to use incentives:

1. Make sure everyone can receive one, whatever the incentive may be (Kendall, 1984).

2. Make the incentives useful and meaningful (Kendall, 1984).

3. Ensure that the incentive ground rules are fair, understandable, and followed by everyone (Kendall, 1984; Chapman 2005).

4. Develop (and refine) a communications plan for the incentives (Chapman, 2005).

5. Make a big deal of awarding the incentive; consider a special meeting or ceremony (Hunnicutt, 2001).

6. Use incentives that are consistent with health promotion philosophies. For example, avoid incentives of alcoholic beverages, high fat or high sugar foods, or other mixed-message prizes.

As a final comment on incentives, several authors (French, Jeffery, & Oliphant, 1994; Jeffery et al., 1993; Matson, Lee, & Hopp, 1993; Price et al., 1992; Robison, 1998) have reported on the effectiveness of using incentives for program participation and behavior change. From these works, it appears that incentives are useful in getting people to participate and change their behavior for a short period of time. Also, more recent studies (Pescatello et al., 2001; Poole, Kumpfer, & Pett, 2001) have shown that incentives have also been useful in changing and maintaining health behavior change over time.

Just as incentives can be used to get people involved in behavior change, **disincentives** can be used to discourage a certain behavior. More formally, disincentives have been defined as "an anticipated negative or undesirable consequence designed to influence the performance of an individual or group" (Chapman, 2005, p. 6). For example, Penner (1989) reports on the use of a surcharge for health insurance to influence the behavior of those who continue to use tobacco products. Another example would be not allowing the use of something because of a certain behavior, such as not allowing employees who smoke to use the employee lounge or company vehicles.

Up to this point, our discussion of incentives and disincentives has been mostly aimed at the intrapersonal, interpersonal, and institutional/organizational levels of influence. However, incentives and disincentives have also been effective when incorporated into the community and public policy levels of influence. "Sustained increases in excise taxes, constraining advertising and marketing, constricting use in public places, and penalizing the sale and distribution to minors have all worked to help drive down the use of tobacco" (McGinnis et al., 2002, pp. 88–89). State legislation to raise the tobacco tax provides a good example of this. Other forms of using incentives and disincentives at the community and public policy levels could include advertising the identity of restaurants in violation of food safety protocols, grants-in-aid to encourage communities to develop bike paths, and economic incentives to encourage health care providers to take a broader perspective for keeping people healthy such as reimbursement for brief interventions to assist smokers to quit or nonexercisers to exercise (McGinnis et al., 2002).

One final note that we need to mention before leaving the topic of incentives and disincentives is the impact that federal legislation has had on incentives and disincentives. As we noted at the beginning of this section, though incentives and disincentives have been used in health promotion programs in a variety of settings, they have been used with great favor in worksite settings. Up until 1996, there were few limitations on how incentive and disincentives were structured (Chapman, 2005) and because of this some employers were creatively tying incentives and disincentives associated with health to individual and group health insurance plans. However, Congress was concerned that employers were being unfair to some employees in order to reduce their health care cost. Thus, with the passage of the Health Insurance Portability & Accountability Act of 1996 (more commonly referred to as HIPAA), new regulations were placed on how incentives and disincentives could be used (Powell & Frank, 2002). More specifically, the legislation has provisions in it that make it illegal for employers to discriminate against their employees because of a "health status related factor" with the outcome of affecting coverage or cost to the employee under a group or individual health plan (Chapman, 2005). That is, those who offer and administer health insurance plans cannot deny health care claim expenses, charge some employees more for their health insurance premiums, or place a surcharge on their premiums because of health status related conditions like high blood pressure, high blood cholesterol, or poor vision. For example, an employer cannot require employees to pay higher premiums than their co-workers because they have high blood pressure. However, the law does not preclude offering incentives—in the form of premium discounts or rebates or modifying applicable co-payments or deductibles—to those who participate in health promotion programs. So an employer could reduce employees' co-payment on a visit to a doctor or on the cost of a prescription medication if the employees participated in the company's employee health promotion program.

Social Activities   The importance of social support for behavior change and its relationship to health have been noted by several researchers (Becker & Green, 1975; Berkman & Syme, 1979; Cohen & Lichtenstein, 1990; Colletti & Brownell, 1982; Horman, 1989; IOM, 2001; Kviz et al., 1994; Kaplan & Cassel, 1977; Cummings, Becker, & Maile, 1980). Many people find it much easier to change a behavior if those around them provide support or are willing to be partners in the behavior change process. One of the major reasons why worksite health promotion programs have been so well received is because of the built-in social support from co-workers (Behrens, 1983).

Reference has already been made to how social support could work as an incentive. That would be one form of a social activity. Other social interventions could include support groups or buddy system, social gatherings, and social networks.

Support Groups and Buddy System.   The importance of support groups as part of comprehensive interventions has been well established. One need only look to the 12-step programs (such as Alcoholics Anonymous, Overeaters Anonymous, and Gamblers Anonymous) and commercial programs (such as Weight Watchers) to realize the importance of people coming together to share their experiences and support one another's efforts. A support group need not be large; it might be as small as just two people. A buddy system is an example of a two-person group. A buddy system can take one of two different forms. In the first, both individuals are trying to change a behavior. In such a relationship, the two individuals support each other, whether this means helping each other stay on a special diet or meeting each other at 6 A.M. for exercise. In the other form, only one of the two is trying to change a behavior. The one not changing the behavior may have already changed (e.g., has already quit smoking or is exercising regularly) and is acting as a mentor to the one trying to change, or may not be trying to change but provides support at regular intervals or as problems arise.

Special elements that can be added to the support group or buddy system are the use of contest or a contract. Contest can take place among individual group members over such things as who can lose the most weight, who can walk/run the most miles, or who can go the longest without a cigarette. Contest could also be based on teams within the priority population (such as two different companies, two schools, or departments within an organization), using similar criteria but now based on group total figures (pounds, miles, or cigarettes). See Chapter 11 for more on contests.

Contracts could be used by having one member of the priority population enter into an agreement with another member or with another person (such as the program facilitator, a friend, or spouse) over a change in some health behavior. The major component of a contract is the contingency. The *contingency* is a statement of what will happen if a contract is met or not met. For example, if a person meets the terms of his contract by losing 10 pounds in 5 weeks, he can then expect to receive something specified (an intangible, such as praise, or a material object) from the person who agreed to the contract. If the terms are not met, then the person for whom the contract was written must forfeit something specified (perhaps time volunteered to a community service or a material object of his own). See Chapter 11 for more on contracts.

Social Gatherings. Social gatherings can be an important type of social intervention. Bringing together people who may be confronting similar problems for the purpose of purely social interaction not related to the problem can indirectly help them deal with the problem. Examples of such activities might be single parents having a cookout or a group of senior citizens attending a play. Although these gatherings do not deal directly with these people's common problems, they do help fill voids in their lives and thus indirectly help with the problem.

Social Networks. Social networks are another type of social intervention. A *network* "is the web of social relationships that surround an individual and the structural characteristics of that web" (IOM, 2001, p. 145). The nature of the structural characteristics can be quite varied, consisting of almost anything that creates a special feeling: need, concern, loyalty, frustration, power, affection, or obligation, to name just a few. When people are "networking," they are said to be looking for relationships that would be useful in helping them with their concerns, such as problem solving, program development, resource identification, and others. As part of a health promotion intervention, social networking may take the form of having program participants trade telephone numbers for the purpose of calling each other when they are trying to resist smoking a cigarette or trying to locate a needed resource to solve a problem.

It should also be noted that although most social support and buddy systems take place between individuals, they can also be established at the institutional level. Like individuals, institutions can be paired up to help one another. For example, if two companies are interested in establishing health promotion programs, they could work together on their programs and share information and resources where appropriate. Or, if one company has a well-established program in place, then that company could "mentor" another company in setting up a program.

Creating Health Promotion Interventions

Once program planners have completed a needs assessment, written program goals and objectives, and considered different types of intervention strategies, they are in a position to begin designing an appropriate intervention.

Criteria and Guidelines for Developing Health Promotion Interventions

There is no one best way of intervening to accomplish a specific program goal that can be generalized to all priority populations. Each priority population has its own needs and wants that must be addressed. Nevertheless, successful and responsible health promotion programs generally adhere to some common set of guidelines, standards, or criteria around which their interventions are planned (Ad Hoc Work Group, 1987). Such guidelines help standardize and ensure the quality of the program, give credibility to a program, help with program accountability, provide a legal defense if a liability situation might arise, and identify ethical concerns that need to be addressed as a part of planning, implementing, and evaluating programs.

In 1987, the American Public Health Association (APHA), in collaboration with the Center for Health Promotion and Education of the Centers for Disease Control (CDC), developed a set of criteria to serve as guidelines for establishing the feasibility and/or the appropriateness of health promotion programs in a variety of settings (industrial, hospital, worksite, voluntary and official agencies) before making a decision to implement them. The criteria were not developed to assure successful programs, but rather to suggest issues that need to be considered in the decision-making process leading to the allocation of resources or the setting of program priorities (Ad Hoc Work Group, 1987, pp. 89–92). The five criteria suggested by the Work Group are:

1. A health promotion program should address one or more risk factors that are carefully defined, measurable, modifiable, and prevalent among the members of a chosen target group, and these factors that constitute a threat to the health status and the quality of life of target group members.

2. A health promotion program should reflect a consideration of the special characteristics, needs, and preferences of its target group(s).

3. Health promotion programs should include interventions that will clearly and effectively reduce a target risk factor and are appropriate for a particular setting.

4. A health promotion program should identify and implement interventions that make optimum use of the available resources.

5. From the outset, a health promotion program should be organized, planned, and implemented in such a way that its operation and effects can be evaluated.

In addition to the criteria set forth by APHA and CDC, other agencies and organizations have suggested criteria and guidelines. The Society of Prospective Medicine has developed the Ethics Guidelines for the Development and Use of Health Assessments (SPMBoD, 1999). Some organizations and professionals have set guidelines, criteria, or **codes of practice** for specific types of health promotion programs. Examples are the criteria set forth by the American College of Sports Medicine (ACSM, 2005) for exercise programs, the guidelines established by the American College of Obstetricians and Gynecologists for exercise during pregnancy, and the clinical practice guidelines for smoking cessation available from the Agency for Healthcare Research and Quality (AHRQ, 2006), as well as those by Bartlett and colleagues (1986). Obviously, these guidelines and criteria are not all that are available. Prudent planners should seek out, through inquiry and networking, other criteria and guidelines that apply to programs they are planning.

Designing Appropriate Interventions

Selection of interventions for a health promotion program should be based on a sound rationale as opposed to chance; a strategy should not be selected just because the planners think it "sounds good" or because they have a "feeling" that it will work. As mentioned earlier, planners should choose an intervention that will be both effective and efficient. Although no prescription for an appropriate intervention has been developed, experience has indicated that the results of some interventions are more predictable than others. In this section, we present eight major questions that planners need to consider when creating health promotion interventions. **Figure 8.4** summarizes these major considerations.

1. **What needs to change?** Designing an appropriate intervention begins by going back to the early steps in the program planning process and examining the results of the needs assessment and reviewing the goals and objectives of the proposed program. The needs assessment identified the behavioral, environmental, and genetic determinants or risk factors of the health problem. [Note: A reminder that because genetic determinants either cannot be changed or often interact with behavior and environment, the planners' focus should be on behavioral and environmental factors.] After the determinants of the health problem were identified, planners then determined the predisposing, enabling, and reinforcing factors that needed to be addressed in the

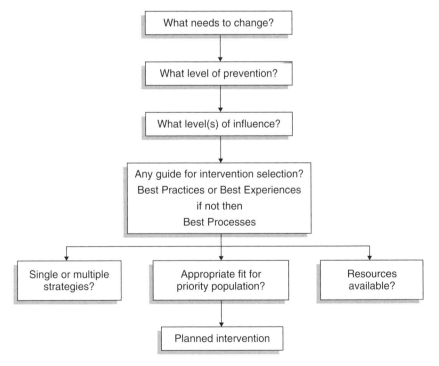

Figure 8.4 Items to consider when creating a health promotion intervention

proposed program. These factors should be reflected in the program goals and objectives. If the single purpose of a program were to increase the awareness of the priority population, the intervention would be very different from what it would be if the purpose were to change behavior.

2. **At what level of prevention will the program be aimed?** Because of the needs and wants of those in the priority population, planners need to consider at which level or levels of prevention—primary, secondary, and tertiary—the program will be aimed. For example, a program aimed at increasing the level of exercise is likely to be received differently by asymtomatic nonexercisers (primary prevention) than by a patient recovering from a heart attack (tertiary prevention).

3. **At what level(s) of influence will the intervention be focused?** Program planners must recognize that those in the priority population "live in social, political, and economic systems that shape behaviors and access to the resources they need to maintain good health" (Pellmar, Brandt, & Baird, 2002, p. 210). As such, planners need to decide at what level or levels of influence they can best obtain the goals and objectives of the program. For example, if the goal of the program is to increase safety belt use, can that best be accomplished by trying to intervene at an intrapersonal level with an individual education program, at the institutional level with a company policy, or at the public policy level with a enhanced state safety belt law?

4. **What types of intervention strategies are known to be effective (i.e., have been successfully used in previous programs) in dealing with the program focus?** Green and Kreuter (2005) have suggested three sources of guidance for selecting intervention strategies—*best practices*, *best experiences*, and *best processes*. **Best practices** refer to "recommendations for an intervention, based on critical review of multiple research and evaluation studies that substantiate the efficacy of the intervention in the populations and circumstances in which the studies were done, if not its effectiveness in other populations and situations where it might be implemented" (p. G-1). Examples of best practices related to health promotion programs are provided in the *Guide to Community Preventive Services* (Zara et al., 2005). A discussion of this document is provided in Chapter 3.

When *best practice* recommendations are not available for use, planners need to look for information on best experiences. **Best experience** intervention strategies are those of prior or existing programs that have not gone through the critical research and evaluation studies and thus fall short of best practice criteria but nonetheless show promise in being effective. *Best experiences* can be found by networking with other professionals and by reviewing the literature.

If neither *best practices* nor *best experiences* are available to planners, then the third source of guidance for selecting an intervention strategy is using *best processes*. **Best processes** intervention strategies are original interventions that the planners create based upon their knowledge and skills of good planning processes including the involvement of those in the priority population and the theories and models presented in Chapter 7 (see **Table 8.4** for a matrix of aligning objectives, program outcomes, methods, theory, intervention strategies, and activities).

Table 8.4 Matrix of type of objectives, program outcomes, methods, theory, intervention strategy, and activities

Type of Objective	Program Outcome	Method	Theory—Construct*	Intervention Strategy	Possible Activities
Learning	• Awareness of risk perception/services/resources	Information	HBM—perceived susceptibility HAPA—motivation to change phase	Health communication	• Informational session • Completion of HRA • Brochure on risks
		Raising awareness	TTM—processes of change SCT—expectations	Health communication	
	• Knowledge	Active learning	SCT—behavioral capability HEM—perceived seriousness HBM—perceived benefits/barriers	Health education	• Classes, seminars, workshops • Printed materials
		Tailoring	HAPA—stages PAPM—stages TTM—stages	Health communication and education	• Classes, seminars, workshops
	• Attitudes	Persuasive communication Processing information	SCT—expectancies TTM—decisional balance ELM—central route TPE—attitude toward the behavior SCT—reinforcement	Health communication and education	• Classes, seminars, workshops • Panel discussions • Guest speakers
		Modeling	SCT/HBM/TTM—self-efficacy TPB—perceived behavioral control	Health communication and education	• Peer educators
	• Skills	Skills training and practice	SCT—self-control SCT—reinforcement		• Classes, seminars, workshops • Simulations
		Modeling Coping response	C-BMRP—self-control	Behavior modification	• Scenarios, role playing

(Table 8.4 continues)

Table 8.4 (continued)

Type of Objective	Program Outcome	Method	Theory—Construct*	Intervention Strategy	Possible Activities
Action/ Behavioral	• Behavior	Reinforcement	HBM—cues to action SRT—punishment/ reinforcement	Incentives Behavior modification	• Determine and provide incentives • 24-hour behavior records
		Counter conditioning	TTM—processes of change	Health communication and education Organizational culture	• keeping journals • classes, seminars, workshops
Environmental	• Physical environment	Facilitation	SCT—reciprocal determinism	Health policy/ enforcement Environmental change	• Regulations/ ordinances
		Barriers	HBM—perceived barriers C-BMRP—high-risk situation		
		Organizational building	CRM—stages	Community mobilization	• Create a coalition
	• Social environment	Social support	TPB—subjective norm	Social activities	• Create networks/ buddies

Abbreviations for theories: C-BMRP=Cognitive-Behavior Model of Relapse Prevention; CRM=Community Readiness Model; ELM=Elaboration Likelihood Model of Persuasion; HAPA=Health Action Process Approach; HBM=Health Belief Model; PAPM=Precaution Adoption Process Model; SCT=Social Cognitive Theory; SRT=Stimulus Response Theory; TPB=Theory of Planned Behavior; TTM=Transtheoretical Model.

5. **Is the intervention an appropriate fit for the priority population?** Intervention strategies need to be designed to "fit" the priority population. Each priority population has certain characteristics that impact how it will receive an intervention. It is important for planners to try to identify these characteristics in order to segment a priority population. **Segmenting** is the process of dividing a broader population into smaller groups with similar characteristics that are likely to exhibit similar behavior/reaction to an intervention (Wright, 1997) (see Box 11.3 for ways by which planners can segment the priority population). Segmentation allows planners to create an intervention to fit the needs and characteristics of a priority audience (Pasick, D'Onofrio, & Otero-Sabogal, 1996). Following are a few examples of how priority population segmentation can be applied. If program planners are developing written materials as part of their intervention, they need to make sure that the materials are written at an acceptable reading level for the priority population. From a developmental stage perspective, it is not reasonable to expect kindergartners to sit still for a one-hour lesson. Interventions also need to "fit" culturally within the priority population (Huff & Kline, 1999; LeMaster & Connell, 1994; Luquis & Perez, 2003; Pahnos, 1992) and be culturally sensitive. Cultural-sensitive interventions are those "that are relevant and acceptable within the cultural framework of the population to be reached" (Frankish, Lovato, & Shannon, 1998).

   If an intervention activity is created specifically for an individual's needs, interests, and circumstances, it is referred to as a **tailored** activity. The rationale for tailoring an intervention activity is based on research that shows people pay more attention to information that is personally relevant to them (NCI, 2002). Tailored intervention activities have been used in a variety of programs including, but not limited to, AIDS (Bakker, 1999), cancer screening (Skinner, Strecher, & Hospers, 1994), exercise (Marcus et al., 1998), immunizations (Kreuter, Vehige, & McGuire, 1996), nutrition (Campbell et al., 1994), smoking cessation (Strecher et al., 1994), and weight loss (Kreuter, Bull, Clark, & Oswald, 1999). See Kreuter and colleagues (2000) for a review of tailoring.

   One final item to consider when thinking about the appropriateness of an intervention strategy for the priority population is to ask if there is any chance that the strategy could cause any unintended effects in the priority population. For example, could the strategy threaten the physical safety or raise undue anxiety in the priority population (CDC, 2003)?

6. **Are the necessary resources available to implement the intervention selected?** Obviously some intervention strategies require more money, time, personnel, or space to implement than others. For example, it may be prudent to provide each person in the priority population with a $100 incentive for participating in the health promotion program, but it may not be possible because of budget limitations.

7. **Would it be better to use an intervention that consists of a single strategy or one that is made up of multiple strategies?** Again, we refer to the principle of multiplicity. A single-strategy intervention would most likely be easier and less expensive to implement and easier to evaluate. There are, however, some real advantages to using several strategies: (1) "hitting" the priority population with a message in a variety of ways; (2) appealing to the variety of learning styles within any priority population; (3) keeping the health message constantly before the priority population; (4) hoping

that at least one strategy appeals enough to the priority population to help bring about the expected outcome; (5) appealing to the various senses (such as sight, hearing, or touch) of each individual in the priority population; and (6) increasing the chances that the combined strategies would help reach the goals and objectives of the program (e.g., communication used to publicize a policy change) (CDC, 2003). Probably the biggest drawback to using multiple strategies is the difficulty of separating the effects of one strategy from the effects of others in evaluating the impact of the total program and of individual components (Ad Hoc Work Group, 1987). However, Glasgow, Vogt, and Boles (1999) have developed an evaluation model titled RE-AIM (acronym for reach, efficacy, adoption, implementation, and maintenance) for use with multistrategy interventions.

SUMMARY

Interventions are strategies used by planners to bring about the outcomes identified in the program objectives. Interventions are also sometimes referred to as *treatments*. Although many times an intervention is made up of a single strategy, it is more common for planners to use a variety of strategies to make up an intervention for a program. In this chapter, intervention strategies were categorized into the following groups:

1. Health communication strategies

2. Health education strategies

3. Health policy/enforcement strategies

4. Environmental change strategies

5. Health-related community service strategies

6. Community mobilization strategies

7. Other strategies

Additionally, this chapter identified the need for program planners to be aware of recommended standards/criteria/guidelines when planning program interventions. Some examples of general, as well as program-specific, guidelines that have been set forth by both professional organizations and individual professionals were reviewed. Finally, this chapter presented questions that planners need to consider when creating health promotion interventions.

REVIEW QUESTIONS

1. What is an intervention?

2. What are the advantages of using a multistrategy intervention (i. e., principle of multiplicity) over one that includes a single strategy? Are there any disadvantages? If so, what are they?

3. What does dose of an intervention mean?

4. What are the major categories of interventions? Explain each.

5. Define each of the following terms as they relate to health education strategies: *curriculum*, *scope*, *sequence*, *unit of study*, *lessons*, and *lesson plans*.

6. State and briefly describe the five stages of Kinzie's (2005) modified framework for instructional design.

7. What is health advocacy?

8. What special issues are there related to incentives with which planners working in the worksite setting need to be concerned?

9. Why should program planners be concerned with program guidelines that have been developed by professional organizations?

10. What are some of the documents and sponsoring groups that have suggested standards, criteria, or guidelines for program development?

11. Briefly discuss the questions set forth in this chapter that should be considered before creating an intervention.

ACTIVITIES

1. Create a multistrategy intervention for a program you are planning.

2. Create a multistrategy intervention for a program that has as its goal "to get third-grade students to wear helmets while riding their bicycles."

3. Create a multistrategy intervention for a program that has as its goal "to eliminate smoking of all employees of Company X."

4. Create a multistrategy intervention for a program that has as its goal "the rehydration of young children in the small village of Y in the Third World country of Q."

5. Design and present on a 8-1/2''× 11'' piece of paper a bulletin board that could be used as part of the multiactivity intervention you are planning. Divide the piece of paper that represents the bulletin board into six equal sections and indicate what you will include in each section.

6. Interview a classmate to find out information about his or her health risks. Then, assuming you are a patient educator in a health clinic, create a one-page *tailored* letter to the person, urging him or her to seek an appropriate screening for the health risk(s).

7. Develop a three-fold pamphlet that can be used as an informational piece for a program you are planning.

8. With other students in your class, write a PSA script for a program you are planning. Then rehearse the script and have it taped/recorded.

9. Write a two-page, double-spaced news release that describes a program you are planning.

10. Write a letter to your state or federal senators or representatives and request their support of a piece of health-related legislation that is currently being considered.

WEBLINKS

1. **http://www.healtheducationadvocate.org**

   Health Education Advocate

   The Health Education Advocate website is sponsored by the Coalition of National Health Education Organizations (CNHEO). It was designed to provide a timely source of advocacy information related to the field of health education and promotion. This site includes a number of items to help health planners with advocacy activities. The site includes, but is not limited to, information about how to identify and contact their senators and congresspersons, the status of specific bills, health resolutions and policy statements of sponsoring agencies, and advocacy resources.

2. **http://www.cdc.gov/healthmarketing/cdcynergy/index.htm**

   CDCynergy

   This is a page at the Centers for Disease Control and Prevention website that presents background information about the CDCynergy health communication planning model. Also, the site provides the latest information on the various editions (i.e., cardiovascular, diabetes) of the CD-Rom program.

3. **http://www.americanheart.org/presenter.jhtml?identifier=2945**

   American Heart Association (AHA)

   This is the advocacy page of the AHA's website. Like most other voluntary health organizations, the American Heart Association has an active advocacy program to support its mission. This site provides an overview of the advocacy work in which the AHA is involved.

4. **http://www.welcoa.org/freesources**

   The Wellness Councils of America (WELCOA)

   This is a page at the WELCOA website that presents free source information on a variety of topics including incentive campaigns offered by the Council.

5. **http://www.thecommunityguide.org/index.html**

   Guide to Community Preventive Services

   This is the webpage for the *Guide to Community Preventive Services* that includes evidence-based recommendations for programs and policies to promote population-based health.

6. http://www.cancer.gov/pinkbook

   Pink Book—*Making Health Communication Programs Work*

   This is the webpage for the *Making Health Communication Programs Work* book. This book is a practical guide to developing specific communication strategies to promote health and prevent disease.

7. http://www.cochrane.org/index.htm

   The Cochrane Collaboration

   This is the homepage for the Cochrane Collaboration. The Cochrane Collaboration is an international not-for-profit and independent organization, which provides up-to-date, accurate information about the effects of healthcare readily available worldwide. It is a source of best practices and best experiences interventions.

Community Organizing and Community Building

After reading this chapter and answering the questions at the end, you should be able to:

- Define *community, community organizing, community building,* and *coalitions.*
- Outline the processes for organizing and building a community.
- Explain the term *mapping community capacity.*
- Provide an overview of PATCH.

active participants	gatekeepers	potential building blocks
bottom-up	grassroots	primary building blocks
citizen-initiated	locality development	secondary building blocks
coalition	mapping community capacity	social action
community		social planning
community building	occasional participants	stakeholders
community organizing	ownership	supporting participants
executive participants	PATCH	

The first eight chapters of this book focused on a number of processes involved in planning health promotion programs. Those processes, for the most part, apply to all health promotion programs. Yet the application of these processes may vary based on a number of circumstances including the level of influence of the ecological perspective at which the program is aimed. That is to say, the processes used by health educators to plan programs are in part predicated on the level of the influence (i.e., intrapersonal, interpersonal, and/or community), and the level of influence is often predicated on the size of the priority population. For example, certain processes are more useful when planning programs for relatively small groups or communities of people such as those found in worksites, clinics, and schools, whereas other processes must be considered when working with larger communities. By community, we do not mean only those groups of people within a certain geographic area, though that could define a community, but more specifically, a **community** is defined as "a group of people who have common characteristics" (Turnock, 2004, p. 383). Israel and colleagues (1994) have stated that communities are characterized by the following elements: (1) membership—a sense of identity and belonging; (2) common symbol systems—similar language, rituals, and ceremonies; (3) shared values and norms; (4) mutual influence—community members have influence and are influenced by each other; (5) shared needs and commitment to meeting them; and (6) shared emotional connection—members share common history, experiences, and mutual support. Thus communities can be defined by location, race, ethnicity, age, occupation, interest in particular problems (e.g., domestic violence), outcomes (e.g., breast cancer survivors), or other common bonds (e.g., people with a disability) (Turnock, 2004).

Although many of the planning processes are applicable regardless of the size of the community, when working with large communities an additional process is needed in order to have a successful program. This additional process is organizing those in the community to come together to work as a group to deal with the needs of the community. This chapter addresses the fundamental elements of organizing communities for action. **Box 9.1** identifies the responsibilities and competencies for health educators that pertain to the material presented in this chapter.

Community Organizing Background and Assumptions

In recent years, there has been a shift in the focus of the work of planners and others in the helping professions. Where once the work of planners focused almost solely on the individual, today the focus is on broadening to the community. *Community-based, community empowerment, community participation*, and *community partnerships* are among the many terms that are being used more frequently by health agencies, outside funders, and policymakers (Minkler, 2005). There are good reasons for the use of these terms and most revolve around the need for communities to organize.

With the evidence to show that interventions aimed at the community level (also referred to as *population-based approaches*) can have a positive affect on the health of a community, it is important that health educators have community organizing skills. In the early history of the United States, a sense of community was inherent in everyday life (Green, 1989). It was natural for communities to pool their resources to deal with shared problems. More recently, the need to organize communities has seemed to increase. Advances in electronics, communications, and increased opportunities for travel have resulted in a loss of the sense of community. Individuals are much more independent than ever before. The days when people knew everyone on their block are past (McKenzie et al., 2008).

Because of these changes in community social structure and the resources necessary to meet the needs of communities, it now takes a concerted effort to organize a community to act for the collective good.

Box 9.1	RESPONSIBILITIES AND COMPETENCIES FOR HEALTH EDUCATORS

Chapter 9 focuses on the fundamental elements of organizing communities. As such, the content presented cuts across several different areas of responsibility for health educators. The responsibilities and competencies related to these tasks include:

Responsibility II: Plan Health Education Strategies, Interventions, and Programs

Competency A: Involve people and organizations in program planning

Competency B: Incorporate data analysis and principles of community organization

Competency F: Select appropriate strategies to meet objectives

Competency G: Assess factors that affect implementation

Responsibility III: Implement Health Education Strategies, Interventions, and Programs

Competency D: Conduct training programs

Responsibility V: Administer Health Education Strategies, Interventions, and Programs

Competency A: Exercise organizational leadership

Competency C: Manage human resources

Competency D: Obtain acceptance and support for programs

Responsibility VI: Serve as a Health Education Resource Person

Competency D: Establish consultative relationships

Responsibility VII: Communicate and Advocate for Health and Health Education

Competency B: Apply a variety of communication methods and techniques

Competency D: Influence health policy to promote health

Source: NCHEC, SOPHE, & AAHE (2006)

"The term *community organization* was coined by American social workers in the late 1880s to describe their efforts to coordinate services for newly arrived immigrants and the poor" (Minkler & Wallerstein, 2005, p. 27). More recently, *community organization* has been used by a variety of professionals, including health educators, and refers to various methods of intervention to deal with social problems. "Community organization is important in health education in part because it reflects one of the field's most fundamental principles, that of 'starting where the people are' (Nyswander, 1956)" (Minkler & Wallerstein, 2005, p. 27). "The health education professional who begins with the community's felt needs, rather than with a personal or agency-dictated agenda, will be far more likely to experience success in the change process and to foster real community ownership of programs and actions than if he or she were to impose an agenda from outside" (Minkler & Wallerstein, 2002, p. 280).

Community organizing has been defined as "a process through which communities are helped to identify common problems or goals, mobilize resources, and in other ways develop and implement strategies for reaching their goals they have collectively set" (Minkler & Wallerstein, 2005, p. 26). It is not a science but rather an art of building consensus within the democratic process (Ross, 1967). (See **Box 9.2** for definitions of related terms.) Although community organization may not be as "natural" as it once was, communities can still organize to analyze and solve problems through collective action. In working toward this end, those who assist communities with organizing must make several assumptions. Ross (1967, pp. 86–92) has stated these as follows:

1. Communities of people can develop the capacity to deal with their own problems.

2. People want to change and can change.

3. People should participate in making, adjusting, or controlling the major changes taking place in their communities.

Box 9.2	TERMS ASSOCIATED WITH COMMUNITY ORGANIZING
Citizen Participation	The bottom-up, grassroots mobilization of citizens for the purpose of undertaking activities to improve the condition of something in the community.
Community Capacity	"The characteristics of communities that affect their ability to identify, mobilize, and address social and public health problems" (Goodman et al., 1999, p. 259).
Community Development	"A process designed to create conditions of economic and social progress for the whole community with its active participation and the fullest possible reliance on the community's initiative" (United Nations, 1955, p. 6).
Empowered Community	"One in which individuals and organizations apply their skills and resources in collective efforts to meet their respective needs" (Israel et al., 1994).
Grassroots Participation	"Bottom-up efforts of people taking collective actions on their own behalf, and they involve the use of a sophisticated blend of confrontation and cooperation in order to achieve their ends" (Perlman, 1978, p. 65).
Macro Practice	The methods of professional change that deal with issues beyond the individual, family, and small group level.
Social Capital	"Relationships and structures within a community that promote cooperation for mutual benefit" (Minkler & Wallerstein, 2005, p. 35).
Participation and Relevance	"Community organizing that 'starts where the people are' and engages community members as equals" (Minkler & Wallerstein, 2005, p. 35).

4. Changes in community living that are self-imposed or self-developed have a meaning and permanence that imposed changes do not have.

5. A "holistic approach" can deal successfully with problems with which a "fragmented approach" cannot cope.

6. Democracy requires cooperative participation and action in the affairs of the community, and that the people must learn the skills that make this possible.

7. Frequently communities of people need help in organizing to deal with their needs, just as many individuals require help in coping with their individual problems.

The Processes of Community Organizing and Community Building

There is no single unified model of community organizing or community building (Minkler & Wallerstein, 2005). In fact, Rothman and Tropman (1987, pp. 4–5) have stated, "We should speak of community organization methods rather than the community organization method." Over the years, several different community organization methods have been used, including revolutionary techniques (Alinsky, 1971). However, the best known categories of community organization were the three put forth by Rothman and Tropman (1987) and include *locality development, social planning*, and *social action*. **Locality development** is most like community development and seeks community change through broad self-help participation from the local community. "It is heavily process oriented, stressing consensus, and cooperation and aimed at building group identity and a sense of community" (Minkler & Wallerstein, 2005, p. 30). **Social planning** "is heavily task oriented, focused on rational-empirical problem solving, usually by an outside expert" (Minkler & Wallerstein, 2005, p. 30). **Social action** "is both task and process oriented. It is concerned with increasing the community's problem-solving ability and achieving concrete changes to redress imbalances of power and privilege between the oppressed or disadvantaged group and the larger society" (Minkler & Wallerstein, 2005, p. 30). Although this model is not used as often as it once was, it was most useful during the civil rights and gay rights movements.

Though the concepts found in community organizing methods proposed by Rothman and Tropman (1987) have been the primary means by which communities have organized over the years, they do have their limitations. One of the greatest limitations is that they are primarily "problem-based and organizer-centered, rather than strength-based and community-centered" (Minkler & Wallerstein, 2002, pp. 284–285). Thus some of the newer models are based more upon collaborative empowerment and community building. Regardless of whether one talks about the "old models" or the "new models," they all revolve around a common theme: The work and resources of many have a much better chance of solving a problem or meeting a goal than the work and resources of a few.

Minkler and Wallerstein (2002) have done a nice job of summarizing the newer perspectives of community organizing with the older models by presenting a typology that incorporates both needs- and strength-based approaches. That typology is presented in **Figure 9.1.** This figure is divided into four quadrants with strength-based and needs-based on the vertical axis and consensus and conflict on the horizontal axis.

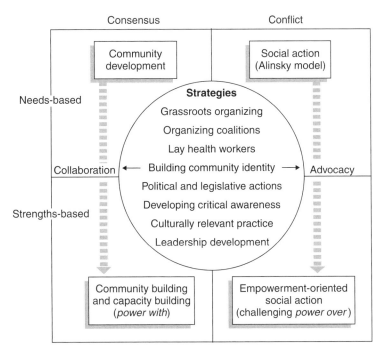

Figure 9.1 Community organization and community-building typology

Source: K.Glanz et al., *Health Behavior and Health Education, 3/e*, p. 287. Copyright © 2002 by John Wiley & Sons, Inc. Used with permission.

Though this typology separates and categorizes the various methods of community organizing and building, Minkler and Wallerstein (2005, pp. 33–34) point out that

> Community organizing and community building are fluid endeavors. While some organizing efforts primarily focus in one quadrant, most incorporate multiple tendencies, possibly starting from a specific need or a crisis and moving to a strengths-based community capacity approach. Different organizing models, such as coalitions, lay health worker programs, political action groups, leadership development, or grassroots organizing, may incorporate needs- or strengths-based approaches at different times, depending on the starting place and the ever-changing social dynamic. It is important, however, that organizing efforts clarify their assumptions and make decisions about primary strategies based on skills of the group members, history of the group, willingness to take risks, or comfort level with different approaches" (Minkler & Wallerstein, 2005, p. 33–34).

Because the purpose of this chapter is to provide an overview of the community organizing and community building processes, and at the risk of oversimplifying the processes, we would like to present a very general or generic approach to community organizing and community building (see **Figure 9.2**). It does not include everything planners need to know about community organizing and community building, but it does present the basic elements.

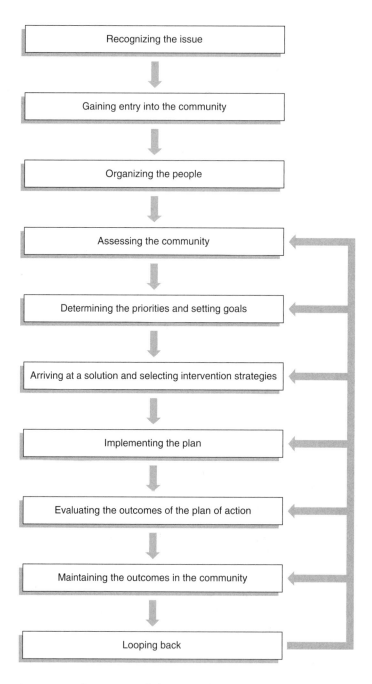

Figure 9.2 Summary of the steps in community organizing and building

For further information about community organizing, refer to any of several references (Minkler, 2005; Minkler & Wallerstein, 2002; Ross, 1967; Rothman & Tropman, 1987; Snow, 2001) that are devoted entirely to the subject. Also, there are several works that deal specifically with the application of community organization to health promotion activities (El-Askari & Walton, 2005; Kumpfer, Turner, & Alvarado, 1991; Maccoby & Solomon, 1981; McAlister et al., 1982; Minkler, 2005b).

Before presenting the generic process for community organizing and community building, we would like to comment on the role of the planner in this process. For many years, the planner was seen as a "leader" of the community organizing effort. However, more often than not, the planner is an "outsider" to the community being organized and, as such, has trouble gaining the credibility to serve as a leader. Yes, he/she may work in the "community" (remember that a community is often defined by something other than geographical boundaries) but often lives outside the "community" where the problem resides. Thus, the role that the planner should take is that of a facilitator or assistant rather than the leader. Experience has shown that it is best if the leaders come from "within" the community. Keep this thought in mind as you read through the general model.

Recognizing the Issue

The processes of community organizing and building begin when someone recognizes that an issue exists in the community and that something needs to be done about it. This recognition may occur as a result of someone reviewing health data on the community and seeing a need (e.g., an unusually high number of teenage pregnancies), by someone actually observing a specific situation in the community that needs attention (e.g., injuries at a particular intersection), or as the result of a community crisis (e.g., lack of resources to deal with a natural disaster). For the purposes of this discussion, assume that the concern is a health problem, but remember that the community organization process may be used with any type of problem found in a community. Concerns can be as specific as trying to get a certain piece of legislation passed or as general as advocating for a drug-free community.

The recognition of an issue can occur from inside or outside the community. A citizen or a church leader from within the community may identify the issue, or it may first be identified by someone outside the community, such as an employee of a local or state health department, a state legislator, or someone from a local voluntary health agency. However, the community organizing efforts that have been most successful have been those that are recognized from the inside. "All historic evidence indicates that significant community development takes place only when local community people are committed to investing themselves and their resources in the effort" (Kretzmann & McKnight, 1993b, p. 11). The primary reason for this is that those within the community are much more likely to take ownership of the effort. It is difficult for someone from the outside coming in and telling community members that they have problems or issues that need to be dealt with and they need to organize to take care of them. When there is internal recognition of the issue or concern, it is referred to as **grassroots**, **citizen-initiated**, or **bottom-up** organizing.

Gaining Entry into the Community

The second step of this generic process of community organizing and community building may or may not be needed. If the issue identified in the previous step is recognized by someone from within the community, then this step of the process will, more than likely, not be needed. We say "more than likely" because those within a community do not need to gain entry into it. But there may be some cases when someone from within a community may identify the issue but has not lived in the community long enough, lacks the political power, or does not know enough about the interactions of the community to proceed with the process. In these later cases, the person may be treated or feel like an "outsider" and may have to proceed as an outsider would.

If the issue is identified by someone from outside the community this becomes a most critical step in the process. Recognition of a concern does not mean that people should immediately set about correcting it. Instead, they should follow a set of steps to deal with it; gaining proper "entry" into the community is the first step. Braithwaite and colleagues (1989) have stressed the importance of tactfully negotiating entry into a community with the individuals who control, both formally and informally, the "political climate" of the community. These individuals are referred to as **gatekeepers.** The term infers that one must pass through the "gate" in order to get at the people in the community (Wright, 1994). These "power brokers" know their community, how it functions, and how to accomplish tasks within it. Longtime residents are usually able to identify the gatekeepers of their community. They may include people such as business leaders, education leaders, heads of law enforcement agencies, leaders of community activist groups, parent and teacher groups, clergy, politicians, and others. Their support is absolutely essential to the success of any attempt to organize a community.

Organizers must approach the gatekeepers on the gatekeepers' terms and "play" the gatekeepers' "game." However, before making this contact, organizers must first be familiar with the community with which they are working. They must (1) know with whom the power lies, (2) know what type of political interactions take place within the community, (3) understand the culture or cultures that exist in the community, and (4) know whether the concern has been recognized before, and, if so, how it was addressed. In other words, community organizers must have a thorough knowledge of the community and the people living there before they try to enter the informal boundaries of the community (Braithwaite et al., 1989). Having a thorough understanding of the community and tactfully approaching its gatekeepers will help community organizers develop credibility and trust with those in the community, and, as noted earlier, it is not easy to bring a concern to the attention of those in the community. Few people are glad to know they have a problem, and fewer still like others to tell them they have a problem. Move with caution, and do not be too aggressive!

When people from outside the community are working to facilitate the organizing efforts, they will find it advantageous to enter the community through an already established, well-respected organization or institution in the community, such as a church, a service group, or another successful local group. Green (1990) has suggested that the academic health center might be the ideal convener to address health services, health protection, or health promotion issues. "It has the deep roots in the community, it is not typically beholden to an out-of-state master, it can cut deals with local organizations, and it can draw upon resources to leverage commitments and resources from other organizations" (p. 175). If those who make up an existing organization/institution in the community can see that a problem exists and that solving the problem will improve the community, it can help smooth the way to gaining entry and achieving the remaining steps in the process.

Organizing the People

Obtaining the support of the community members to deal with the concern is the next step in the process. It is best to begin with those individuals who are already interested in addressing the concern. This is not the time to try to convert people to the cause or to make sure that all the key players of the community are involved. The initial group must be made up of those people most affected by the problem and who want to see change occur. For example, if the identified problem is teenage drug use, then teens needed to be included in the group. If the issue is housing for low income individuals, then those low income individuals need to be included. If the problem is something that a community agency or organization (i.e., the local health department, or a social service agency) has dealt with for a period of time but is unable to solve, then this group should be involved. Or, if a group of parents, or another defined group, has been struggling with the problem without resolution, then its leaders should be invited to participate. More often than not, this core group will be small and consist of people who are committed to the resolution of the concern, regardless of the time frame. Brager and colleagues (1987) have referred to this core group as **executive participants.** From among the core group, a leader or coordinator must be identified. If at all possible, the leader should be someone with leadership skills, good knowledge of the concern and the community, and most of all, someone from within the community. One of the early tasks of the leader will be to help build group cohesion.

Not everyone is cut out to be an organizer or a leader. Researchers have found that good organizers are successful because of a combination of skills and attributes. These skills and attributes fall into three main areas: change vision attributes, technical skills, and interactional or experience skills. *Change vision attributes* are closely aligned with the organizer's view of the world political terms. These people see a need for change and are personally dedicated and committed to seeing the change occur—so much so that they are willing to put other priorities aside to see the project through (Mondros & Wilson, 1994).

Technical skills include two areas: those related to efficacy on issues and those related to organizational health and effectiveness. The former includes being able to analyze issues, opponents, and power structure; develop and implement change strategies; achieve goals; and have outstanding communication and public relation skills. Organizational health and effectiveness skills include building structures for the recruitment and involvement of others, forming and maintaining task groups, and implementing skills of fundraising and organizational management (Mondros & Wilson, 1994).

The third characteristic of a good organizer is possessing *interactional* or *experience skills.* These include an ability to respond with empathy, to assess and intervene with individuals and groups, and to be able to identify, develop, educate, and maintain organizational members and leaders (Mondros & Wilson, 1994).

With the core group and leader in place, the next step is to expand the group to build support for dealing with the concern—that is, to broaden the constituency. Brager and colleagues (1987) have noted that other group participants will include *active, occasional*, and *supporting participants*. The **active participants** (who may also be executive participants) take part in most group activities and are not afraid to do the work that needs to be done. The **occasional participants** become involved on an irregular basis and usually only when major decisions are made. The **supporting participants** are seldom involved but help swell the ranks and may contribute in nonactive ways or through financial contributions. When expanding the group, look for others who may be interested in helping, and ask current group members for names of people who might be interested. Look for people who may already be dealing with the concern, affected by the problem through their present work, or who have resources to contribute. This search should include existing social groups, such as voluntary health agencies, agricultural extension services, church groups, hospitals, health care providers, political officeholders, policymakers, police, educators, lay citizens, or special interest groups. (See **Box 9.3** on tips for understanding the diversity in a working group.)

Box 9.3   UNDERSTANDING DIVERSITY

Members of a group come from many different backgrounds. Some members may be much older or much younger than other members; some may represent different cultural, racial, or ethnic groups; some may represent different educational levels and abilities. Extra awareness and flexibility are required for the facilitator and other group members to remain sensitive to different backgrounds. Below we suggest a few ways to improve your awareness of differences. In general, new information is acquired so that different perspectives can be understood and appreciated.

- Become aware of differences in the group by asking questions and getting involved in small-group discussions.
- Seek involvement and input and listen to persons of different backgrounds without bias, and avoid being defensive.
- Learn the beliefs and feelings of specific groups about particular issues.
- Read about current and emerging issues that concern different groups, and read literature that is popular among different groups.
- Learn about the language, humor, gestures, norms, expectations, and values of different groups.
- Attend events that appeal to members of specific groups.
- Become attuned to cultural cliches, stereotypes, and distortions you may encounter in the media.
- Use examples to which persons of different cultures and backgrounds can relate.
- Learn the facts before you make statements or form opinions about different groups.

Source: Centers for Disease Control and Prevention (no date), p. A2–15.

Over the last few decades, in many communities the number of people interested in volunteering their time has decreased. Today, if you ask someone to volunteer, you may hear the reply, "I'm already too busy." There are two primary reasons for this response. First, there are many families in which both husband and wife work outside the home. Between 1970 and 2006, the proportion of married women with preschool-aged children who were in the labor force more than doubled, from 30.3% to 64.7%. Also during this same period of time, the proportion of married women with children of school age who were in the labor force jumped from 49.2% to 66.8%. In 2006, 66% of married couples with children reported that both husband and wife were employed outside the home (USDL, 2007). Second, there are more single-parent households. Today, they constitute almost one-fifth (22%) of all family households with children, and most (18% vs. 4%) are headed by women (USCB, 2006). (See **Box 9.4** for tips on working with volunteers.)

Sometimes these expanded community groups become *coalitions*. A **coalition** can be defined as a "formal, long-term alliance among a group of individuals representing diverse organizations, factors, or constituencies within the community who agree to work together to achieve a common goal" (Butterfoss & Whitt, 2003, p. 354) often, to compensate for deficits in power, resources, and expertise. The underlying concept

---

| **Box 9.4** | TIPS ON WORKING WITH VOLUNTEERS |

Volunteers work for self-satisfaction, personal growth, fun, and other intangible rewards. Each volunteer should be treated as a colleague and recognized as an official part of the team. However, offer volunteers more flexibility than you can to employees, and adjust your expectations accordingly. For example, because volunteers cannot contribute as much time as paid, full-time workers do, they cannot complete tasks as quickly. When scheduling activities, be realistic about how long a busy participant will need to complete it.

Get to know each volunteer personally so that you can learn about special abilities and limitations and match responsibilities to skills. Vary responsibilities as desired by volunteers.

Be sure to assign specific and clearly defined tasks and to explain procedures and expectations. Develop a work plan or job description for the volunteer to help ensure that roles and responsibilities are understood. Provide training and give credit for work done. Give lots of feedback, encouragement, and signs of appreciation. Be willing to change the placement of volunteers, if that seems appropriate, or even dismiss a volunteer if necessary.

Keep in mind the following key points of working with volunteers. They want to be

- appreciated for the work that they do.
- busy with worthwhile and varied tasks.
- provided with clear communication about tasks and expectations.
- developed through training.

Source: Centers for Disease Control and Prevention (no date), p. A2–17.

behind coalitions is collaboration, for several individuals, groups, or organizations with their collective resources have a better chance of solving the problem than any single entity (see **Box 9.5** for characteristics of successful coalitions). "Building and maintaining effective coalitions have increasingly been recognized as vital components of much effective community organizing and community building" (Minkler, 2005, p. 16). For those wanting more information about coalition development, Butterfoss and Whitt (2003) and Wandersman, Goodman, & Butterfoss (2005) have provided nice overviews on the processes of building and sustaining coalitions.

Assessing the Community

Earlier in this chapter reference was made to the Rothman and Tropman's (1987) typology of community organization: locality development, social planning, and social action. Each of these community organizing strategies operates "from the assumption that problems in society can be addressed by the community becoming better or differently 'organized,' with each strategy perceiving the problems and how or whom to organize in order to address them somewhat differently" (Walter, 1997, p. 69). In contrast to these strategies is community building. **Community building** "is an orientation to community that is

---

Box 9.5	CHARACTERISTICS OF SUCCESSFUL COALITIONS

- Continuity of coalition staff, in particular the coordinator position.
- Ownership of the problem by coalition members and the community.
- Community leaders support the coalition and its efforts.
- Active involvement of community volunteer agencies.
- High level of trust and reciprocity among members.
- Frequent and ongoing training for coalition members and staff.
- Benefits of membership outweigh the costs.
- Active involvement of members in developing coalition goals, objectives, and strategies.
- Development of a strategic action plan rather than a project-by-project approach.
- Consensus is reached on issues instead of voting.
- Productive coalition meetings.
- Large problems are broken down into smaller, solvable pieces.
- Steering committee of elected leaders and staff guides coalition.
- Task or work groups of members design and implement strategies.
- Rules and procedures are formalized.
- Local media are actively involved.
- Coalition and its activities are evaluated continuously.

Source: R. J. Bentley et al., *Community Health Education Methods*, 2nd edition, p. 329. Copyright © 2003 Jones and Bartlett Publishers, Sudbury, MA. Reprinted with permission.

strength based rather than need based and stresses the identification, nurturing, and celebration of community assets" (Minkler, 2005, p. 4). Asset-based community building is intended to affirm the strong community-rooted traditions, and to build upon the good work already going on in communities (Kretzmann & McKnight, 1993b). One of the major differences between community organization and community building is the type of assessment that is used to determine where to focus the community's efforts. In the community organization approach, the assessment is focused on the needs of the community, whereas in community building, the assessment focuses on the assets and capabilities of the community. A clearer picture of the community will be revealed, and a stronger base will be developed for change, if the assessment includes the identification of both the needs and assets, and involves those who live in the community. Hancock and Minkler (2005, p. 139) provide this illustration:

> For example, a narrowly defined needs assessment designed and conducted by outside experts as a means of justifying and providing raw data for organizing around a predetermined community health need may be effective in achieving its objectives. But by failing to meaningfully involve community members in determining the goals of the assessment process, by focusing solely on needs rather than identifying and building on community strengths, and by failing to make empowerment of people a central goal of the assessment process, such an approach would fail to meet several critical criteria of community organizing and community building practice.

You may recall in Chapter 4 we outlined the procedures for conducting a needs assessment and described how the resulting needs could be placed on a map (i.e., *mapping*) to provide a visual representation of the needs of a community. **Figure 9.3** provides an example of such a map. However, an assessment that focuses entirely on needs/deficiencies presents only half of the information that is needed in community organizing and building (McKnight & Kretzmann, 2005). Organizers also need to know the capacities and assets. McKnight and Kretzmann (2005) point out "communities have never been built upon deficiencies. Building community has always depended on mobilizing the capacities and assets of a people and place" (p. 170).

In order to map community assets (a process referred to as **mapping community capacity**), McKnight and Kretzmann (2005) have categorized assets into three different groups based on their availability to the community and refer to them as *building blocks*. **Primary building blocks** are the most accessible assets (see **Figure 9.4**). They are located in the neighborhood and are largely under the control of those who live in the neighborhood. Primary building blocks can be organized into the assets of individuals and those of organizations or associations (see **Box 9.6** for examples of each). The next most accessible building blocks are **secondary building blocks,** which are assets located in the neighborhood but largely controlled by people outside (see Box 9.6). The least accessible assets are referred to as **potential building blocks.** They are located resources originating outside the neighborhood and controlled by people outside (see Box 9.6). Figure 9.4 presents an example of an asset map using the three types of building blocks. Knowing both the needs and assets of the community, organizers can work to identify the true concerns of the community and the capacity to deal with them.

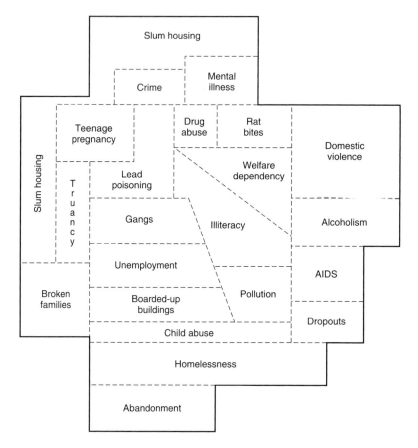

Figure 9.3 Neighborhood needs map

Source: Adapted from J. L. McKnight et al., "Building Blocks of Communities," in M. Minkler, *Community Organizing and Community Building for Health.* Copyright © 1997. Reprinted by permission of the authors.

Determining Priorities and Setting Goals

Once the community has been assessed, the community group is ready to develop its goals. The goal-setting process includes two phases. The first phase consists of identifying the priorities of the group—what the group wants to accomplish. The priorities should be determined through consensus rather than through formal voting (see **Box 9.7** for tips on how to reach consensus). The second phase consists of using the priority list to write the goals. To help ensure that the ideals of community organization take hold, the **stakeholders** (those in the community who have something to gain or lose from the community organizing and building efforts) must be the ones to establish priorities and set goals. This may sound simple, but in fact it may be the most difficult part of the process. Getting the stakeholders to agree on priorities takes a skilled group facilitator because there is sure to be more than one point of view.

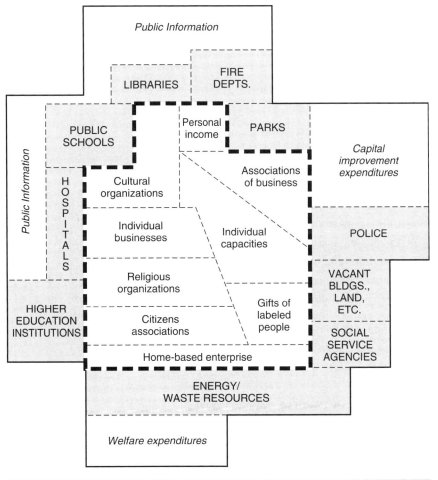

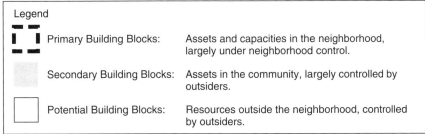

Figure 9.4 Neighborhood assets map

Source: Adapted from J. L. McKnight et al., "Building Blocks of Communities," in M. Minkler, *Community Organizing and Community Building For Health.* Copyright © 1997. Reprinted by permission of the authors.

When working with coalitions and task forces, one is likely to face some challenges (Clark, Friedman, & Lachance, 2006). One challenge that may surface when determining priorities and setting goals is *turf struggles* (disagreements over the control of resources and re-

Box 9.6	BUILDING BLOCKS (ASSETS) OF COMMUNITIES

Primary Building Blocks

Individual assets

- Skills and abilities of residents
- Individual businesses
- Home-based enterprises
- Personal income
- Gifts of labeled (disabled) people

Organizational assets

- Associations of businesses (e.g., Chamber of Commerce)
- Citizens' associations (e.g., neighborhood watch)
- Cultural organization (e.g., Old West End Festival, British Club)
- Communications organizations (e.g., newspapers, TV, radio)
- Religious organizations
- Financial institutions

Secondary Building Blocks

Private and nonprofit organizations

- Higher education institutions
- Hospitals
- Social service groups (e.g., United Way)

Public institutions and services

- Public schools
- Police and fire departments
- Libraries
- Parks

Physical resources

- Vacant land, vacant commercial and industrial structures, vacant housing
- Energy and waste resources

Potential Building Blocks

Welfare expenditures

Public capital-information expenditures

Public information

Source: Adapted from J. L. McKnight et al., "Building Blocks of Communities," in M. Minkler, *Community Organizing and Community Building For Health*. Copyright © 1997. Reprinted by permission of the authors.

Box 9.7	REACHING CONSENSUS

Groups sometimes find it hard to reach a consensus, or general agreement. Remind participants of the following guidelines to group decision making.

- Avoid the "one best way" attitude; the best way is that which reflects the best collective judgment of the group.
- Avoid "either, or" thinking; often the best solution combines several approaches.
- A majority vote is not always the best solution. When participants give and take, several viewpoints can be combined.
- Healthy conflict, which can help participants reach a consensus, should not be smoothed over or ended prematurely.
- Problems are best solved when participants try to both communicate and listen.

If a group has trouble reaching consensus, consider using some special techniques such as brainstorming, the nominal group process, and conflict resolution.

Source: Centers for Disease Control and Prevention (no date), p. A2–12.

sponsibilities). Even though individuals or representatives of their organizations have come together to solve a problem, many people will still be concerned with finding specific solutions to the problems faced by their organization. For example, in the case of drug abuse in the community, consensus may indicate that the majority of people believe the concerns lie in the educational system, but people who work in the treatment centers may believe that they lie in the treatment of drug abuse. The facilitator will need special skills to keep these treatment center people involved after the priority-setting process does not identify their concern as a problem the group will attack. One means of dealing with this is to have subgoals that can be worked on by special interest subcommittees. Such an arrangement will allow the subcommittee to have a feeling of **ownership** in the process.

Miller (as cited in Minkler & Wallenstein 2005, p. 39) has identified five criteria that community organizers need to consider when determining priorities and setting goals. The concern/issue/problem: (1) must be winnable, ensuring that working on it does not simply reinforce fatalistic attitudes and beliefs that things cannot be improved; (2) must be simple and specific so that any member of the organizing group can explain it clearly in a sentence or two; (3) must unite members of the organizing group and involve them in a meaningful way in achieving concern/issue/problem resolution; (4) should affect many people and build up the community; and (5) should be a part of a larger plan or strategy to enhance the community.

Arriving at a Solution and Selecting Intervention Strategies

To achieve the goals that it has set, the group will need to identify alternative solutions and—again, through consensus—choose a course of action. Most community problems/issues/concerns can be dealt with in any of several ways; however, each alternative has advantages and disadvantages. The group should examine the alternatives in terms of probable outcomes, acceptability to the community, probable long- and short-term effects on the community, and the cost of resources to solve the problem (Archer & Fleshman, 1985). Most of the intervention strategies discussed in Chapter 8 are means by which the group can address the problem/issue/concern.

Much of the work to identify the appropriate solution(s) can be accomplished through subcommittees. Subcommittees can complete specific tasks that will contribute to the larger plan of action. Their work should yield specific strategies that are culturally sensitive and appropriate for the community. The plan of action is usually written in a proposal format and will be given final approval at a meeting of the full committee or coalition. It is important to take care in putting together this proposal; as many as possible of the ideas of the various subcommittees should be included. This will help to ensure approval of the entire plan. In the end, the real test of the course of action selected is whether it can provide whatever it is the people are seeking (Brager et al., 1987).

Final Steps in the Community Organizing and Building Processes

The final four steps in community organizing and building processes include implementing the plan, evaluating the outcomes of the plan of action, maintaining the outcomes in the community, and, if necessary, "looping" back to the appropriate point in the process to modify the steps and restructure the work plan. Implementation of the intervention strategy includes identifying and collecting the necessary resources for carrying out the solution and creating an appropriate time line for implementation. Oftentimes the resources can be found within a community and thus horizontal relationships (the interaction of local units with one another) are needed (Warren, 1963). Other times the resources must be obtained from units located outside the community and in this case vertical relationships (those where local units interact with extra-community systems) are needed (Warren, 1963). An example of this latter relationship is the interaction between a local chamber of commerce and its state affiliate. Chapter 12 provides more detailed information on implementation.

The evaluation step of the community organizing and building process includes two types of evaluation: process and summative evaluation. Briefly, process evaluation deals with the measurement of the process used to improve the quality of the effort, whereas summative evaluation focuses on comparing the outcomes of the process to the earlier stated goals (see Chapters 13 and 14 for more on evaluation). When reporting on the work of coalitions, Clark and her colleagues (2006) stated "process evaluation was the easier type of assessment to conduct. Effective tools are more available, data collection is more immediate, and problems of association and correlation are less daunting than those associated with outcome evaluation. Outcome evaluation requires time, patience, and the willingness to accept that in complex community settings, definitive conclusions are elusive" (p. 152S).

Maintaining or sustaining the outcomes may be one of the most difficult steps in the entire process. Maintaining or sustaining the outcomes are challenged by (1) the energy and effort necessary to stay organized, (2) continuing the interest and involvement of the members (Clark et al., 2006), (3) continuing need for funding to sustain the efforts, and (4) "ensuring the lasting impact of their work through policies, cross-facility agreements, standardized protocols, and so on" (Clark et al., 2006, p. 151S). At this point organizers need to seriously consider the need for long-term capacity for a lasting solution.

Through the steps of implementation, evaluation, and maintenance/sustainability of the outcomes, organizers may see a need to "loop back" to a previous step in the process to rethink or rework before proceeding onward in their plan. And finally, once the work of the group has been completed (that is, either the issue has been solved or community empowerment achieved), the group can either disband or reorganize to deal with other issues.

Other Models Used for Community Organizing and Building

So far, this chapter has described a generic step-by-step approach for organizing and building a community. As has been noted throughout the description of this approach, there is much overlap in the processes of planning a health promotion program for smaller priority populations and organizing and building a community to deal with the needs of a larger group of people. Several planning models have been created to deal specifically with larger populations that also include components that assist with community organizing and building. A couple of these models (Mobilizing for Action Through Planning and Partnerships [MAPP] and Healthy Communities) were presented as planning models in Chapter 2. However, one other that has received considerable use and attention in the area of health promotion is the Planned Approach to Community Health, better known by its acronym, **PATCH** (Kreuter et al., 1985) (see **Figure 9.5**). The concept of PATCH emerged in 1983 as the response of the Centers for Disease Control and Prevention (CDC) to the shift in the federal policy regarding the distribution of money to states via categorical (block) grants

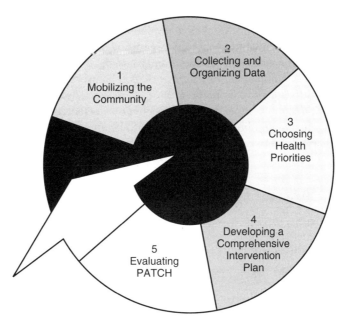

Figure 9.5 The five phases of PATCH

Source: Centers for Disease Control and Prevention (no date). *Planned Approach to Community Health.* Retrieved May 26, 2007 from www.cdc.gov/nccdphp/publications/PATCH/index.htm

(Kreuter, 1992). PATCH was designed using the PRECEDE model and was created "to strengthen state and local health departments' capacities to plan, implement, and evaluate community-based health promotion activities targeted toward priority health problems" (Kreuter, 1992, p. 135). Since its development, PATCH has proved to be a useful process with a good "track record for facilitating collaborative, community-based programs" (Speers, 1992, p. 132). The use of PATCH also led to the inspiration for PROCEED (Green & Kreuter, 1992). (See the *Journal of Health Education*, April 1992, for accounts of some of the success stories.) The essential elements of PATCH include community organization with local support, participation, and leadership; community members using local health data to determine the health problems, prioritize the health problems, and set goals and objectives; carrying out interventions; and evaluating the results (Speers, 1992). PATCH is a team approach in which the people of the community make the decisions (via a consensus process) and do the work, with technical assistance from the state and local health departments and the Centers for Disease Control and Prevention. These team members not only facilitate the necessary work but also provide financial support for the project.

Boxes 9.3, 9.4, and 9.7 presented in this chapter have come from the "PATCH Guide for the Local Coordinator" (USDHHS, CDC, no date). For more information on PATCH see the *Weblinks* at the end of the chapter.

SUMMARY

Community organization refers to various methods of intervention whereby individuals, groups, and organizations engage in planned collective action to deal with social concerns. The literature on community organizing and building is not distinct; it is often intertwined with such terms as *community-based, community empowerment, community participation*, and *community partnerships*. The process of community organization has been used for many years in the area of social work, but its history in the area of health promotion is much more recent. This chapter presented generic processes for community organizing and building, which should be an adequate introduction to the process, as well as a brief overview of the PATCH model.

REVIEW QUESTIONS

1. What is meant by the term *community?*

2. How does community organization relate to community empowerment?

3. Community organization originated out of what discipline?

4. What is the underlying concept of community organization?

5. What are some of the assumptions under which planners work when organizing a community?

6. What are the basic steps in the community organizing and building processes?

7. What is meant by the term *gatekeepers?*

8. What is the difference between a needs assessment and a capacities and assets assessment?

9. What is meant by *mapping community capacity?*

10. What are the differences among primary, secondary, and potential building blocks (assets)?

11. What does the acronym PATCH stand for? What are the major components of this process?

ACTIVITIES

1. Assume that a core group of individuals have come together to deal with the concern of a high rate of teenage pregnancy in the community. Identify (by job title/function) others who you think should be invited to be part of the larger group. In addition, provide a one-sentence rationale for inviting each. Assume that this community is large enough to have most social service organizations.

2. Provide a list of at least 10 different community agencies that should be invited to make up an antismoking coalition in your home town. Provide a one-sentence rationale for including each.

3. Assume that you want to make entry into a community with which you are not familiar in order to help to organize and build the community. Describe such a community, and then write a two-page paper to tell what steps you would take to gain entrance into the community.

4. If you wanted to find out more about your community's resources regarding exercise programs, with whom would you network? Provide a list of at least five contacts, and provide a one-sentence rationale for why you selected each.

5. Ask your professor if he or she is aware of any community organizing or building efforts in a local community. If such exists, make an appointment along with some of your classmates to interview the organizers. Ask the organizers to respond to the following questions:

   a. What is the concern being tackled?

   b. Who identified the initial concern?

   c. Who makes up the core group? How large is it?

   d. Did the group complete an assessment?

   e. What type of intervention is being used?

   f. What type of community organizing or building model was used?

6. To get a feel for the process of mapping community capacity, obtain a map of your college/university and "map" the health-related assets on your campus. Try to identify the assets in terms of primary, secondary, and potential building blocks for the campus as defined by McKnight and Kretzmann (2005). After your map is complete, analyze what you have found. Where are most of the assets located? Did the results surprise you? If your campus were going to increase its health capacity, what would you recommend? Why?

7. The most common form of community organizing efforts found in most communities are coalitions. Ask your professor if he or she is aware of any coalitions in the community. If such exists, with some of your classmates make an appointment to interview the coordinator of the coalition. Find out about the general functioning of the coalition and specifically ask about the challenges the coalition has faced and how its members dealt with them. If possible, also attend a coalition meeting. Summarize your results in a three-page paper.

WEBLINKS

1. http://www.northwestern.edu/ipr/abcd/abcdtopics.html

   Asset-Based Community Development (ABCD) Institute, Northwestern University

   This is the web page of the Asset-Based Community Development Institute (ABCD) established in 1995 at Northwestern University's Institute for Policy Research. The ABCD was built on the community development research of John Kretzmann and John L. McKnight. The website provides background information on many of the projects sponsored by the ABCD Institute.

2. http://ctb.ku.edu/index.jsp

   The Community Tool Box (CTB), University of Kansas

   The CTB provides practical information to support work in promoting community health and development. This website is created and maintained by the Work Group on Health Promotion and Community Development at the University of Kansas in Lawrence, Kansas, in collaboration with AHEC/Community Partners in Amherst, MA. The core of the CTB is the "topic sections" that include practical guidance for the different tasks necessary to promote community health and development. Each section includes a description of the task, advantages of doing it, step-by-step guidelines, examples, checklists of points to review, and training materials.

3. http://www.nhlbi.nih.gov/health/prof/heart/obesity/hrt_n_pk/cm_gde.pdf

   National Heart, Lung, and Blood Institute (NHLBI)

   This is the site at the web page of the NHLBI where the *Community Mobilization Guide*, developed by the NHLBI and the National Recreation and Park Association, can be found. The guide was created to assist planners at the community level with implementing a Hearts N' Parks program that is aimed at promoting heart-healthy lifestyles and changes such as increased physical activity and heart-healthy eating among children and adults. The guide provides all the necessary tools for implementing this program including background information and materials, techniques for creating and delivering heart-healthy activities to participants, tools and strategies for reaching targeted groups, forming partnerships, and working with the media, as well as assessment tools to measure program performance.

4. http://www.cdc.gov/nccdphp/publications/PATCH/index.htm

   Planned Approach to Community Health (PATCH)

   This is the web page for PATCH. Visitors to this site can download the PATCH guide and supporting visual materials. The PATCH Guide is designed to be used by the local coordinator and contains "how to" information on the process, things to consider when adapting the process to your community, and sample overheads and handout materials.

5. www.nfg.org/cotb/index.htm

   Community Organizing Toolbox: A Funders Guide To Community Organizing

   This is a web page from the site of the Neighborhood Funders Group (NFG). NFG is a national network of foundations and philanthropic organizations that support community-based efforts to improve economic and social conditions in low-income communities. Visitors to this site will find a workbook that provides a step-by-step approach to community organizing presented by using case studies from community organizing efforts.

PART II

IMPLEMENTING A HEALTH PROMOTION PROGRAM

The chapters in this section present information used in implementing a health promotion program. The chapters identify important components related to implementation and address the challenges one may face during the implementation process. The chapters and topics presented in this section are:

Identification and Allocation of Resources

After reading this chapter and answering the questions at the end, you should be able to:

- Define *resources*.
- List the common resources used in most health promotion programs.
- Identify the tasks to be carried out by program personnel.
- Explain the difference between *internal* and *external* personnel.
- Define *culturally competent*.
- Explain what is meant by the term *canned health promotion programs*.
- Identify questions to ask vendors when they are selling their programs, products, and services.
- List and explain common means of financing health promotion programs.
- Define *budget*.
- Identify and explain the major components of a grant proposal.

budget	hard money	request for proposals (RFPs)
canned program	in-house materials	resources
culturally competent	in-kind support	seed dollars
curriculum	internal personnel	sliding-scale fee
external personnel	ownership	soft money
flex time	peer education	speaker's bureaus
grant money	profit margin	vendors
grantsmanship	proposal	

For a program to reach the identified goals and objectives, it must be supported with the appropriate resources. **Resources** include the "human, fiscal, and technical assets available" (Johnson & Breckon, 2007, p. 296) to plan, implement, and evaluate a program. The quantity or amount of resources needed to plan, implement, and evaluate a program depends on the scope and nature of the program. Most resources carry a "price tag," which planners must take into account. Thus planners face the task of securing the financial resources necessary to carry out a program. However, several different resources are provided by organizations, mostly voluntary or governmental health organizations, that are free or inexpensive. This chapter identifies, describes, and suggests sources for obtaining the resources commonly needed in planning, implementing, and evaluating health promotion programs. **Box 10.1** identifies the responsibilities and competencies for health educators that pertain to the material presented in this chapter.

Box 10.2 lists the major categories of resources and accompanying questions that need to be answered in order to have the necessary resources to plan, implement, and evaluate a program. If you are currently planning a health promotion program, take a few minutes to read through the list and attempt to answer the questions as they pertain to the program you are planning prior to reading the remainder of the chapter.

Box 10.1	RESPONSIBILITIES AND COMPETENCIES FOR HEALTH EDUCATORS

Chapter 10 focuses on identifying and allocating the resources needed to plan, implement, and evaluate a program. Because resources are needed for all aspects of the program, Chapter 10 cuts across several different areas of responsibility. The responsibilities and competencies related to these tasks include:

Responsibility II: Plan Health Education Strategies, Interventions, and Programs

Competency F: Select appropriate strategies to meet objectives

Responsibility III: Implement Health Education Strategies, Interventions, and Programs

Competency D: Conduct training programs

Responsibility V: Administer Health Education Strategies, Interventions, and Programs

Competency B: Secure financial resources

Competency C: Manage human resources

Responsibility VI: Serve as a Health Education Resource Person

Competency C: Select resource materials for dissemination

Responsibility VII: Communicate and Advocate for Health and Health Education

Competency B: Apply a variety of communication methods and techniques

Source: NCHEC, SOPHE, & AAHE (2006)

Box 10.2   APPLICATION — WHAT RESOURCES ARE NEEDED TO PLAN, IMPLEMENT, AND EVALUATE A PROGRAM?

Personnel

- Who is needed to plan the program? Professionals? Advisory committee?
- Who is needed to implement the program? Facilitators? Support staff? Will you use a vendor?
- Who will evaluate the program? Someone associated with the program? Someone from outside?

Curriculum and other instructional resources

- What educational materials are needed to implement the program? Will the planners create them? Will they be purchased? Will they be donated?
- Will a canned program be used?

Space

- What space is needed to implement the program? How will you obtain the space? Will there be a charge for the space? Will it be donated? If donated, are there hidden costs like paying for custodial services?

Equipment

- What equipment is needed to plan the program? Is office equipment such as computers and copy machines needed?
- Is equipment needed for implementation such as table and chairs, instruction equipment (e.g., computer and projector), exercise equipment, etc.?

Supplies

- What supplies are needed for planning the program such as typical office supplies? Are postal and mailing supplies needed?
- What supplies are needed for implementation? Who will provide them? Planners? Participants? Outside group?

Financial resources

- How will the program be paid for? Will the planning group pay for it? Will the program participants pay for it? Will some third party pay for it (i.e., sponsoring group or agency, grant funded)? Or will it be paid for by a combination of sources?

Personnel

The key resource of any program is the individuals needed to carry out the program. Instead of trying to identify all the individuals necessary to ensure the program's success (because many times the same person is responsible for several different program components), planners should focus on the tasks that need to be completed by the program personnel. These tasks include planning; identifying resources; advertising; marketing; conducting the program, including having the necessary interpreters for those who speak a different language than the one in which the program is offered and accommodating those with disabilities; evaluating the program; making arrangements for space and program materials; handling clerical work; and keeping records (for program sign-up, collection of fees, attendance, and budgeting).

In some cases, the program participants themselves constitute a program resource. For example, in the case of a worksite health promotion program, planners will need to find out whether the employees will participate on company time, on their own time before or after work hours, on a combination of company time and employee time, or on their own anytime during the work day as long as they put in their regular number of work hours. (This last option is known as **flex time.**) The current trend in worksite health promotion programs is to ask the employees to participate at least partially on their own time. The reasoning behind this trend is that this investment by the participant helps to promote a sense of program **ownership** ("I have put something into this program, and therefore I am going to support it") and thus build loyalty among participants.

Internal Personnel

When identifying the personnel needed to conduct a program, planners have three basic options. One, referred to as **internal personnel,** uses individuals from within the planning agency/organization or people from within the priority population to supply the needed labor. These individuals may be hired specifically to serve as program personnel or existing employees may be trained to handle specific tasks. An example of using internal personnel would be when a local health department was planning a health promotion program in a community, the employees of the health department might handle the planning, implementation, and evaluation of the program. If that same health department was planning a health promotion program for the faculty and staff of a school district, there would likely be many school employees (i.e., school nurse, health educator, physical education instructor, family and consumer science teacher) who have the expertise (knowledge and skills) to carry out much of the program. If the department was planning a worksite program, there would probably be some employees who would be qualified to conduct at least a portion of the program (for example, an employee who is certified to teach first aid or cardiopulmonary resuscitation).

Another internal resource that health promotion planners are using successfully in a variety of settings, especially in schools (from kindergarten to college), is **peer education.** The process is simple: Individuals who have specific knowledge, skills, or understanding of a concept help to educate their peers. For example, college students may work with other college students to help educate them about the dangers of drinking and driving. The major advantages of peer education are its low cost and the credibility of the instructor. Children, for example, are greatly influenced by slightly older peers.

External Personnel

A second source of personnel for a program is to bring in individuals from outside the planning agency/organization or the priority population to conduct part or all of the program. Such individuals are considered **external personnel.** Typically, these individuals are brought in when it is found that there is a gap between what can be provided internally and what ultimately must be provided to accomplish the program goals and objectives (Harris, 2001). Many companies now offer or sell programs, services, or consulting to groups wanting health promotion programs. These companies are referred to as **vendors.** Some vendors are for-profit groups—such as hospitals, consulting agencies, health promotion companies, or related businesses—whereas others are nonprofit organizations—such as voluntary health agencies, YMCAs, YWCAs, governmental health agencies, universities/colleges, extension services, or professional organizations.

Planners must be careful when using vendors because the quality of vendors can vary greatly. **Figure 10.1** provides a checklist (Harris & McKenzie, 2004) that can be used to assist planners in screening vendors. It should be noted that the checklist has not been standardized and there is no set score that will assure that a vendor will be a good supplier of health promotion services. However, vendors who receive "yes checks" in a vast majority of the questions are likely to be highly qualified. Those who have a large number of "no checks" should be viewed skeptically (Harris, McKenzie, & Zuti, 1986).

An often untapped inexpensive source of personnel for health promotion programs is experts available through **speaker's bureaus.** Most local offices of voluntary health agencies, hospitals, and other health-related organizations maintain speaker's bureaus. The services of these experts are usually available at little or no cost to groups. With some inquiry and a little networking, it is not difficult for planners to identify organizations that have individuals available to speak on a variety of health-related topics, or health care organizations willing to send their medical experts into the community to share their knowledge. The speaker's bureau is a win-win concept for both the group offering the service and the one receiving it. Groups that take advantage of a speaker's bureau gain access to expert information, but those delivering the information gain in terms of public relations and recognition.

There are advantages and disadvantages connected with using either internal or external personnel to conduct health promotion programs. **Table 10.1** lists the pros and cons of each.

Combination of Internal and External Personnel

The third option for obtaining personnel to carry out a program is a combination of internal and external personnel. This option is the one most commonly used because it allows the program planners to make use of the advantages of the first two options and avoid many of the disadvantages. In fact, in worksite health promotion there is evidence (Elliott, 1998) to support the use of both internal and external personnel by those in best-practice (i.e., the most successful) organizations.

One special concern associated with personnel, regardless of whether they are internal, external, or a combination of the two, is to remember the importance of culture in planning, implementing, and evaluating health promotion programs. Cultural factors arise from guidelines (both explicit and implicit) that individuals "inherit" from being a part of a particular society, racial or ethnic group, religious community, or other group. In order for planners to be effective, they need to strive to be culturally competent

Checklist for Selecting Health Promotion Vendors

Developed by John Harris, M.Ed., FAWHP and James F. McKenzie, Ph.D, M.P.H.

> **CODE:**
> Yes = Yes, the vendor does/did this
> No = No, the vendor does not/did not do this
> NA = Not applicable
> NS = Not sure

1. Initial Experience with the Vendor

A. Did the vendor present a good professional image?
Yes ☐ No ☐ NA ☐ NS ☐

B. Did the vendor do the necessary homework on your company prior to the initial meeting?
Yes ☐ No ☐ NA ☐ NS ☐

C. Is the vendor's philosophy of health promotion consistent with your company's philosophy?
Yes ☐ No ☐ NA ☐ NS ☐

D. Can the vendor explain why and how its product/service can meet the needs of your company?
Yes ☐ No ☐ NA ☐ NS ☐

E. Did the vendor appear responsive to your company's needs?
Yes ☐ No ☐ NA ☐ NS ☐

F. Was the vendor willing to listen to you or was its representative too busy trying to sell?
Yes ☐ No ☐ NA ☐ NS ☐

G. Is the vendor willing to make a proposal or presentation to your company?
Yes ☐ No ☐ NA ☐ NS ☐

H. Did the vendor demonstrate expertise with regard to the product/service?
Yes ☐ No ☐ NA ☐ NS ☐

I. Did the vendor provide you with a reference list of other customers?
Yes ☐ No ☐ NA ☐ NS ☐

J. Did the vendor leave written materials that summarize its product/service?
Yes ☐ No ☐ NA ☐ NS ☐

K. Does the vendor enjoy a good reputation in the field?
Yes ☐ No ☐ NA ☐ NS ☐

2. Product Quality

A. Did the vendor provide an overview of its product/service content?
Yes ☐ No ☐ NA ☐ NS ☐

B. Did the vendor provide careful documentation of its product/service health or cost impact?
Yes ☐ No ☐ NA ☐ NS ☐

C. Does the vendor have evaluative data to support the product/service?
Yes ☐ No ☐ NA ☐ NS ☐

D. Does the vendor have data to compare success rates of its products/services to those of its competitors?
Yes ☐ No ☐ NA ☐ NS ☐

E. Can the vendor provide data that show the adequacy of its products/services with a population similar to yours?
Yes ☐ No ☐ NA ☐ NS ☐

F. Does the vendor have a written continuous quality improvement plan?
Yes ☐ No ☐ NA ☐ NS ☐

G. Does the vendor demonstrate sensitivity to the culture of your organization?
Yes ☐ No ☐ NA ☐ NS ☐

H. Can the vendor provide several different integrated products/services or does it just specialize in one area?
Yes ☐ No ☐ NA ☐ NS ☐

I. Did the vendor explain the art and or science that produces the results associated with its products/services?
Yes ☐ No ☐ NA ☐ NS ☐

J. Will the vendor "customize" the product to meet the needs of your company?
Yes ☐ No ☐ NA ☐ NS ☐

K. Can the vendor offer products/services which meet the special needs of your employees (e.g., reading levels, various levels of health status, languages, cultural diversity,etc.)?
Yes ☐ No ☐ NA ☐ NS ☐

L. If written informational materials are provided, are they written clearly and presented in an attractive way?
Yes ☐ No ☐ NA ☐ NS ☐

M. Are the products/services of the vendor up-to-date with current research, technologies, industry trends, etc.?
Yes ☐ No ☐ NA ☐ NS ☐

3. Professionals Involved with Delivery

A. What type of education and training do the professionals involved with the product/service delivery have?
Yes ☐ No ☐ NA ☐ NS ☐

B. Do the professionals involved in product/service delivery belong to recognized professional associations?
Yes ☐ No ☐ NA ☐ NS ☐

C. Are the professionals involved certified by a professional and/or health organization?
Yes ☐ No ☐ NA ☐ NS ☐

D. Are the professionals involved required to update their training periodically?
Yes ☐ No ☐ NA ☐ NS ☐

E. Is training specific to the products/services the professional delivers provided by the vendor?
Yes ☐ No ☐ NA ☐ NS ☐

F. Are the professional-to-participant ratios reasonable?
Yes ☐ No ☐ NA ☐ NS ☐

G. Is the performance of professionals delivering products/services audited by the vendor for effectiveness, efficiency,accuracy, etc?
Yes ☐ No ☐ NA ☐ NS ☐

Figure 10.1 Checklist for selecting health promotion vendors

Source: J. H. Harris, "Selecting the right vendor for your health promotion program," *Absolute Advantage* I(4), pp. 4–5, 2001.
Absolute Advantage is a publication of the Wellness Councils of America (www.welcoa.org).

4. Product/Service Delivery And Customer Satisfaction

A. Can the vendor clearly state in writing the products/services that will be provided?
Yes ☐　No ☐　NA ☐　NS ☐

B. Can the vendor clearly state in writing the roles and responsibilities of both parties in product/service delivery?
Yes ☐　No ☐　NA ☐　NS ☐

C. Is the vendor willing to establish a contract with your organization?
Yes ☐　No ☐　NA ☐　NS ☐

D. Is the vendor willing to help market the product inside your company as part of its service?
Yes ☐　No ☐　NA ☐　NS ☐

E. Does purchase of the product include measurement, evaluation, and reporting?
Yes ☐　No ☐　NA ☐　NS ☐

F. Can the vendor appropriately serve the size of your company's population?
Yes ☐　No ☐　NA ☐　NS ☐

G. Can the vendor provide the product/service at all sites desired?
Yes ☐　No ☐　NA ☐　NS ☐

H. Can the vendor provide the product/service at the times desired?
Yes ☐　No ☐　NA ☐　NS ☐

I. Does the vendor provide you with an "account manager" who will take full responsibility for your complete customer satisfaction?
Yes ☐　No ☐　NA ☐　NS ☐

J. Does the vendor have a track record of providing similar services effectively to other organizations similar to yours?
Yes ☐　No ☐　NA ☐　NS ☐

K. Has the vendor been in business/providing the product/service for at least five years?
Yes ☐　No ☐　NA ☐　NS ☐

L. Is the vendor's company well managed and financially sound?
Yes ☐　No ☐　NA ☐　NS ☐

5. Vendor Technological Capability

A. Does the vendor possess the technology necessary for the delivery of the product/service?
Yes ☐　No ☐　NA ☐　NS ☐

B. Is the vendor up-to-date with the technology it uses?
Yes ☐　No ☐　NA ☐　NS ☐

C. Is the computer system and software of the vendor compatible with yours?
Yes ☐　No ☐　NA ☐　NS ☐

D. Does the vendor utilize Web-based applications in the delivery of its products/services?
Yes ☐　No ☐　NA ☐　NS ☐

E. Are Web-based applications personalized, interactive, easy to navigate, and secure?
Yes ☐　No ☐　NA ☐　NS ☐

F. Does the vendor have an adequate "Information Services" department to support the products/services provided?
Yes ☐　No ☐　NA ☐　NS ☐

6. Evaluation and Reporting

A. Does the vendor collect adequate and accurate data on the product/service activity and outcomes?
Yes ☐　No ☐　NA ☐　NS ☐

B. Is the data the property of the vendor or the customer?
Yes ☐　No ☐　NA ☐　NS ☐

C. Does the vendor have written procedures to protect the integrity and confidentiality of the data (including HIPAA compliance)?
Yes ☐　No ☐　NA ☐　NS ☐

D. Can the vendor adequately convert data into meaningful reports?
Yes ☐　No ☐　NA ☐　NS ☐

E. Can the vendor provide reports and other aggregate data to the customer in appropriate electronic formats?
Yes ☐　No ☐　NA ☐　NS ☐

F. Can the vendor accommodate customized data and reporting requests?
Yes ☐　No ☐　NA ☐　NS ☐

7. Product Cost and Value

A. Is the cost of the product/service competitive with the cost of other vendors?
Yes ☐　No ☐　NA ☐　NS ☐

B. Will the vendor participate in a competitive bidding process?
Yes ☐　No ☐　NA ☐　NS ☐

C. Is pricing all-inclusive (no hidden costs)?
Yes ☐　No ☐　NA ☐　NS ☐

D. Does the cost per unit go down when the volume of work increases?
Yes ☐　No ☐　NA ☐　NS ☐

E. Does the cost per unit go down if additional products/services are purchased from the same vendor?
Yes ☐　No ☐　NA ☐　NS ☐

F. Will the vendor agree to performance guarantees (where costs to the customer are reduced if set standards are not met)?
Yes ☐　No ☐　NA ☐　NS ☐

G. Do the results of the product/service justify the price? (Is there an adequate value proposition?)
Yes ☐　No ☐　NA ☐　NS ☐

8. General Concerns

A. Does the vendor carry adequate liability insurance (as determined by the customer's Risk Management professionals)?
Yes ☐　No ☐　NA ☐　NS ☐

B. Does the vendor provide "added value" assistance such as reasonable consulting with senior professionals, without the customer incurring additional charges?
Yes ☐　No ☐　NA ☐　NS ☐

C. Is the "chemistry" good between the staff of the vendor and the staff of the customer?
Yes ☐　No ☐　NA ☐　NS ☐

For more information contact John Harris at Harris HealthTrends, Inc. at 419-885-5100

Figure 10.1 (continued)

Table 10.1 Advantages and disadvantages of using internal and external personnel

	Advantages	Disadvantages
Internal Program Personnel	1. Reduced costs. 2. Internal arrangements can be made to free needed personnel from their work schedules. 3. More control over those involved.	1. Limited by the interest and abilities of those on staff. 2. May have to train personnel or be limited by the expertise of those on staff. 3. Might spend more time developing the program than implementing it, thus reaching fewer people.
External Program Personnel	1. Known expertise. 2. The responsibility for conducting the program becomes the work of another. 3. Can request product (program) guarantees. 4. Sometimes external personnel are more respected than internal personnel just because they are from the outside. 5. Bring global knowledge to the program because they have worked with a variety of entities and cultures (Harris, 2001). 6. Have the resources for sophisticated tools and programs because they can spread the cost across many clients (Harris, 2001). 7. Can reach a priority population that is geographically dispersed (Harris, 2001).	1. Often more costly than using internal personnel. 2. Subject to the limitations of any given vendor. 3. Sometimes less control over the program.

(Davis & Rankin, 2006; Luquis, Pérez, & Young, 2006; Selig, Tropiano, & Greene-Moton, 2006). Being **culturally competent** means having the ability "to understand and respect values, attitudes, beliefs, and mores that differ across cultures, and to consider and respond appropriately to these differences in planning, implementing, and evaluating health education and health promotion programs and interventions" (Joint Committee, 2001, p. 99). Luquis and Pérez (2003) have provided a discussion of some of the issues surrounding cultural competence and some strategies by which planners can become more culturally competent. One strategy is becoming familiar with Standards for Culturally and Linguistically Appropriate Services (CLAS) presented by the Office of Minority Health (OMH, 2001) (see *Weblinks* at the end of this chapter for the website). In addition, if planners are not familiar with the culture of those in the priority population we would recommend that they work with indigenous health workers and/or those who are well trained and are bilingual and bicultural.

Curricula and Other Instructional Resources

In Chapter 8, the word **curriculum** was defined as a written plan outlining what those in the priority population will be taught (a course of study) (ASCD, 2007). When it comes to selecting the curriculum and other instructional materials that will be used to present the content of the program, planners can proceed in four ways: (1) by developing their own materials (in-house) or having someone else develop custom materials for them; (2) by purchasing or obtaining various instructional materials from outside sources; (3) by purchasing or obtaining entire "canned" programs from outside vendors; or (4) by using any combination of in-house materials, materials from outside sources, and canned program materials.

Developing **in-house materials** or having someone else develop custom materials has the major advantage of allowing the developers to create materials that match very closely the needs of the priority population. The more "unique" the priority population, the more important this approach may be—especially if the priority population possesses cultural differences. Materials must be relevant and culturally appropriate to the priority population (Kline & Huff, 1999). However, a serious drawback is the time, money, and effort necessary to develop an original curriculum and other instructional materials. The exact amount of time necessary would obviously depend on the scope of the program and the expertise of those doing the work. No matter who does the work, however, the commitment of time and resources is sure to be considerable. In putting together an in-house program, planners should be aware of several different sources from which they can obtain free or inexpensive materials to supplement the ones they develop. Planners might also find that there is no need to create in-house materials because of the wide array of materials available. For example, most voluntary and governmental health agencies have up-to-date pamphlets on a variety of subjects that they are willing and eager to give away in quantity. Also, most communities have a public library with a video/DVD section that includes some health videos and DVDs. If the public library does not carry health videos and DVDs, almost all local and state health departments offer such a service. Planners who are unsure about what sources of information are available in their community can begin by checking the Yellow Pages of the local telephone directory.

Planners need to remember that just because a piece of instructional material exists it may not be appropriate for the priority population with which they are working. To help insure that the materials are suitable for the priority population, we would recommend the use of SAM: a suitability assessment of materials instrument (Doak, Doak, & Root, 1996) (see **Figure 10.2**). This validated instrument "was originally designed for use with print material and illustrations, but it has also been applied successfully to video- and audiotaped instructions. For each material, SAM provides a numerical score (in percent) that may fall in one of three categories: superior, adequate, or not suitable" (Doak et al., 1996, p. 49). Here are the steps for using SAM (Doak et al., 1996):

1. Read through the SAM factor list and the evaluation criteria.

2. Read the material (or view the video) you wish to evaluate and write brief statements as to its purpose(s) and key points.

3. For short materials, evaluate the entire piece. For long materials, select samples that are central to the purpose of the document to evaluate.

2 points for superior rating
1 point for adequate rating
0 points for not suitable rating
N/A if the factor does not apply to this material

FACTOR TO BE RATED	SCORE	COMMENTS
1. CONTENT		
(a) Purpose is evident	_____	_____
(b) Content about behaviors	_____	_____
(c) Scope is limited	_____	_____
(d) Summary or review included	_____	_____
2. LITERACY DEMAND		
(a) Reading grade level	_____	_____
(b) Writing style, active voice	_____	_____
(c) Vocabulary uses common words	_____	_____
(d) Context is given first	_____	_____
(e) Learning aids via "road signs"	_____	_____
3. GRAPHICS		
(a) Cover graphic shows purpose	_____	_____
(b) Type of graphics	_____	_____
(c) Relevance of illustration	_____	_____
(d) List, tables, etc. explained	_____	_____
(e) Captions used for graphics	_____	_____
4. LAYOUT AND TYPOGRAPHY		
(a) Layout factors	_____	_____
(b) Typography	_____	_____
(c) Subheads ("chunking") used	_____	_____
5. LEARNING STIMULATION, MOTIVATION		
(a) Interaction used	_____	_____
(b) Behaviors are modeled and specific	_____	_____
(c) Motivation—self-efficacy	_____	_____
6. CULTURAL APPROPRIATENESS		
(a) Match in logic, language, experience	_____	_____
(b) Cultural image and examples	_____	_____

Total SAM score: _____

Total possible score: _____ , Percent score: _____%

Figure 10.2 SAM scoring sheet

Source: C. C. Doak et al., *Teaching Patients With Low Literacy Skills, 2nd edition,* © 1996 C. C. Doak. Reprinted by permission.

4. Evaluate and score each of the 22 SAM items, rating them as "superior" and assigning a score of two, "adequate" and assigning a score of one, "not suitable" and assigning a score of zero, or marking an item "N/A" if the factor does not apply to the material.

5. Calculate the total suitability score by summing the scores from the rated items and dividing by the total number of items rated. Do not include the items marked N/A. Multiply the score by 100 to get a percentage.

    70–100% = superior material
    40–69% = adequate material
    0–39% = not suitable material

6. Decide on the impact of deficiencies of the material and what action to take about whether to use or not use the material.

Purchasing or obtaining entire canned programs from vendors has become very popular in recent years because of the time and money needed to create programs. A **canned program** is one that has been developed by an outside group and includes the basic components and materials necessary to implement a program. Because some vendors are for-profit groups whereas others are nonprofit organizations, the cost of these programs can range from literally nothing at all to thousands of dollars.

Most canned programs have five major components:

1. A participant's manual (printed material that is easy to follow and read and is handy for participants)

2. An instructor's manual (a much more comprehensive document than the participant's manual, which includes the program content, background information, and lesson and unit plans with ideas for presenting the material)

3. Audiovisual materials that help present the program content (usually including videotapes/DVDs and audiotapes, PowerPoint© presentations charts, or posters)

4. Training for the instructors (a concentrated experience that prepares individuals to become instructors)

5. Marketing (the "wrapping" that makes the program attractive to both the participants and the planners who will purchase it to market to the participants)

The advantages and disadvantages of these canned programs are just the opposite of those for materials developed in-house. No time is spent on development; however, the program may not fit the needs or the demographic characteristics of the priority population. For example, using the same canned smoking cessation program with middle-aged adults who realize the long-term hazards of cigarettes and with teenagers who are required to attend a smoking cessation program for disciplinary reasons may not be advisable. Most adults who enter smoking cessation programs are there because they do not want to smoke. Obviously, this is not the case with teenagers who have been caught smoking. The approaches taken with these two programs would have to be very different if both are to be successful. Another example of when use of a canned program would not be advisable is use of a program that was designed for upper-middle-class suburban adults in a program for low-income inner-city populations. The lifestyles of the two groups are just too different for the same program to be appropriate in both situations. Because of the possible mismatch between the needs and peculiarities (i.e., age, culture, ethnicity, norms, race, sex, socioeconomic status) of a particular priority population, planners are urged to move with caution when deciding on the use of a canned program. Make sure there is a good fit.

Canned programs often come attractively packaged and seemingly complete, but this does not mean that they are well conceived and effective programs. Before adopting canned programs for use, planners should consider the following questions:

1. Is the program based on best practices? If not, why not?

2. Does the program include a long-term behavior modification component? There are no "quick fixes" with regard to many health behavior changes. If behavior modification is used, it should be based on sound health behavior practice over an appropriate time frame.

3. Is the program educationally sound? Not only should the program be based on sound psychological and sociological theory but it should also be based on valid educational theory.

4. Is the program motivational? Health behavior change is not easy to accomplish, and so all programs need to include activities that motivate people to get and stay involved.

5. Is the program enjoyable? Planned programs should be enjoyable. Some people like hard work, but it is difficult to sustain hard work for a long time without some enjoyment.

6. Can the program be modified to meet the specific needs and peculiarities of the priority population? As mentioned earlier, not all populations have the same needs, beliefs, traditions, and ways of approaching a problem.

Space

Another major resource needed for most health promotion programs is sufficient space—a place where the program can be held. Depending on the type of program and the intended audience, space may or may not be readily available. For example, an employer may make space available for a worksite program, or a school system may furnish space for a school program. If space is a problem, planners may locate inexpensive space in local schools, colleges and universities, religious facilities, and in "community service rooms" (rooms that are available free of charge to community groups as a community service) of local businesses. In addition, planners may find educational institutions and local businesses that are willing to cosponsor programs and thus contribute the space necessary to conduct the program. It may also be possible to obtain space by trading for it. For instance, a planner might trade expertise, such as serving as consultant for a program, in return for the use of suitable space. Or it might be possible to trade one space for another, such as trading the use of classrooms for time in the local YMCA/YWCA pool.

One final note of caution about space: Even if space is provided free of charge for a program, make sure to ask if there are any associated costs for the "free space." It is not uncommon for an organization offering the space (e.g., a school district) to do so with the obligation to pay for the custodial time to clean up the space once it has been used. Thus, a charge such as two hours of overtime pay for the custodial staff may be an obligation in order to use the free space.

Equipment and Supplies

Most health promotion programs will need both equipment and supplies in order to be planned, implemented, and evaluated. While oftentimes the words "equipment" and "supplies" are used to mean the same thing, from planning and budgeting perspectives they are usually considered two different types of commodities, and not all organizations define the words the same. Some organizations define equipment and supplies by costs. That is, equipment may be anything costing more than $500, whereas supplies are anything costing between $1 and $499. Thus, a computer may be equipment, while paper or even a chair may be a supply. These same organizations usually have a dollar amount definition for major equipment items (sometimes referred to as *capital expenditures* or *capital equipment*) as anything costing more than so many thousands of dollars depending on the nature of the organization. Other organizations may define equipment and supplies based on the "life" of the commodity. For example, equipment may be anything that will last three years or more, and supplies anything that lasts fewer than three years. Thus, under this type of classification a computer may be considered a supply. Or, an organization may define equipment as something that is not consumable, like a desk, and a supply to be something that is consumable like photocopy paper. It is not so important how the words are defined, but planners need to know how they are defined and work within those parameters.

Some programs may require a great deal of equipment and supplies. For example, first aid and safety programs need items such as CPR mannequins, splints, blankets, bandages, dressings, and video equipment. Other programs, such as a stress management program, may need only paper and pencils. Whatever the kinds and amounts of equipment and supplies required, planners must give advance thought to their needs so as to:

1. Determine the necessary equipment and supplies to facilitate the program.

2. Identify the sources where the equipment and supplies can be obtained.

3. Find a way to pay for the needed equipment and supplies.

Financial Resources

To hire the individuals needed to plan, implement, and evaluate a health promotion program and to pay for the other resources required, planners must obtain appropriate financial support. Most programs are limited by the financial support available. In fact, few programs are financed at such a level that planners would say they have all the money they need. Because of this, the planners are often faced with making decisions about how to allocate the funds that are available. Some typical financial questions that planners generally must address are the following:

1. Is it better to run an adequately financed program for a few people or to run a poorly financed program for more people?

2. If funds are limited where is the first place we should cut?

3. Should we start a program knowing that we will be short of funds, or should we wait until we have appropriate funding before we begin?

4. Is it better to have fewer instructors or to make do with fewer supplies?

Programs can be financed in several different ways. Some sources of financial support are very traditional, whereas others may be limited only by the creativity and imagination of those involved. Following are several established ways of financing programs.

Participant Fee

This method of financing a program requires the participants to pay for the cost of the program. Depending on whether the program is offered on a profit-making basis, this fee may be equal to expenses or may include a **profit margin**. Participant fees not only are a means by which programs can be financed but they also help motivate participants to stay involved in a program. If people pay to participate in a program, then they may be more likely to continue to participate because they have made an investment—that is, a commitment. This concept has also been referred to as *ownership*. Many participants who pay a fee feel like they are part "owners" of the program. However, it should be noted that not everyone shares in the ownership concept. There are some participants who still would prefer a free or almost free program that has been paid for by others. An example of the ownership and cost issue is the participant fees associated with smoking cessation programs. If planners were looking for vendors of smoking cessation programs, they would find that the costs of such programs range from zero (i.e., American Cancer Society's *FreshStart* program) to modest (i.e., American Lung Association's *Freedom from Smoking* program) to expensive (i.e., those offered by private health promotion companies).

Deciding to finance a program through a participant fee may sound easy, but planners need to give serious thought to how much they will charge and who will be charged. Often, those most in need of a health promotion program are the least able to pay. Planners do not want to create a barrier to program participation by charging a fee or setting the fee too high. If a fee is necessary, then planners should consider creating a fee structure on "ability to pay." One form of this is a **sliding-scale fee**—that is, the less one's income, the lower the participant fee. Or, planners may want to consider offering "scholarships" to those unable to pay.

Third-Party Support

Most individuals are familiar with insurance companies acting as third-party payers to cover the costs of health care. Although health insurance companies do not often pay for health promotion programs, others can be third-party payers. Third-party means that someone other than participants (the first-party) or planners (the second-party) is paying for the program. Third-party payers that may cover the cost of health promotion programs are:

1. Employers that pick up the cost for employees, as is often the case in worksite health promotion programs

2. Agencies other than the groups sponsoring the program—for example, when local service or civic groups "adopt" a pet program

3. A professional association or union that financially supports a program

The money used by third-party payers can be generated from a special fund-raising event, from sale of concessions, or with money saved from reduced health care costs, absenteeism, or the remodeling of employee benefit plans.

Cost Sharing

A third means of financing a program is a combination of participant fee and third-party support. It is not unusual to have an employer pay 50% to 80% of a program's costs and let the employee pay the remaining 50% to 20%. Or, an employer may have a reimbursement policy for program participation. With such policies, employees are responsible for paying the participation fee, and then based upon either attendance at the program (e.g., the employee must attend at least 80% of the program sessions) or completion of the program (e.g., employee must produce a certificate of completion), the employer reimburses the employee for either all or a portion of the participant fee. Such arrangements have the advantages of both ownership and a fringe benefit.

Organizational Sponsorship

Many times, the sponsoring organization (health department, hospital, or voluntary agency) bears the cost of the program as a part of its programming or operating budget. For example, the American Cancer Society offers its smoking cessation program free of charge. That is, program materials are provided free and an American Cancer Society volunteer conducts the program. The program is paid for with the society's community service funds.

Grants and Gifts

Another means of financing health promotion programs is through gifts and grants from other agencies, foundations, groups, and individuals. This source of money is often referred to as **grant money**, external money, or **soft money**. The term *soft money* refers to the fact that grants and gifts are usually given for a specific period of time and at some point will be taken away. This is in contrast to **hard money,** which is an ongoing source of funds that is part of the operating budget of an organization from year to year.

Grant money has become an important source of program funding, especially for those working in voluntary or governmental health agencies. It thus becomes necessary for planners to develop adequate **grantsmanship** skills. These skills include (1) discovering where the grant money is located, (2) finding out how to get (apply for) the money, and (3) writing a proposal requesting the money.

Locating Grant Money There are four basic types of grant makers: foundations, corporations, voluntary agencies, and government. These grant makers are found at three different levels: local, state, and national. They are not the only grant makers, however. Planners may also find a variety of local organizations (such as service groups like the Lion's Club or the Jaycees, or a community group like the United Way) that may be willing to support specific local causes through a grant. Philanthropic foundations are not-for-profit organizations that award grants to serve the public interest. A number of large national foundations support health promotion (e.g., Robert Wood Johnson Foundation, Rockefeller Foundation, W. K. Kellogg Foundation), but planners may also find state and local foundations too.

Not all corporations have giving programs, but many do as a part of a community service or public relations program. Planners will need to contact the corporations to "ask who is in charge of charitable giving, what subjects they consider for grants, and how the company giving program operates" (Guyer, 1999, p. 1). Library or Internet searching will possibly help answer these questions.

Voluntary health agencies also have grant programs. Though most grants from voluntary organizations at the national level are specified for research efforts, planners may find the local or state offices of these organizations are willing to provide **seed dollars** (start-up dollars) or **in-kind support** (such as providing free materials or other resources) for local programs.

Government is the largest grant maker. Government, at all three levels—local, state, and federal—makes grants for many purposes. With the other three grant makers (foundations, corporations, and voluntary agencies), planners can ask them to fund any project. However, with the government, only grants that are in one of the subjects specified by the government have a chance of being funded (Guyer, 1999).

When looking for grant makers, planners need to look for a pattern in giving by asking key questions: Has this funder made grants in the past for subject areas like mine? In my geographic area? In the amount I need? For the things I need funded? (Guyer, 1999). The answers to these questions, often found at Internet websites of the grant makers, will indicate whether it is a good idea to contact the funder. After doing the initial "research," planners should call or write funding sources to ask questions and to obtain any guidelines, grant request forms or applications, and printed material about their grant making. This contact will also help establish a relationship with the funder. Planners not only can obtain needed information but they can also introduce their organization to the funder. This can be done by sending publications about the planners' organization, making personal contacts, and staying in touch (Guyer, 1999).

Planners can identify possible funding sources in several different ways. The first is by networking with others who have been successful in obtaining grant funding in the past. Because seeking grant funding is a competitive process, planners may have to network with others who are not seeking funding from the same grant maker. A second means of identifying funding sources is through library "research." A variety of books on grants may be found in college and university libraries as well as many larger public libraries. For example, there are directories of grant makers for foundations and corporations, and there is usually a directory that lists grant funders that are specific to a state. Most of these books are indexed by subject area.

Three good places to begin searches for government grants are the *Catalog of Federal Domestic Assistance* (CFDA), the *Federal Register*, and *GRANTS.GOV* (see the

Weblinks at the end of the chapter). The CFDA, which is updated biweekly, is an online *catalog* "database of all Federal programs available to State and local governments (including the District of Columbia); federally-recognized Indian tribal governments; Territories (and possessions) of the United States; domestic public, quasi-public, and private profit and nonprofit organizations and institutions; specialized groups; and individuals" (GSA, 2007, ¶. 1). The *CFDA* allows planners to search the database for programs meeting their needs and for which they are eligible. However, to apply for one of the programs, planners need to contact the office that administers the program they are interested in.

The *Federal Register* "is the official daily publication for rules, proposed rules, and notices of Federal agencies and organizations, as well as executive orders and other presidential documents" (U.S. GPO, 2004, ¶. 1). It would list the latest grant opportunities. *GRANTS.GOV* is a website where planners can find and apply for federal government grants. The site was created in 2002 to "allow applicants to apply for and ultimately manage grant funds online through a common website, simplifying grants management and eliminating redundancies" (USDHHS, 2007c, ¶. 1). At this website planners will find over 1,000 grant programs from 26 federal grant-making agencies.

A third way of identifying funding sources is through the Internet. There are several advantages to using the Internet for seeking grant makers: convenience, time saving, and being able to reach several grant makers at the same time. Planners do not have to leave their office to conduct a search; thus much "leg work" of finding out whether a grant maker is a "good fit" with the planner's organization can be found almost instantaneously. In addition, some websites permit an applicant to complete one form for grant consideration at several different funders (Breen, 1999).

The fourth way of identifying grant makers is the least difficult. Planners should be alert for **requests for proposals,** known as **RFPs.** Many times some funding agency would like to have a project conducted for it, so the group will issue an RFP. If you feel qualified to do the work, you can submit a proposal.

Submitting Grant Proposals   As noted in the previous section, most funding agencies have specific guidelines outlining who is qualified to submit a proposal (perhaps only nonprofit groups can apply, or only practitioners who hold certain certifications) and the format for making an application. Those seeking money can request or apply for the money by writing a proposal. A **proposal** can be thought of as a written document that represents a request for money. A good proposal is one that is well written and explains how the needs of the funding agency can be met by the group wishing to receive the money. To increase their chances of writing a good proposal, planners should call the funding agency first and speak with the grant officer to find out specifically what he or she is looking for and the format desired.

Because there is a great deal of competition for grant money, it is more than likely that proposals will be read by a busy, impatient, skeptical person who has no reason to give any one proposal special consideration and who is faced with many more requests than he or she can grant, or even read thoroughly. Such a reader wants to find out quickly and easily the answers to these questions:

1. What do you want to do, how much will it cost, and how much time will it take?

2. How does the proposed project relate to the sponsor's interests?

3. What will be gained if this project is carried out?

4. What has already been done in the area of the project?

5. How do you plan to do it?

6. How will the results be evaluated?

7. Why should you, rather than someone else, conduct this project?

As noted, funding agencies request proposals in a variety of different forms. However, several components are contained in most proposals no matter what the funding agency. **Box 10.3** presents these components.

A Combination of Sources

It should be obvious that planners should not be limited to any single source for financing a health promotion program. In fact, it is more than likely that most programs will be funded via a variety of sources—that is, any combination of the sources listed previously.

Box 10.3 THE COMPONENTS OF A GRANT PROPOSAL

1. **Title (or cover) page.** When writing the title, be concise and explicit; avoid words that add nothing.

2. **Abstract or executive summary.** Provides a summary of the proposed project. May be the most important part of the proposal. Should be written last and be about 200 words long.

3. **Table of contents.** May or may not be needed, depending on the length of the proposal. It is a convenience for the reader.

4. **Introduction.** Should begin with a capsule statement, be comprehensible to the informed layperson, and include the statement of the problem, significance of the program, and purpose of the program.

5. **Background.** Should include the proposer's previous related work and the related literature.

6. **Description of proposed program.** Should include the objectives, description of intervention, evaluation plan, and time frame.

7. **Description of relevant institutional/agency resources.** Should identify the resources the proposer's organization will bring to the project.

8. **List of references.** Should include references cited in the proposal.

9. **Personnel section.** Should include the résumés of those who are to work with the program.

10. **Budget.** Should include budget needs for personnel (salaries and wages), equipment, materials and supplies, travel, services, other needed items, and indirect costs.

Preparing and Monitoring a Budget

Simply put, a **budget** is a "formal statement of the estimated revenues and expenditures" (Johnson & Breckon, 2007, p. 170) for a program. A budget represents the decision makers' intentions and expectations by allocating funds to achieve desired outcomes (program goals and objectives) (Finkler, 1992; Shim & Siegel, 1994).

A budget can be prepared for any length of time. When programs are planned, budgets are usually created for the entire length of the program. However, when a program is projected to last longer than a year, the overall program budget is typically broken down into 12-month periods.

"Developing a budget is an essential part of the planning process" (Johnson & Breckon, 2007, p. 174). Typically, a program budget is developed by those planning the program and any other key decision makers who control resources that will be used in the program. The process begins by examining the financial objective of the program. From a financial standpoint, programs can make money (a profit), lose money, or break even. If a program must make money, the revenue will have to be greater than the expenditures, and the intended profit (*profit margin*) will need to be included in the budgeting process. **Figure 10.3** presents a sample budget sheet that lists line items that are often included in health promotion program budgets.

Once the financial objective of the program is known, planners can then turn their attention to the estimated revenues of the program. In other words, from where will the income come? If a program is being paid for by a grant, gift, or contributions from sponsors, the planners may know exactly how much money they will have to work with. However, if the revenue for a program is coming, either in part or whole, from participant fees, an estimate will have to be made of how many participants are expected to take part. At this point budgeting becomes a bit more complicated. Hopefully, there may be some history from previous programs to guide planners in estimating participation and thus estimate revenue, but sometimes planners may have to make decisions based on "best guesses." Whether revenue is estimated based on previous programs or "best guesses," it is not uncommon to see a budget line in the revenue portion of the budget for participants' fees as: 22 participants @ $50 each = $1,100.

After the revenue for the program is determined, planners need to estimate what expenditures are necessary for the program. The categories of expenditures will vary from program to program based on program needs. The level of detail in a budget will also vary depending on the organization for which the program is being planned. Some organizations may require that the budget expenditures just be broken down into major categories (i.e., personnel, curriculum materials, equipment), whereas others will want more detail under each of these categories. Oftentimes, the largest expenditure for any program is for personnel, and because the salaries and wages are often included in a budget, the detail required to show personnel involved in a program may be very involved. For example, when including the cost of personnel, planners may have to account for: the salary or wage, Social Security taxes, and fringe benefits (i.e., health and disability insurance, vacation days, sick days). Oftentimes the exact dollar amount of fringe benefits is not calculated for a budget, but rather a percent of an employee's salary or wage is used to express the cost of fringe benefits. Thus, a fringe benefit line of a budget may read: 0.30 of $30,000 = $9,000. This means that the person preparing the budget estimates that the value of providing fringe benefits to a full-time employee making $30,000 per year is an additional

Revenue	Amount	
Contribution from sponsors	_____	
Gifts	_____	
Grants	_____	
Participant fee	_____	
Sale of curriculum material	_____	
	Total income	_____
Expenditures		
Curriculum materials	_____	
Equipment	_____	
Incentives	_____	
Marketing	_____	
Print advertising	_____	
Other media	_____	
Meetings	_____	
Personnel	_____	
For planning	_____	
Program facilitators	_____	
Clerical	_____	
Evaluator(s)	_____	
Participants	_____	
Postage	_____	
Space	_____	
Supplies	_____	
Travel	_____	
	Total expenses	_____
	Balance	_____

Figure 10.3 Sample budget sheet

$9,000. Another complicating factor in calculating personnel expenditures for a program is that a person may not be dedicated full time to a program, but the program is just one of many duties assigned to the employee. In this case, it is not uncommon to see a salary budget line presented as: 0.20 FTE of $40,000 = $8,000. This means that 20% of a full-time equivalent (FTE) employee who makes $40,000 a year is being charged to the program. Regardless of the format used to create a budget, the budget should be put together in sufficient detail that all revenue and expenditures are accounted for.

After the program is up and running, the budget must be monitored. This duty often falls to the person who oversees the financial resources of those planning the program. It may be one of the program planners, but will more than likely be a person who has financial responsibilities for the planning organization. This person may be responsible for both preparing and distributing the financial reports. At a minimum, those receiving the reports should include the decision makers and those responsible for the day-to-day operation of the program. The financial reports are usually generated and distributed on a regular basis (i.e., monthly, bimonthly, quarterly), and each report usually includes actual revenue and expenditures for the period, year-to-date totals on actual revenue and expenditures, and year-to-date budgeted revenue and expenditures. Such data allows decision makers and planners to know exactly where they are with regard to financial resources.

SUMMARY

This chapter identified and discussed the most often used resources for health promotion programs: personnel, curriculum and other instructional materials, space, equipment and supplies, and funding. In addition, information was presented on how to secure and allocate resources, how to obtain funding, and how to create and monitor a budget.

REVIEW QUESTIONS

1. What are the major categories of resources that planners need to consider when planning a health promotion program?

2. What are the advantages and disadvantages of using internal personnel? External personnel?

3. Define the terms *ownership*, *flex time*, *vendor*, and *canned programs*.

4. What are some key questions that planners should ask vendors when they try to sell their product?

5. How might program planners obtain free or inexpensive space for a program?

6. What is the SAM? What is it used for?

7. List and explain the different means by which health promotion programs can be funded.

8. What is meant by the term *profit margin*?

9. What is a budget? What are the major components of a budget?

ACTIVITIES

1. Identify and describe the resources you anticipate needing to carry out a program you are planning. Be sure to answer the following questions that apply to your program:
   a. What personnel will be needed to carry out the program? List the individuals and the duties to be carried out.

b. What curriculum or educational materials will you use in your program? Why did you select it or them?

c. What kind of space allocation will your program require? How will you obtain the space? How much will it cost?

d. What equipment and supplies do you anticipate using? How will you obtain them?

e. How do you anticipate paying for the program? Why did you select this method?

2. Visit the local office of a voluntary agency and find out what type of resources it makes available to individuals planning health promotion programs. Ask for a sample of the materials. Also, ask if the agency offers any canned programs. If it does, find out as much as you can about the programs and ask for any available descriptive literature.

3. Collect information on a single type of canned health promotion program (for example, smoking cessation or stress management) from vendors. Then compare the strengths and weaknesses of the programs.

4. Through the process of networking and using the local telephone book, find where in your community there is free or inexpensive space available for health promotion programs.

5. Call three different voluntary agencies and one hospital in your community and find out if they have a speaker's bureau. If they do, find out how to use the bureaus and what topics the speakers can address.

6. Prepare a mock grant proposal for a program you are planning. Make sure it includes all the components noted in Box 10.3.

7. Outline the major sources of income and expenses that would be associated with the program you are planning by preparing a budget sheet.

WEBLINKS

Note to readers: Because this chapter focuses on the resources necessary to conduct a program additional *Weblinks* are provided.

1. http://www.cancer.org/

American Cancer Society (ACS)

This is the home page for ACS. The site presents the most up-to-date information on cancer including treatment and prevention. The site also provides information about the ACS and the resources it can provide for cancer survivors and program planners.

2. http://www.americanheart.org

   American Heart Association (AHA)

   This is the home page for the AHA. It provides planners with a wealth of information and materials about many of the cardiovascular diseases and stroke.

3. http://www.lungusa.org

   American Lung Association (ALA)

   This is the home page for the ALA. It provides a variety of information about various lung diseases including asthma, chronic obstructive pulmonary disease (COPD), and lung cancer.

4. http://www.plannedparenthood.org

   Planned Parenthood Federation of America, Inc.

   This is the home page for the Planned Parenthood. It is the world's largest voluntary reproductive health care organization. Planners working on programs aimed at reproductive health should find it useful.

5. http://www.welcoa.org

   The Wellness Councils of America (WELCOA)

   This is the home page for the WELCOA. This site provides a variety of resources for those interested in worksite wellness programs.

6. http://www.aarp.org

   AARP

   This is the home page of the AARP. AARP is a nonprofit membership organization dedicated to addressing the needs and interests of persons 50 and older. This site has a lot of information that would be applicable to those planning programs for seniors. This site also has a special section on health and wellness.

7. http://www.nationaldairycouncil.org

   National Dairy Council (NDC)

   This is the home page for the NDC. The site provides a wealth of information about nutrition and weight management.

8. http://www.nih.gov/

   National Institutes of Health (NIH)

   This is the home page of the NIH. It not only includes information about NIH and links to all the institutes, centers, and offices, but it also includes health information, grant opportunities, and scientific resources.

9. http://www.cdc.gov/

   Centers for Disease Control and Prevention (CDC)

   This is the home page of the CDC. It includes information for the lay public (i.e., traveler's health and emergency preparedness) as well as information to assist health promotion planners (i.e., health topics A-Z, CDC recommendations, *MMWR*, and special funded initiatives).

10. http://www.healthfinder.gov/

healthfinder®

This is the home page of healthfinder®. Of all the *Weblinks* provided in this chapter, this one includes information on the greatest variety of health topics. It includes information on prevention, wellness, diseases, health care, and alternative medicine. It also includes medical dictionaries, an encyclopedia, journals, and more.

11. http://cdcnpin.org/scripts/index.asp

CDC National Prevention Information Network (NPIN)

This is the home page for the NPIN. This site houses the nation's largest collection of information and resources on HIV/AIDS, STD, and TB prevention.

12. http://12.46.245.173/cfda/cfda.html

The Catalog of Federal Domestic Assistance (CFDA)

This is the web page for the CFDA that provides information on federal grants. The site deals with all types of assistance, not just financial aid. The site uses "Assistance Program" as a generic term rather than speaking specifically about grant, loan, or another sort of program.

13. http://www.grants.gov

Grants.gov

This site allows planners to electronically find and apply for competitive grant opportunities from all federal grant making agencies. The site provides all the information planners need to apply for a grant and walks them through the process, step by step to their preferred practice setting.

14. http://www.gpoaccess.gov/fr/about.html

Federal Register (FR)

This is the main page of the FR. Published by the Office of the Federal Register, National Archives and Records Administration (NARA), the FR is the official daily publication for rules, proposed rules, and notices of Federal agencies and organizations, as well as executive orders and other presidential documents.

15. http://www.omhrc.gov/

Office of Minority Health (OMH)

This is a web page of the OMH that presents information on cultural competence. The OMH was mandated by the U.S. Congress in 1994, via P.L. 101–527, to develop the capacity of healthcare professionals to address the cultural and linguistic barriers to healthcare delivery and increase access to healthcare for limited English-proficient people. This site provides many different resources including, but not limited to, standards, materials, and links to other websites to assist health professionals to become more culturally competent.

CHAPTER 11

Marketing
Making Sure Programs Respond to the Wants and Needs of Consumers

After reading this chapter and answering the questions at the end, you should be able to:

- Define *market, marketing*, and *social marketing*.
- Explain the "exchange" process.
- Explain the purposes of segmentation.
- List and explain the factors that are used to segment an audience.
- Explain the diffusion theory.
- Explain how the diffusion theory can be used in marketing a health promotion program.
- Explain the functions involved in the marketing process as outlined by Syre and Wilson (1990).
- Explain the relationship between a needs assessment and a marketing program.
- Explain the marketing mix or four Ps of marketing.
- List and explain techniques for motivating program participants to continue in a program.

barriers	incentives	price
benefit	innovators	product
brand	laggards	promotion
contingencies	late majority	segmentation
diffusion theory	market	social marketing
early adopters	marketing	social support
early majority	marketing mix	
exchange	place	

In Chapter 2, you read about social marketing, the SMART model, and other marketing concepts. **Social marketing** attempts to change behavior for improved health or social outcomes. In contrast, commercial **marketing** that is defined by the American Market Association as ". . . a set of processes for creating, communicating, and delivering value to customers . . ." is concerned with financial profit. Regardless of the intended outcome, the key marketing principles that will ensure success are the same. One fundamental principle is a continual focus on the wants and needs of the consumers in a predetermined priority population. Other key principles include making sure that you: have a product that meets the consumer's need and offers a benefit that they value, offer the product at a price the consumer can afford, make the product available in places that are convenient, and promote it in a way that attracts the consumer's attention and prompts them to action.

This chapter discusses these basic marketing principles and how to apply them to developing a marketing strategy that results in the priority population purchasing your product (health promotion intervention). **Box 11.1** identifies the responsibilities and competencies for health educators that pertain to the material presented in this chapter.

Market and Marketing

Different types of items can be marketed: goods, services, events, experiences, persons, places, properties, organizations, information, ideas (Kotler & Keller, 2007), or behaviors. For the purpose of this chapter, we are marketing health promotion interventions as described in Chapter 8. These interventions may include information (best-practice guidelines for worksite health promotion programs), ideas (recycling), goods (bicycle helmet), services (breastfeeding class for new mothers), events (walk-a-thon for multiple sclerosis), or behaviors (wearing a safety belt while riding as a passenger in a car). Products will be discussed in further detail later in the chapter.

Box 11.1	RESPONSIBILITIES AND COMPETENCIES FOR HEALTH EDUCATORS

Responsibility I: Assess Individual and Community Needs for Health Education

    Competency B: Collect health-related data

Responsibility II: Plan Health Education Strategies, Interventions, and Programs

    Competency A: Involve people and organizations in program planning

    Competency B: Incorporate data analysis and principles of community organization

    Competency G: Assess factors that affect implementation

Responsibility VII: Communicate and Advocate for Health and Health Education

    Competency B: Apply a variety of communication methods and techniques

Source: NCHEC, SOPHE, & AAHE (2006).

The basic idea of marketing is that there are sellers who have a product and buyers who want to purchase or obtain the product. In health promotion, the priority population is the buyer, also called the consumer, target audience, or market. Kotler and Clarke (1987, p. 108) define **market** as "the set of all people who have an actual or potential interest in a product or service." As the seller (program planner) you have a product that meets a consumer's need and provides a benefit that they value. Your goal is to make it possible for the consumer to get the product at a reasonable cost and with minimal effort. This process is referred to as the **exchange**. Said another way, "strip away all the fancy language, and marketing comes down to offering benefits that an identified group of potential consumers will pay a price for and be satisfied with" (Novelli, 1988, p. 7). The process of marketing operates on this underlying concept of exchange theory.

Applying the definition of marketing to health promotion suggests that planners would like to have an exchange with the priority population where the program planner offers benefits that the priority population values (through an intervention) in exchange for the priority population giving some financial or nonfinancial cost. For the exchange to occur between the buyer and seller, the benefits offered by the product must be greater than what it costs the consumer to obtain the product. Additionally, the benefits must be outcomes that are important to and of value to the priority population. For example, women will breastfeed their children because it provides an opportunity to bond with their child (Kotler, Roberto, & Lee, 2002). This outcome is of more importance than other benefits program planners often promote, such as "your baby will be healthier," or "breastfeeding will cost less money." Although those benefits are true, the outcome or benefit that matters most to women is "bonding with my child."

To successfully facilitate the exchange, planners must have an understanding of marketing principles. Unfortunately, many health promotion planners have had to learn the hard way—by planning a program and then not have anyone engage in the behavior, attend a seminar, call a telephone number, or sign up to participate in a program. For example, one of the authors was asked to provide a one-hour presentation on heart disease for college-age women at a local university. On the day of the presentation only one person showed up—and that person was not a college-age woman. In retrospect, the topic was not relevant to the priority population (the seminar on getting adequate sleep had over 100 participants), the time of day was wrong (there was typically a weekly, campus-wide event at that same time), and the advertising was poorly executed.

Marketing principles are not difficult to learn, but their application to health promotion can be challenging. One of the challenges in social marketing is that instead of exchanging money for a tangible item and the related benefits, we are often exchanging a product and its benefits (that may not be received for a long time) for costs that are greater than money. For example, we are not offering a pair of shoes and looking cool for 50 dollars. Instead, we are offering a weight loss class and the benefit of reduced heart disease in exchange for consumers giving up the cooking methods they have used for years and were learned from their grandmother. In sum, applying marketing principles to a health promotion program is not as easy as applying them to the latest model of a car or a new line of clothing. **Box 11.2** illustrates a few general marketing elements and how marketing a tangible commercial item differs from social marketing a behavior. However,

Box 11.2	MARKETING A COMMERCIAL MARKETING TANGIBLE VERSUS A SOCIAL MARKETING INTANGIBLE

Elements	Tangible	Intangible
Product	Specific item	Behavior
Price	Money	Time, effort, discomfort, etc.
Measure of success	Number of items sold	Number of people who change behavior
Competition	Other businesses that offer the same product or similar versions of the same product	Other behaviors that give more pleasure or satisfaction
Decision	One-time choice to buy product	Ongoing choices to do the behavior

once learned and appropriately applied, a program or intervention that is based on marketing principles has the potential to be more effective than traditional practitioner-developed programs (Neiger & Thackeray, 2002).

The Marketing Process and Health Promotion Programs

If everyone in a given population recognized their health needs and took the appropriate steps to get involved in the programs that could address their needs, there would be no need for marketing the programs. However, because that is not the case, program planners must understand the marketing process and be able to apply its principles. Keys to understanding the marketing process are understanding the priority population, knowing how to segment the priority population, and having a good understanding of the diffusion theory. Each of these items is discussed below.

The Consumer and Segmentation

The most important part of the marketing process is knowing and understanding the priority population. All marketing-related programmatic decisions, including the type of intervention that is developed, how it is offered, how much it will cost, and how you promote it, should be based on what you know about the priority population. If you are making decisions without knowing who is in the priority population and something about them, including things such as how they see the world, what makes them tick, how they spend their time, and what is important to them, then you are not doing marketing. A good example of how critical this principle is to marketing can be found in the tobacco industry documents that describe, in detail, who their customer segments are and how they are going to market tobacco to them (see the Legacy Tobacco Documents Library at http://legacy.library.ucsf.edu/).

As a program planner you may think that everyone can benefit from your health promotion interventions, so you should try to reach everyone. However, not everyone is interested, ready, or even willing to respond. **Segmentation** is a way to divide the priority population into smaller, more homogeneous or similar groups. Segmentation is important because it helps you narrow and focus your marketing strategy and develop the right product. It also helps you be more effective and efficient, because you are able to identify groups of consumers who have similar needs and will respond to your marketing strategy in a similar way. This helps you to make the best decisions in terms of where to offer your program, how to make the price affordable, and how to tailor your promotional strategy including messages and communication channels to the priority population.

Segmentation permits planners to develop programs that will meet the specific needs and desires of the priority population, thus greatly increasing the chances for an exchange between the two parties. For example, a segmentation process discovered that among women who did not regularly receive mammograms, a lack of knowledge about how often they should get a mammogram was a key factor. One group did not know that they should have an annual mammogram, while the other one did (Forthofer & Bryant, 2000). Therefore, your marketing communication strategy among those who know about the guidelines would focus on reducing barriers to and making it easy for them to do the behavior. Among those who were not aware, a main strategy would be increasing their awareness that mammograms are available and how often they should get one.

Factors or variables on which to base segmentation include demographics, geographics, geodemographics, lifestyle/psychographics, benefits sought, and behavioral (readiness to change, knowledge, attitudes, beliefs, or behaviors) (see **Box 11.3**). Planners will need to experiment with several variables to determine what works best for them. You want to choose factors that will distinguish how the priority population will respond to your intervention. For example, just because people share similar demographics (e.g., college-age males) does not mean that they will engage in the same behavior of binge drinking on the weekend. However, how they prefer to spend their time and the perceived benefits or reasons for drinking may be more important.

Generally you use not just one factor, but multiple variables to identify audience segments. For example, in a study of African-American and white adults in St. Louis, researchers found that using demographics (i.e., age, race, sex, income, and years of education) was only slightly better at helping them identify a homogenous segment than doing no segmentation at all. They were able to get groups that were more similar when they used health status factors (i.e., general health status, number of chronic diseases, and whether the participant had been advised by a doctor or nurse to exercise more) or psychosocial variables (i.e., barriers to physical activity and the self-efficacy, intrinsic motivation, and social support scales). However, the best segmentation happened when they combined all three variables—demographics, health status, and psychosocial (Boslaugh, Kreuter, Nicholson, & Naleid, 2005)

There is no right or wrong way to identify population segments. The segmentation process you develop for the priority population must be useful to you and your program planning decisions. Planners can segment groups of people before surveying them (*a priori*) or afterwards (*a posteriori*). With the a priori approach, planners most often start with demographic variables such as age, gender, income, marital status, occupation, religion, ethnicity, and socioeconomic status. However, these do not always explain why

| **Box 11.3** | SEGMENTATION CATEGORIES AND VARIABLES |

1. Geographic segmentation
   a. Nations
   b. States
   c. Regions
   d. Service areas
   e. Counties
   f. Cities, towns, villages
   g. Neighborhoods

2. Demographic segmentation
   a. Age
   b. Stage of life cycle
   c. Disease or diagnostic category
      • Health history
      • Risk factors
   d. Gender
   e. Health insurance
   f. Income
   g. Education
   h. Religion
   i. Race/ethnicity

3. Psychographic segmentation
   a. Social class
      • Upper upper (less than 1% of population)
      • Lower upper (2%)
      • Upper middle (12%)
      • Lower middle (30%)
      • Upper lower (35%)
      • Lower lower (20%)
   b. Lifestyle
   c. Attitudes
   d. Values
   e. Personality
      • Self-image
      • Self-concept

4. Behavioral segmentation
   a. Purchase occasion
   b. User status
   c. Usage rate
   d. Loyalty status
   e. Stages of buyer readiness
   f. Health behavior

5. Benefits sought

6. Constructs of behavior theories

Source: Adapted from Hertoz et al., 1993; Kotler & Clarke, 1987; Romer & Kim, 1995; Williams & Flora, 1995.

people engage in behaviors or predict whether they will respond to your marketing efforts. Variables related to consumers' motives, personality attributes, and lifestyles can be "the most powerful segmentation variables in social marketing" (Slater, Kelly, & Thackeray, 2006, p. 171).

A planner conducts a posteriori segmentation after surveying the priority population and collecting data, such as those listed above, including psychographics (attitudes, values, and lifestyle), risk factors, health history, or personal health behaviors. For example, the National Cancer Institute (NCI) personnel used attitudes and lifestyle to identify different segments of the priority population for communications about cancer. They found that one group, which they called the naive optimists, were generally optimistic, self-involved, and complacent about their health. They did not make any effort to stay healthy or seek health information and did not worry about their health. This group of people was young with high incomes and made up about 12% of the population (Freimuth & Mettger, 1990). Segmentation could thus be most helpful in developing a market plan for this group of people.

Once you have identified potential segments, you have to choose on which segments to focus. There is not a right or wrong way, or simple and easy way, to choose segments. You have to combine the data with your organization's ability and your goals or what you are trying to achieve and make the best decision. One approach you can take is this—once you have identified all the possible segments, review your segments by considering the following five criteria (Kotler & Keller, 2007).

Measurable. With this criterion you consider how many people are in the segment and whether important characteristics (or factors) can be measured. The segmentation process for mammography discussed earlier actually resulted in seven segments, but they found that the majority of the population was in only two of the segments (Forthofer & Bryant, 2000).

Substantial. This criterion includes whether the segment is large enough and profitable enough, meaning will you be able to reach enough people with your intervention to make a difference. Will your efforts be effective and efficient? **Figure 11.1** shows the concept of audience segmentation, identifying African-American teenagers for a dietary excess intervention. This figure illustrates that the priority population, African-American teenagers, is a unique but potentially small segment when considering the total population and all of its health problems.

Accessible. This criterion helps you assess whether or not you will be able to reach the segment and then deliver the services. Perhaps your product is a mobile mammography unit. One segment identified is located in a remote area of your state. Due to time and distance factors you are not able to reach them to deliver the service.

Differentiable. Are the segments unique or different enough so that each segment responds in its own way to your marketing strategy? If the segments will respond the same, then they are really not unique groups. In developing a program to increase use of folic acid by women of childbearing age, planners found that women 18–24 were not receptive to messages about pregnancy whereas older women were more amenable to discussing the possibility of becoming pregnant (Lindsey et al., *in press*). A marketing strategy for these two groups would be clearly different and unique.

Actionable. Here you decide whether or not programs could be developed that would attract and serve segments. Because of segment characteristics or organizational

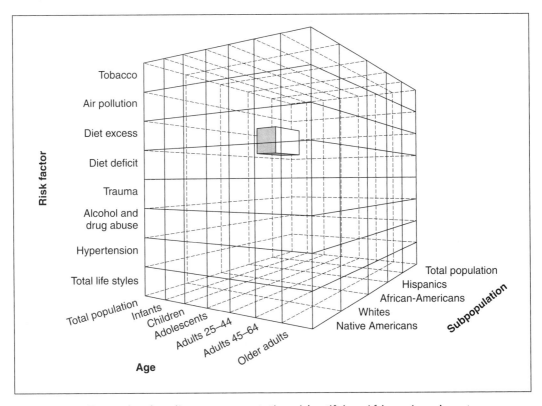

Figure 11.1 Example of audience segmentation, identifying African American teenagers for a dietary intervention

Source: U.S. Dept. of Health and Human Services (1986a), p. 41

abilities, you may not be able to create a product that adequately meets the needs or benefits that a segment wants. Planners in the United Kingdom learned that one of the main reasons that low-income people smoked was that smoking was a way to cope with stress and anxiety and it was one of their only "pleasures" in life (MacAskill, Stead, MacKintosh, & Hastings, 2002). In evaluating this segment, you would have to decide whether you could develop a smoking cessation intervention that would be appealing and provide a benefit that helped them cope with stress and gave them greater pleasure.

Another alternative is to use the criteria suggested by Andreasen (1995) that shares similar items: segment size, problem incidence, problem severity, defenselessness, reachability, general responsiveness, incremental costs, response to marketing mix, and organizational capability.

Marketing and the Diffusion Theory

A theory that may be helpful in segmenting the priority population is the **diffusion theory** (Rogers, 1962). The theory provides an explanation for the diffusion of innovations (something new, such as a product) in populations; stated another way, it provides an explanation for the pattern of adoption of the innovations. If one thinks of a health promotion program as an innovation, the theory describes a pattern the priority population will follow in adopting the program. The pattern of adoption can be represented by the normal bell-shaped curve (Rogers, 2003) (see **Figure 11.2**). Therefore those individuals who fall in the portion of the curve to the left of minus 2 standard deviations from the mean (this would be between 2% and 3% of the priority population) would probably become involved in the program just because they had heard about it and wanted to be first. These people are called **innovators.** They are venturesome, independent, risky, and daring. They want to be the first to do things, though they may not be respected by others in the social system.

The second group of people to adopt something new are those represented on the curve between minus 2 and minus 1 standard deviations. This group, which composes about 14% of the priority population, is called **early adopters.** These people are very interested in the innovation, but they are not the first to sign up. They wait until the innovators are already involved to make sure the innovation is useful. Early adopters are respected by others in the social system and looked upon as opinion leaders.

The next two groups are the **early majority** and the **late majority.** They fall between minus 1 standard deviation and the mean and between the mean and plus 1 standard deviation on the curve, respectively. Each of these groups comprises about 34% of the priority population. Those in the early majority may be interested in the health promotion program, but they will need external motivation to become involved. Those in the early majority will deliberate for some time before making a decision. It will take more

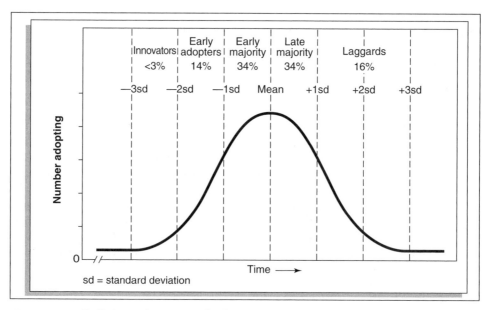

Figure 11.2 Bell-shaped curve and adopter categories

work to get the late majority involved, because they are skeptical and will not adopt an innovation until most people in the social system have done so. Planners may be able to get them involved through a peer or mentoring program, or through constant exposure about the innovation.

The last group, the **laggards** (16%), are represented by the part of the curve greater than plus 1 standard deviation. They are not very interested in innovation and would be the last to become involved in new health promotion programs, if at all. Some would say that this group will not become involved in health promotion programs at all. They are very traditional and are suspicious of innovations. Laggards tend to have limited communication networks, so they really do not know much about new things.

Figure 11.3 presents an *s*-shaped curve showing the cumulative prevalence of adopters at successive points in time. At first, only a few people adopt (innovators). However, over time, the curve begins to climb as additional individuals decide to adopt the innovation (early adopters, early majority, and late majority). The curve then levels off as adoption of the innovation ceases, leaving a few who have not adopted (laggards) (Goldman, 1998; Rogers, 2003).

The real advantage of using the diffusion theory when trying to market a health promotion program is that "the distinguishing characteristics of the people who fall into each category of adopters from 'innovators' to 'early adopters' to middle majority categories to 'late adopters' [laggards] tend to be consistent across a wide range of innovations" (Green, 1989). Therefore different marketing techniques can be used depending on the type of people the planners are trying to reach with a program. For

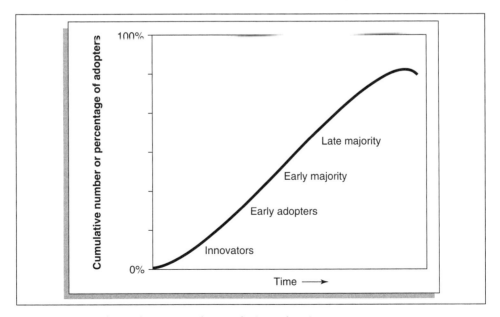

Figure 11.3 *S*-shaped curve and cumulative adoption

example, program planners want rapid diffusion of innovations. They know that although innovators will adopt the program or product first, the key subgroups of the priority population are the early adopters and early majority. It is especially important to identify the early adopters (opinion leaders) as soon as possible in the implementation process since, according to diffusion theory, the sooner they adopt the innovation the sooner the rest of the population will follow. The challenge is how to identify and reach the early adopters.

The application of the diffusion theory to health promotion programs is quite common now (Haider & Kreps, 2004). To learn more about the concept and its application to health promotion programs, review some of the following references to see how they have applied the concept in a variety of health promotion and health education settings (Backer & Rogers, 1998; Bertrand, 2004; Berwick, 2003; Borras, Fernandez, Schiaffino, Borrell, & La Vecchia, 2000; Ferrence, 1996; Goldman, 1998; Hallfors & Godette, 2002; Murphy, 2004; Rogers, 2002; Ruof, Mittendorf, Pirk, & von der Schulenberg, 2002; Svenkerud & Singhal, 1998; Taylor, Elliott, & Riley, 1998).

One of the more interesting uses of the diffusion theory has been its use to "conceptualize the transference of health promotion programs from one locale to another" (Steckler et al., 1992). Steckler and colleagues (1992) developed a series of six questionnaires to measure the extent to which health promotion programs are successfully disseminated. Planners should refer to this work if they are interested in using and measuring diffusion.

A Marketing Process

Syre and Wilson (1990) have identified five distinct functions of the marketing process as they relate to the healthcare field. These functions are also applicable to health promotion.

1. Using marketing research to determine the needs and desires of the present and prospective clients from the priority population.

2. Developing a product that satisfies the needs and desires of the clients.

3. Developing informative and persuasive communication flows between those offering the program and the clients.

4. Ensuring that the product is provided in the appropriate form, at the right time and place, and at the best price.

5. Keeping the clients satisfied and loyal after the exchange has taken place.

Next, each of these functions will be discussed.

Using Marketing Research to Determine Needs and Desires   This particular function involves conducting formative research as discussed in Chapter 2. Because the needs assessment process was discussed in detail in Chapter 4, that discussion will not be repeated here. However, the focus of formative research as performed in social marketing is a bit different than that of a traditional needs assessment for a program. The types of data planners try to uncover in formative research are, as described in the SMART Model, related to consumer analysis (wants, needs, and preferences of the priority population), market analysis (defining the market mix, described later in this chapter, and identifying competing behaviors, messages, and programs), and channel analyses (communication and promotion strategies). Some formative research can be conducted as part of a regular needs assessment, such as collecting information that would help segment the market (see the next section for a discussion of market segmentation) or finding out how best to position a program for a specific audience. Still other components, such as pretesting and pilot tests, are also considered formative research techniques.

Planners conducting formative research as part of primary data collection, including a program needs assessment, may want to consider asking the following type questions.

1. What would make it easy for the priority population to obtain the product or respond to the intervention?
2. What makes it difficult for or keeps the priority population from responding to the intervention?
3. What benefit does the priority population desire as a result of responding to the intervention?
4. What would the priority population be willing to give up to obtain the product and accompanying benefits?

For service-related interventions, specific questions may include:

1. What type of health promotion programs would the priority population participate in if they were offered in the community?
2. Where would the priority population like the program offered?
3. On what days of the week would the priority population like the program offered?
4. At what time of the day would the priority population like the program offered?
5. Would the priority population prefer individual attention or small group participation?
6. How much would the priority population be willing to pay to attend the program?
7. What is the best way to communicate information to the priority population about the program?
8. Do members of the priority population think other members of their family would like to participate in these programs? If yes, which members?

Developing a Product That Satisfies the Needs and Desires of Clients   The steps involved in developing a high-quality, marketable product (health promotion intervention) were discussed in earlier chapters. One key to developing a marketable product is knowing as much as possible about the priority population (i.e., conducting formative research) as mentioned previously. One of the primary things you should learn from formative research is what the consumer's needs are and what they value. Your goal with formative research is to know enough about the priority population that you can create a product that meets the consumer's needs and provides a benefit they value.

When making purchasing decisions about tangible objects, people decide to buy certain products for their functional use and because of what the product represents, and the value or **benefit** the product provides. For example, you are probably less likely to buy a generic brand of jeans or running shoes and more likely to buy a well-recognized brand because of what the product represents or symbolizes (e.g., serious runners wear Nike brand shoes). It is the same with health-related behaviors. People will choose to do certain behaviors (or not do them) because of the value it provides. For example, people will choose to engage in physical activity or exercise not only because it will reduce their risk of heart disease (a long-term benefit), but if they do exercise, then they will be thinner, they can wear certain clothes, and ultimately be more attractive (short-term benefits). Weinreich (1999) refers to this as the ladder of benefits (see **Box 11.4**).

Developing Informative and Persuasive Communication Flows   This function, which is closely associated with product promotion (discussed later) relates to the creative strategy and message strategy (Kotler & Keller, 2007). That is, what avenues will planners use to get the "message" out about their product as well as what will the message say and what visual images will go with the messages.

The creative strategy requires that planners identify appropriate channels to communicate messages and promote their programs. Marketing communication channels can include personal or nonpersonal channels or, as described in Chapter 2, interpersonal, small group, organizational, community, and mass media outlets. To select the right channel or combination of channels, planners must understand the tendencies and preferences of the priority population as identified in formative research.

Several authors (Kline & Huff, 1999; Lefebvre & Flora, 1988; Rice & Atkin, 1989) have made suggestions on items that planners should consider when developing the communication message and flow:

1. What are the media habits of the priority population?

2. What medium (electronic or print, visual or auditory, combination of several) should be used?

3. What are the costs of each medium versus the benefits?

4. Can the medium's capability build on or multiply the effects of another medium?

5. Will the message reach a significant portion of the priority population?

6. Can the message be sent through several different channels?

7. Is the message culturally appropriate?

8. Through how many intermediaries must the message travel to reach the priority population?

9. How frequently should the message be delivered?

10. Can a medium be overused to the point that it will "turn off" the priority population to the message?

| Box 11.4 | BENEFIT LADDER: WHAT ARE THE ATTRIBUTES AND BENEFITS OF PHYSICAL EXERCISE (THE PRODUCT) THAT WE CAN USE TO APPEAL TO THE PRIMARY POPULATION? |

Attribute ⟶	Benefit ⟶	Benefit ⟶	Benefit
Increase heart rate	Lose weight	Look better	Be sexier
Helps to burn fat and increase metabolism		Feel better about yourself	
Increase high-density lipoproteins	Lowers cholesterol level		
	Lowers risk of heart disease	Live a longer and healthier life	Watch your grandchildren and great-grandchildren grow up
Decrease blood pressure	Lowers risk of stroke Lowers risk of heart disease		
Produces endorphins	Reduce your stress levels	Feel more energetic	Feel more in control of your life Get more done in your day
Builds muscle strength	Become stronger	Be more independent in your daily activities	Have more freedom
Can be done with other people	Spend time with your family and friends	It is an opportunity to socialize	Have fun
Can be done alone	Spend time for yourself	Get away from it all	You deserve to have private time
Many people do it	Join the trend toward exercise	You will fit in	People will approve of you

Source: N. K. Weinreich, *Hands on social marketing: A step by step guide.* Copyright © 1999. Reprinted by permission of Sage Publications.

In order for planners to develop effective message strategy, planners must know what may be motivating the priority population. They must know how to frame the message so that it will cut through the clutter, capture the priority population's attention, and motivate them to action. Key parts of the message should be that the product will offer a benefit that the priority population desires, that the product costs less than the benefits it provides, and how they can obtain the product.

For example, after performing formative research related to diet and physical activity among a group of public employees, planners learned that preferences for message content included "helping employees understand that the desired changes could be inexpensive, fun and easy, and that changes would require only a minimal amount of time." Based on these preferences, messages through electronic mail, public announcements, posters, and direct supervisor contacts (all preferred channels), were successfully used to recruit a large group of participants in a successful intervention (Neiger et al., 2001).

Another example of this concept was the segmentation process that resulted from focus groups conducted with teenage girls as part of a physical activity project (Staten, Birnbaum, Jobe, & Elder, 2006). The process resulted in seven main segments that described the girls: athletic, preppy, quiet, rebel, smart, tough, and other. In addition, they discovered preferences for the types of images that would be best for communication materials.

> Respondents provided the following suggestions: (a) For athletic girls, pictures should show girls participating in organized, competitive activities; (b) for preppy girls, pictures might show girls cheerleading, well-dressed individuals, groups of friends being active, girls being active with boys watching (with positive affect, not leering or jeering), and organized sports with "cute" uniforms; (c) for quiet girls, pictures should show girls alone or in small groups doing activities (don't focus on competitive sports); (d) for rebel girls, pictures might include girls on skateboards, perhaps with some visible body piercing, girls wearing dark clothes, images implying dancing to punk rock music; and (e) for smart girls, pictures should show girls who are not too muscular or strong being active in small groups, and positive attitudes and neat but not trendy dress may be appealing. Small group images that show some smart girls and some preppy girls being active together may be appealing. And (f) for tough girls, pictures might show girls doing stepping or hip-hop dance or girls playing basketball (not necessarily in uniform; show street games, pick-up games). Images of girls should not be conservative. Groups of friends would be appealing. (p.76)

The process for developing appropriate messages is both an art and a science. Many communication theories and models can be used to develop effective messages. A good place to start is with consumer-based health communications, as described in the National Cancer Institute's book *Making Health Communication Programs Work*, otherwise known as the "Pink Book" (See http://www.nci/cancer.gov/pinkbook).

Ensuring That the Product Is Provided in an Appropriate Manner The fourth marketing function outlined by Syre and Wilson (1990) can best be explained by marketing's traditional four Ps: *product, price, place,* and *promotion.* The particular blend of these four marketing variables that planners use to achieve their objective(s) is referred to as the **marketing mix.** To realize the greatest effect in a marketing strategy, there must be a combination of all market mix components, including promotion (Belch & Belch, 2007).

Product. The **product** is what you are offering that will meet the customer's needs. As noted earlier, in health promotion you can market several products. In fact, with any health promotion program, you may have more than one product that you are selling. For example, you have a program where you are trying to reduce the prevalence of heart disease in a community. To do so, you may provide various products for your priority population.

Behavior: 30 minutes of physical activity

Good or Tangible Item: a pedometer to keep track of their steps

Service: a walking-buddy program

Event: a health fair at the community center during physical fitness and sport month (May)

Information. Information is a common health promotion product. Health promoters want to get the most accurate and reliable information to the consumers so they can make informed decisions. This type of information varies depending on the priority population. For example, the *Guide to Community Preventive Sources* (Zara et al., 2005) conducts evidence-based reviews about best practices for public health. Their priority population for this information is public health practitioners and policy makers. The value it provides is that practitioners and policy makers can be confident that they are making the best programmatic decisions and offering the best programs for their priority populations. An example of information for the general public would be guidelines for when to have your child immunized. The benefit this product provides is that parents will have a healthy, happy child.

Ideas. Ideas are another common type of health promotion product. You may be trying to convince people to adopt a certain way of thinking. For example, babies should be put to sleep on their back, motorcyclists should wear a helmet when riding, people should not talk on their cellular phone while driving a car, etc. One social marketing campaign aimed to get people to adopt the idea of fertilizing their lawn in the fall instead of the spring. This idea was based on the fact that spring water runoff contaminated with chemicals affected water quality in the Chesapeake Bay. In exchange for adopting this idea and the subsequent behavior, planners offered the benefit that "delicious Bay blue crab and other seafood would continue to grace the plates of people in greater D.C." (Landers, Mitchell, Smith, Lehman, & Conner, 2006, p. 19). Ideas will often become the behaviors that you want the priority population to do.

Goods. Goods are also called tangible items or products. Tangible items often help support a behavior change. The consumer may have to pay money to obtain this product. Examples of goods in health promotion is a health department offering bicycle helmets at a reduced cost to increase usage or supplying people with diabetes glucose meters to monitor their blood sugar.

Services. Services include screening, counseling, education programs, self-help and support groups, telephone hotlines, health care, and social welfare assistance, to name a few. In Texas, social marketers promoted the WIC program which provided mothers with nutrition education, supplementary foods, and referral to social services (Bryant et al., 2001).

Events.   Events are occurrences in which you want the priority population to participate. Common events are health fairs, walk-a-thons, or activities related to National Health Observances such as National Heart Month, National School Lunch Week, and Public Health Week.

Behavior.   A behavior is an action that you want the priority population to either start, continue, or stop doing. Behavior change is what health promotion is all about. The examples are endless and you can think of many yourself.

Price.   **Price** is what it costs the priority population to obtain the product and its associated benefits. It is what they have to "give up." In other words, price is the sum of costs the consumer must accept to engage in the exchange process (Neiger & Thackeray, 1998). The cost to the priority population may be financial, but often with health promotion interventions the costs are something other than financial (see **Box 11.5**). Nonfinancial costs are often social, mental, emotional, behavioral, or psychological. For example, consumers may pay a price in terms of the time and energy they spend in acquiring new information or in developing a new personal health habit, discomfort while doing a behavior, or the loss of friends because old habits were stopped.

In designing the marketing strategy, the planner must make sure that the benefits the priority population receives are greater than what it costs them to obtain the product. Even if they are not actually less, you have to make them seem less than what they are getting in return. For example, for a mother to bring her child in to be immunized it might cost her time away from other tasks, time to drive to the clinic, the effort to get to the clinic, and being willing to put up with a cranky baby for a few hours after the immunization is received. In communicating about this product (immunizations), the health promoter has to convey that the benefits of a healthy child are greater than a few minor inconveniences (her cost).

Price is not the same thing as barriers. **Barriers** are what keep people from responding to an intervention or doing a behavior. The cost or price of the behavior may be one factor that keeps them from doing (or not doing) the behavior. But there may be other factors as well. Planners in the Marshall Islands found that barriers to people making healthy food choices included a lack of choices at the local supermarket, the perception that a can of meat (e.g., Spam) could feed more people than a piece of fresh fish, that fresh meat cost too much money and took too long to prepare and then cook, and a lack of skills for cooking foods in different ways. These were all barriers. The price it would cost them to do the behavior (choose healthier alternatives) was the cost of the food, but also time—they would have to give up time to prepare and cook the food (Gittelsohn et al., 2006).

When planners asked people why they would not attend a nutrition education class, they said that a major reason was that they lacked transportation and there was nobody to baby-sit their children (John, Kerby, & Landers, 2004). These are barriers but not costs. The people do not have to give up transportation or childcare to participate in the exchange. However, it will keep them from obtaining the product. They would have to give up money for transportation or to pay a sitter. In designing your

| **Box 11.5** | OTHER PRICES OF PARTICIPATION IN A HEALTH PROGRAM |

Behavioral

What am I going to have to stop doing in order to start doing the new behavior? What will I have to do to obtain the product? For example, am I willing to stop eating a candy bar each afternoon in order to eat a healthier choice?

Time

How much time am I willing to give in order to obtain the product? For example, am I willing to take personal leave time from work to attend the WIC clinic and receive nutrition education as well as food vouchers?

Effort

What am I willing to do to get the product? For example, am I willing to make the effort to go the gym every day after work to exercise?

Physical

What am I willing to endure to obtain the product or engage in the behavior? For example, am I willing to be sore for a few days after I start exercising? Am I willing to sacrifice my comfort for a mammogram? Am I willing to give up my safety to get to a location where the product is offered?

Psychological/Emotional

What am I willing to endure mentally or emotionally to obtain this product? For example, if I stop watering my lawn to conserve water, am I willing to be criticized by my neighbors for a brown lawn? If I go in for an AIDS test, am I ready to accept the results?

Social

What am I willing to give up in terms of my friends or family to obtain this product? For example, am I willing to lose my friends if I quit smoking?

product or intervention, you have to make sure that you reduce the barriers and lower the cost—both for the same purpose—to make it easy for people to engage in the behavior, participate in your program, or respond to an intervention.

From an economic standpoint, *price* refers to charging the appropriate amount for the product (program) being provided. As was mentioned in Chapter 10, there are many ways to finance a program. If you are "selling" participation in the program, then the price must match the participants' ability and willingness to pay. When considering the amount to be charged for a product (program), planners should determine:

1. Who are the clients?

2. What is their ability to pay?

3. Are copayers involved?

4. Is the program covered under an insurance program?

5. What is the mission of the planner's agency?

6. What are competitors charging?

7. What is the demand for the program?

The price of a program and who pays for it help determine how a program should be marketed. Whether the program is intended to make a profit will have a great impact on the price. Does the program have to make money? Break even? Or can it lose money? It is a real art not to overprice or underprice the program. Demand and location (*place*) will also influence price. If a program is in high demand, obviously the price can be raised. For example, a stress-management program in a large metropolitan area may be able to command a higher price than one located in a small rural area.

Not only do the demand and the location influence the amount one might charge for a program, but so can the psychological mindset of those in the priority population. Some individuals would not participate in a free or inexpensive program because they question how such a program could be any good. Others believe they have to spend a lot of money to get anything of worth. Also, sometimes when programs are offered free of charge, people may be less likely to attend regularly because they have not "invested" financially in the program. On the other hand, there are some people who, if given the choice of a free program versus one with a cost, will always take the free program, even if they are financially able to pay. Being able to segment the priority population with regard to these economic issues can help set the right price.

Place. The third marketing variable is **place**, which can be thought of as where the priority population has access to the product or where they may engage in the desired behavior. When considering place, you want to make it easy for the consumer to participate or obtain the product. In addition, when placing an intervention it is important to avoid areas where people do not normally go or places where they would not feel comfortable or safe. For example, a local health department decided that they would make it easy for the senior-aged population to get their influenza vaccination. To do so, they offered a "drive-up" service where on a Saturday morning people could drive their cars to the health department parking lot and get a vaccination. Another example was a partnership between bar owners and public health researchers who aimed to make it easier for people to get a taxi cab home, thereby discouraging drinking and driving. They provided taxi cab drivers at a special spot to wait (which also guaranteed them passengers). The area was also well-lit, covered, and in a generally safe place, all important things to the customers (Bhatt, 2006).

When the product is offered it is closely associated with its place. If the priority population has to go to a specific location to obtain the product, you might think about when it will be most convenient for the priority population to do so. For example, if consumers have to come to the local health department to have their car seat checked to ensure that it is properly installed, having that service available at times that are convenient for the priority population will reduce a barrier and make it more likely that the consumer will take action to obtain the product. If it is a program, then you might consider what time of day the program would be best offered. If a worksite program were offered in the evenings, so that the workers had to return to the worksite after dinner, that probably would not be much different from driving across town from work to attend a program. Offering a program right after a shift or on a lunch hour would be much more appealing to most workers. Obviously, planners should be concerned about placing their program in a desirable locale (where they are wanted and needed) at the best possible time.

Promotion. The fourth marketing variable is **promotion.** Promotion is what most people think of when they hear the word "marketing." But promotion is just one component of the overall marketing mix. Promotion is your communication strategy for letting the priority populations know about your product and how to obtain or purchase it. Promotion, also referred to as marketing communications, has three primary purposes (Kotler & Keller, 2007): (1) increase product awareness or inform consumers, (2) persuade people to purchase the product, or (3) remind them that the product exists. There are various tools that you can use to promote your program and achieve these purposes, including advertising, direct marketing, Internet/interactive marketing, sales promotion, personal selling, and publicity/public relations (Belch & Belch, 2007).

Advertising is marketing communication that is paid and nonpersonal, meaning it is not trying to reach one person but rather large groups of people. Common tools for advertising have included mass media (print, radio, and television) and outdoor signage. The national 5-a-day campaign used point-of-purchase advertising in grocery store produce departments to remind people to eat five servings of fruits and vegetables. Local coalition members developed a summer VERB program where they increased the number of places in the community for tweens to be active. They developed a card where tweens could keep track of places they went to be physically active. Advertising space was paid for in the local newspaper, in a local family magazine, and on the radio. In addition, they got free publicity from the local media outlets and word of mouth from program partners and coalition members (Courtney, 2004). The National Bone Health Campaign used advertising including print ads and 30-second radio spots (Lefebvre, 2006).

Direct marketing involves communicating directly with the consumer about a product with the purpose of getting a response from the consumer (Belch & Belch, 2007). Common tools for direct marketing include direct mail, direct selling, or telemarketing. Direct contact with specific groups that might be at high risk and in need of the programs (contacting recent heart attack patients about a program on the need to eat in a "heart healthy" manner), distributing mailbox stuffers or door-to-door flyers, or inserts with employee paychecks are examples of direct marketing. One of the most common ways that healthcare providers in the United States informed patients about the safety and effectiveness of genetic tests was through distributing pamphlets (Cho, Arruda, & Holtzman, 2006).

Internet or interactive marketing uses technology to reach and communicate with the target audience. This form of promotion can generate a great deal of interest in the product for a relative low cost and in a short period of time. The availability of electronic media including the Internet, cell phones, MP3 players, or personal digital assistants has expanded promotional alternatives. For example, social marketers can use podcasts, PDA downloads, and the Internet to promote their products. Websites are probably the most common form of interactive marketing in public health. The National Bone Health campaign developed a website specifically for teen girls (Lefebvre, 2006), and they placed banner ads on other websites that the priority population often visited.

Personal selling refers to person-to-person interaction with the intent to persuade the customer to buy the product. Personal selling is used regularly in healthcare marketing. Pharmaceutical companies have representatives who meet with healthcare providers one-on-one for the purpose of convincing them to use a certain prescription drug. Another example of personal selling is the use of lay health workers, or promotoras. In rural South Carolina, promotoras were used to give information, assistance, and referral to services (Sherrill et al., 2005). One way these lay health workers could engage in personal selling is by going to individual homes and encouraging people with diabetes to attend the health clinic screening and have their blood glucose tested.

Sales promotions are incentives that entice the consumer to try the product. Types of sales promotion include coupons, premiums (e.g., prizes with purchase), contests and sweepstakes, rebates, or samples (Clow & Baack, 2007). This tool is probably used less often in social marketing. However, a common tactic would be to use sales promotions for services such as a coupon for a reduced-cost mammogram, a coupon for a free bike helmet, or a reduced fee at the local fitness center. Sales promotions could also be part of the incentive strategy (discussed later in the chapter). For example, program participants are given a chance to win a prize if they successfully complete a behavior change program.

Finally, public relations, also called publicity, represents both internal and external marketing communications. The media coverage that external public relations activities generate is typically not paid for by the organization (as compared with advertising). Typical public relations tools include the use of ongoing media outreach and sponsorship of large events that draw attention and exposure such as a special kickoff, countdown, ribbon-cutting, or health party to get a program started. Public relations activities can also be used to increase awareness about new products. When the National Cancer Institute personnel released results from the Prostate Cancer Prevention Trial, one of their strategies was to hold a press conference and provide video news releases. This resulted in hundreds of news stories reaching millions of viewers (Croker et al., 2004).

Depending on the product, where it is offered, the purpose of the promotion, your priority population, and the message, the promotional tools you choose will vary. Most importantly, when choosing your promotional tools you should consider the priority population's preferences. For example, formative research for a disaster preparedness campaign in Vietnam found that the majority of respondents owned a radio, fewer people owned a television, and almost nobody had subscriptions to the newspaper or magazines (Ramaprasad, 2005). Therefore, in selecting a promotional strategy and materials, you probably would not place an advertisement in the newspaper, but may consider a radio spot. The National Bone Health Campaign found that the most common ways for girls grade 6–12 to stay in touch with their friends was through text messages, instant messaging, and cell phones. In addition, the most popular magazines were *Seventeen* and *Teen People* (Lefebvre, 2006).

An important component of any marketing strategy is ensuring that you have a strong brand. A **brand** is "a name, term, design, symbol, or any other feature that identifies one seller's good or service as distinct from those of other sellers" (American Marketing Association, 2007). Your brand can be considered your image, reputation, or how you want people to think or feel when they hear about or see your brand (Kotler & Lee, 2006). A strong brand can increase your competitive advantage. This means that when given a choice, the consumer is more likely to choose your product (participate in your program) because of what they associate with your brand. Elements that contribute to your brand include your logo, tag line, colors, images, and even the product name. For example, when you are planning a vacation and think about lodging options, what words, images, or feelings come to your mind when you hear "Motel 6" or "Days Inn." In contrast, what comes to mind when you hear "Marriott" or "Hilton." Each of these has a distinct brand.

The choice of a program name is an important element in its promotion, since the name can make a difference in whether someone from the priority population will be interested in the program. Creating a name is part of the marketing process used to develop informative and persuasive communication flows between the providers of a program and those in the priority population. More likely than not, a program name will be the first contact that someone in the priority population will have with the product (health promotion program). A program name is analogous to the headline of a newspaper article. When most people read a newspaper, they do not read every article; rather, they skim the headlines of the articles and then read those articles that appeal to them. It is the headlines that grab their attention. The same concept applies in advertising a product. A good headline ought to compel members of the priority population to read the rest of the message (Granat, 1994), or, in the case of a health promotion program, create enough interest that those in the priority population want to find out more about the program.

In addition to creative names, acronyms are useful in bringing attention to a program. For example, Foldcraft, a company in Minnesota, uses the acronym H.E.A.L.T.H. as the name of its health program. It stands for "Hey Everyone Always Learns The Hardway." Program titles and acronyms seem to be limited only by the planners' creativity. **Box 11.6** shows additional examples of past and current program names.

Keeping Clients Satisfied and Loyal Keeping existing customers is easier than trying to get new ones. Maintaining your customers means keeping them satisfied by continuing to offer products that meet their needs better than something else that they could choose instead (the competition). Customers always have a choice.

Keeping clients satisfied and loyal has two main advantages. The first is that satisfied and loyal clients can add much to future marketing efforts by providing word-of-mouth advertising. They can provide a lot of favorable advertising, free of charge. Second, and more important, is the value of keeping those in the priority population involved in the health-enhancing behavior that they began as a result of being involved in the health promotion program.

For products that are services such as classes or other eductional-based offerings, becoming involved in a program is important, but maintaining a health-enhancing behavior is a more important objective. There is strong evidence that people are not very

Box 11.6	SAMPLE PROGRAM NAMES
Title (topic)	**Organization/Company**
A Plan for Life (general health)	IBM
Awakening the Spirit (diabetes program for Native Americans)	American Diabetes Association
Freedom from Smoking (smoking cessation)	American Lung Association
FreshStart (smoking cessation)	American Cancer Society
Health e Strategies (e-health)	Wellness Councils of America
Health Track (general health)	Union Pacific
Heart at Work (cardiovascular health)	American Heart Association
Hey everyone always learns the hardway	Foldcraft (Minnesota)
Live for Life (general health)	Johnson & Johnson
Live Well—Be Well (general health)	Quaker Oats
STEPS to a Healthier U.S.	U.S. Department of Health and Human Service
Time Out for Life (general health)	Colonial Life and Accident Insurance Company
Total Life Concept (general health)	AT&T
United Way at Work (general health)	United Way
StayWell (general health)	Control Data
Up with Life (general health)	Dow Chemical

likely to maintain health behavior change over a long period of time. The problem of recidivism to past behaviors, such as substance abuse, has been known for quite a while (Hunt, Barnett, & Branch, 1971). In addition, researchers have warned health education and health promotion program planners of recidivism and dropout problems associated with exercise (Dishman, 1988; Dishman, Sallis, & Orenstein, 1985; Horne, 1975), weight loss (Davis & Addis, 1999; Jeffery et al., 2000), and smoking cessation (Burns & Warner, 2004; USDHHS, 2000a). (Further discussion of relapse can be found in Chapter 7.)

Why do people behave the way they do? Why do some people begin and continue with health promotion programs, whereas others make a strong start but drop out, and still others never begin? Research has shown that the reasons are many and varied. Participation in health promotion programs may be influenced by a variety of factors—including demographic, behavioral, and psychosocial variables—and program structure. "Lack of time, failure to recognize significance of participation, inconvenience to the participant, failure to achieve personal goals, and lack of enjoyment of participation are some of the reasons why individuals drop out of wellness [health promotion] programs" (Bensley, 1991, p. 89). Said another way, the product fails to provide a benefit that the priority population values. Proper motivation is one way of preventing dropouts.

Motivation   A key element for initial involvement and continued participation in a health promotion program seems to be motivation, which has been described as a concept that is both simple and complex. "The concept of motivation . . . is simple because the behavior of individuals is goal-directed and either externally or internally induced. It is complex because the mechanism which induces behavior consists of the individual's needs, wants, and desires and these are shaped, affected, and satisfied in many different ways" (Rakich, Longest, & O'Donovan, 1977, p. 262). Feldman (1983) suggests a variety of ways in which participants may be motivated to adopt a new health behavior. These means are seldom independent of each other, but from a planning standpoint, they are usually viewed separately. The key to motivation is matching the means of motivating with those things that seem to reinforce the individual program participants. What motivates one individual may not be motivating to another individual, and vice versa.

Two approaches are commonly used. The first is to include questions about motivation as part of a needs assessment when planning the program. For example, if the planners are surveying a priority population regarding their needs, they could include questions on reinforcers, such as "What incentives would entice you to participate in the exercise program?" or "What would it take to get you to participate in this program?" or "What would it take to keep you involved in a program?" The responses to these questions should provide some direction concerning the type of reinforcers that would be most useful for the priority population. The second is the "shotgun" approach based on a planner's previous experience or the experience reported by others. Using the shotgun approach, a program planner would offer a variety of reinforcers to meet the needs of a large percentage of the program's priority population. The former approach is recommended, particularly if you are using a consumer-focused marketing approach to program planning. In addition to making sure that you have the right product for the priority population, there are some tactics you can use to help enhance the likelihood that the consumer will be successful at modifying their behavior. The remaining portions of this chapter provide ideas for motivating program participants.

Using Contracts to Motivate.   A *contract* is an agreement between two or more parties that outlines the future behavior of those parties. Contracts are a common part of everyday living. People enter into contracts when they sign a lease for an apartment or a residence hall agreement, take out an insurance policy, borrow money, or buy something over a period of time. The same concept can be applied to getting and keeping people motivated in health promotion programs. Each program participant would enter into a contract with another person (the program facilitator, a significant other, or a fellow participant) and then work toward an objective or agreement specified in the contract. The contract would also specify **contingencies**—that is, what happens as a result of the contract's either being met or not being met.

For an exercise program, this system might work as follows. The program participant and program facilitator would draw up a contract based on the participant's present status in the program (e.g., exercising for 30 minutes once a week) and on what would be a reasonable goal for the near future (e.g., eight weeks). Thus the contract might state that the participant will exercise for 30 minutes twice a week for the first week, 30 minutes three times a week for the second week, and so forth, building up gradually to the final goal of exercising for 60 minutes most days of the week at the end of eight weeks. The outcome should focus on a behavior that can be maintained at the end of the contract period. For a weight loss program, the goal might be written as eliminating snacking in the evening, increasing fruits and vegetables in the diet to five servings per day, and walking for 30 minutes three times a week. These are behaviors that can reasonably be maintained after the weight loss.

The parties to the contract then decide on what the contingencies will be. Thus the participant might offer to make a contribution to some local charity or state that she will continue in the program for another eight weeks if she does not meet the contract goal. The facilitator might promise the participant a program tee-shirt if she fulfills the contract during the specified eight-week period. Other ideas for contingencies might include granting a kickback on fees for completing a certain percentage of the classes, or earning points toward products or services. No matter what the contingencies are, it seems to help if the contract is completed in writing.

Using Social Support to Motivate.   It has long been recognized that whatever the behavior may be, it is almost always easier to do if people have the support of those around them. Long-standing examples of the concept of **social support** in the area of health promotion are programs such as Weight Watchers and Alcoholics Anonymous. They are based on the support of others who are experiencing the same behavior change. One of the key reasons why worksite health promotion programs are so effective is that the working environment lends itself to social support. Being around other individuals who are engaging in the same behavior change provides a good support system.

Another means of helping program participants develop the necessary support system might be to pair them with other participants in a "buddy" arrangement. People find it harder to let others down than to disappoint themselves. Another technique that is being used increasingly is to incorporate the help of family members or significant others to provide the needed motivation. It is easier for someone to quit smoking if all members in the household try quitting at the same time, than to "go it alone" while others in the household continue to smoke.

Using Media to Motivate.   Another technique for keeping people motivated to continue in a health promotion program is to recognize them publicly through some medium available to those in the program. Examples of such media include organization newsletters or newspapers, community newspapers, local television and radio stations, bulletin boards at the location where the program is being offered or public bulletin boards elsewhere, and letters sent to the significant others of the participants (family members, job superiors, etc.) noting the participants' progress in the program.

It is important for planners to exercise caution when recognizing people through the different types of media. Not everyone likes to see their name publicized. Before you publicly acknowledge individual participants, make sure they do not mind if you do so.

Using Incentives to Motivate.   In Chapter 8, **incentives** were discussed as an intervention strategy, but they are also useful in keeping people involved in programs (Jason et al., 1990). Dunbar, Marshall, and Howell (1979) state that reinforcement may be any consequence that would increase the probability of a behavior's being repeated. Wilson (1990, p. 33) defines incentive as "some reward for achieving a level of performance or goal." It has been reported (Frederiksen, 1984) that incentives seem to be most effective if they are provided in small quantities, are frequent in nature, are tailored to those in the priority population, address behaviors over which the individual has control, and do not conflict with any organizational policies.

A Contest as a Means of Motivating.   Wilson (1990, p. 33) reports that contests (or competitions) have been a useful means of "introducing and promoting health promotion programs and achieving significant initial participation rates." A contest can be described as a challenge between two teams (groups) or individuals in which the object is to try to outperform the other competitor. In a health promotion context, this could mean competing to lose the most pounds, smoke the fewest cigarettes, walk the most miles, swim the most laps, or plan the most nutritious meals. Contests are a good method of introducing a health promotion program, but they are probably not useful as an ongoing recruitment tool (Wilson, 1990).

Final Comment on Marketing

Planners who intend to use a canned program should be sure to ask the vendor if there is a marketing plan that goes along with the program. The good programs will usually include some useful marketing strategies, if not an entire plan. A word of caution about the marketing materials: like the canned programs themselves, they are usually aimed at a general population, not one that has been segmented. Therefore they may have to be tailored to meet local needs.

SUMMARY

An important aspect of any health promotion program is being able to design a product (an intervention) that will attract the priority population initially and keep them involved once they have started the program or begun a behavior. All products must provide a benefit or outcome that the priority population values. Using marketing principles can help you develop successful programs. Understanding the consumers, including their wants and needs, is at the heart of the marketing process. An important step in the process is identifying segments that share similar characteristics. The marketing mix should take into account the four Ps of marketing: product, price, place, and promotion. These elements together become the basis for your marketing strategy that will facilitate the exchange between you as the marketer and your priority population as the customer. Once people are enrolled in a program, they need to be motivated to remain involved. Strategies of contracts, social support, media recognition, incentives, and contests can be most helpful in motivating people to continue their participation in a program.

REVIEW QUESTIONS

1. Define the following terms: *market, marketing,* and *social marketing.*

2. What is the relationship between marketing and needs assessment?

3. How does segmenting your priority population help you?

4. What are some factors to use when segmenting your priority population? Which ones are most important?

5. How does the diffusion theory relate to marketing a program?

6. What are the five different groups of people described in the diffusion theory? When would each group most likely join a health promotion program?

7. What has to happen in order for an exchange to take place between the planner and the priority population?

8. What are the differences between marketing a tangible product and an intangible product?

9. What are the four Ps of marketing? Explain each one.

10. What are the five techniques for motivating people to stay involved in a health promotion program?

ACTIVITIES

1. Respond to the following statements/questions with regard to a program you are planning:
   a. Describe your product. What benefit is it providing to your customer?
   b. Describe your segmented population. What segmentation factors did you use?
   c. What will it cost the priority population to obtain the product? If you are providing a service or tangible item, how much money will you charge? Explain the rationale on which you based your decision.
   d. Where will the product be placed? What is your reason for placing it this way? If you have a service product, when will it be offered (location, days, and time)?
   e. What promotional tools will you use to promote your program? How, when, and where will you advertise?

2. Create a promotional piece that could be used to promote your program through advertising, direct marketing, personal selling, sales promotions, or Internet marketing. This promotional piece should include both text and graphics.

3. Give an example of how you could use each of the five methods described in the chapter for motivating program participants to stay in a program.

WEBLINKS

1. http://www.aed.org/socialmarketingandbehaviorchange/

   Academy for Educational Development

   The Academy for Educational Development has done extensive work in social marketing, particularly as it relates to development and health in global settings. This website is a good resource for social marketing, health communications, and health promotion in general.

2. http://www.mapnp.org/library/mrktng/mrktng.htm

   All About Marketing

   This site provides an overview of program design and marketing for nonprofit organizations. It includes valuable insight into marketing in general, market planning, positioning programs, pricing, naming and branding, advertising and promotions, and public and media relations.

3. http://www.marketingpower.com/welcome.php

   American Marketing Association

   The American Marketing Association is one of the largest professional associations for marketers. This site provides best practices related to marketing strategies including marketing tools and templates and marketing services directories.

4. http://ctb.ku.edu/

   Community Tool Box

   The site provides excellent resources on promoting participation and social marketing. Topic sections include step-by-step instruction, examples, checklists, and related resources.

5. http://www.social-marketing.org/index.html

   Social Marketing Institute

   The mission of the Social Marketing Institute is to advance the science and practice of social marketing. This site provides a comprehensive library of success stories in social marketing, papers, conferences, employment listings, and related sites.

6. http://www.hc-sc.gc.ca/ahc-asc/activit/marketsoc/index_e.html

   Social Marketing Network

   This site provides the latest information on social marketing and lessons learned by Health Canada's Marketing and Creative Services Division. Current case studies provide step-by-step instructions for the marketing process.

7. http://www.sophe.org/

   Society for Public Health Education

   Under the link, Publications and Journals, view *Social Marketing Resource Guide*. This guide provides information on social marketing in general, audience segmentation, message development, planning tools, and health communications. [Note: Purchase is required to view this document]

8. http://www.social-marketing.com

   Weinreich Communications

   This site contains social marketing-related articles, resources, conference calendar, and extensive lists of links to pertinent sources of information.

9. http://www.turningpointprogram.org/Pages/socialmkt.html

   Turning Point

   This website is dedicated to social marketing training and resources. It includes several social marketing resource guides and other campaign development tools.

10. www.health.gov/communication

    Prevention Communication Research Database (PCRD)

    This site contains full-text audience research reports on key prevention issues such as asthma, cancer, diabetes, and substance abuse. Sponsored by the Department of Health and Human Services, the PCRD website provides information for shaping audience communications programs.

Implementation
Strategies and Associated Concerns

After reading this chapter and answering the questions at the end, you should be able to:

- Define *implementation*.
- Identify the different phases for implementing health promotion programs.
- List and briefly describe the concerns that need to be addressed before implementation can take place.

act of commission	implementation	pilot testing
act of omission	informed consent	program kick off
anonymity	key activity chart	program launch
beneficence	management	program rollout
confidentiality	negligence	prudent
critical path method	news hook	Task Development Time Line
ethical issues	nonmaleficence	Type III errors
Gantt chart	PERT	
HIPAA	phased in	

In Chapters 1–10 of this book we discussed the steps necessary to plan a solid health promotion program. In Chapter 11, we presented information that would assist planners in marketing the program they planned. As a part of the marketing process we presented information on the process of program adoption using the diffusion theory (Rogers, 2003). It is the adoption of a program (or stated differently, the decision to participate) by those in the priority population that is the beginning of the program implementation process. Yet many other things need to be considered in the implementation process that are critical

Box 12.1	RESPONSIBILITIES AND COMPETENCIES FOR HEALTH EDUCATORS

Chapter 12 focuses on program implementation. Because implementation is a culmination of all the preparation and planning that has come before it, several of the responsibilities and competencies for health educators apply. The responsibilities and competencies related to these tasks associated with implementation include:

Responsibility II: Plan Health Education Strategies, Interventions, and Programs
Competency G: Assess factors that affect implementation

Responsibility III: Implement Health Education Strategies, Interventions, and Programs
Competency A: Initiate a plan of action
Competency B: Demonstrate a variety of skills in delivering strategies, interventions, and programs
Competency C: Use a variety of methods to implement strategies, interventions, and programs
Competency D: Conduct training programs

Responsibility IV: Conduct Evaluation and Research Related to Health Education
Competency D: Carry out evaluation and research plans

Responsibility V: Administer Health Education Strategies, Interventions, and Programs
Competency C: Manage human resources

Responsibility VI: Serve as a Health Education Resource Person
Competency B: Respond to requests for health information

Responsibility VI: Communicate and Advocate for Health and Health Education
Competency B: Apply a variety of communication methods and techniques

Source: NCHEC, SOPHE, & AAHE (2006)

to a successful program. The eventual impact of a program will be judged not only by the effectiveness of the interventions but also by the quality of the implementation (Parcel, 1995). In fact, Timmreck (2003) has stated "implementation is the most critical part of the planning process; a plan that is not implemented is no plan at all" (p. 171). In this chapter, we present the key phases in implementing a program and identify the many concerns that must be addressed as implementation unfolds. **Box 12.1** identifies the responsibilities and competencies for health educators that pertain to the material presented in this chapter.

Defining Implementation

In the simplest terms, implementation means to carry out. Timmreck (1997) defined **implementation** as the "the act of converting planning, goals, and objectives into action through administrative structure, management activities, policies, procedures, regulations, and organizational actions of new programs" (p. 328). Keyser and colleagues (1997) summarized implementation as the setting up, managing, and executing of a project.

While Bartholomew, Parcel, Kok, and Gottleib (2006) indicated that implementation is one of the three stages of program diffusion with the other two being *adoption* and *sustainability*. Let's look now at the phases in the implementation process.

Phases of Program Implementation

The phases of implementation that we present here are a combination of some of our own ideas with those of Parkinson and Associates (1982), Hayden (2000), Bartholomew and colleagues (2006), and Johnson and Breckon (2007). It should be noted that the resulting generic phases presented are flexible in nature and can be modified to meet the many different situations and circumstances faced by planners.

Phase 1: Adoption of the Program

Because the adoption process was presented at length in Chapter 11, it will not be repeated here. However, we do want to remind planners that great care must go into the marketing process to ensure that a relevant product (i.e., the health promotion program) is planned so that those in the priority population will want to participate in it.

Phase 2: Identifying and Prioritizing the Tasks To Be Completed

In order for a program to be implemented, planners will need to identify and prioritize a number of smaller tasks. Even though many of these tasks are small in nature, they cannot be overlooked if planners want a smooth implementation. Reserving space where the program is to be held, making sure audiovisual equipment is available when requested, ordering the correct number of participant education packets or manuals, and arranging for interpreters when working a diverse population are examples of tasks that are important to the success of a program. Other implementation tasks are presented later in this chapter in the section titled "Concerns Associated with Implementation."

To assist planners in identifying and prioritizing these tasks, it is recommended that the planners use some form of a planning timetable or timeline. Planning timetables can assist in "the defining of tasks, the laying out of plans over the life of the project, and the monitoring of progress so that midcourse corrections can be made, if needed" (McDermott & Sarvela, 1999, p. 72). Planning timetables that are commonly used include: key activity charts (McDermott & Sarvela, 1999), Task Development Time Lines (TDTLs) (Anspaugh, Dignan, & Anspaugh, 2000), Gantt charts, PERT charts, and the critical path method (CPM). A **key activity chart** may be the simplest of the tools. It includes three components, a listing of all the key activities or tasks to be carried out, an estimate of the dates when the activities will take place, and the time allocated to complete the activities.

Task Development Time Lines and Gantt charts all are very similar. They are both comprised of rows and columns. The rows on the left-hand side of the chart represent the tasks or activities to be completed, while the columns represent periods of time. In the examples presented in **Figures 12.1** and **12.2**, the columns represent months, but

Tasks Year 1	Months											
	J	F	M	A	M	J	J	A	S	O	N	D
Develop program rationale	✔	✔										
Conduct needs assessment			✔									
Develop goals and objectives				✔								
Create intervention					✔							
Conduct formative evaluation						✔						
Assemble necessary resources						✔						
Market program						✔	✔					
Pilot test program								✔				
Refine program									✔			
Phase in intervention #1										✔		
Phase in intervention #2											✔	
Phase in intervention #3												✔

Tasks Year 2	Months											
	J	F	M	A	M	J	J	A	S	O	N	D
Phase in intervention #4	✔											
Total implementation		✔	✔	✔	✔	✔	✔	✔	✔	✔	✔	✔
Collect and analyze data for evaluation			✔									
Prepare evaluation report				✔								
Distribute report					✔							
Continue with follow-up for long-term evaluation						✔	✔	✔	✔	✔	✔	✔

Figure 12.1 Sample task development time line for program planning, implementation, and evaluation

	Mar.	April	May	June	July	Aug.	Sept.	Oct.	Nov.	Dec.
Hire and train program facilitators	▬▬▬	▬▬▬								
Pilot test program			▬▬▬	▬▬▬						
Revise program based on pilot					▬▬▬					
Promote the program					▬▬▬	▬▬				
Prepare for program ¡kick off"						▬▬▬				
Phase in program							▬▬▬	▬▬▬		
Full implementation								▬▬▬	▬▬▬	
Evaluate program									▬▬▬	▬▬▬
Write final report										▬▬▬

▬▬▬ = planned time frame

——— = completed

Figure 12.2 Sample Gantt chart for program implementation and evaluation

they could just as easily represent weeks or for that matter days if the chart were being used for a short-term project. The major difference between a TDTL and a Gantt chart is in the detail presented. A **Task Development Time Line** identifies the tasks that need to be completed and the time frame in which the tasks will be completed (Anspaugh et al., 2000) using "Xs" or "Us" (see Figure 12.1). A **Gantt chart**, developed in 1917 by Henry Gantt as a production control tool (TechTarget, 2007), does the same plus provides an indication of the progress made toward completing the task by using different size lines to distinguish between the projected time frame for a task and the progress toward completing the task. In addition, a Gantt chart uses a marker above the columns to indicate the current date (Timmreck, 2003) (see the check mark above the month of August in Figure 12.2). Thus if using a Gantt chart, planners would update their progress regularly on the chart.

PERT is an acronym for program evaluation and review technique. PERT charts are more complex than Gantt charts and have not been used as much with health promotion programs (Timmreck, 2003). PERT charts are comprised of two components, a diagram and a timetable (Breckon, 1997). The diagram presents a visual representation of the relationship between and among the tasks to be completed. The diagram also indicates the order by sequentially numbering the tasks to be completed. This means that tasks identified with lower numbers must be completed prior to taking on tasks identified with higher numbers (TechTarget, 2007a). The timetable of a PERT chart is similar to the key activity chart but also includes three estimates of time for each task. Included in the estimates are an optimistic, pessimistic, and a probabilistic timeframe. The complexity of PERT puts a detailed explanation beyond the scope of this textbook. If readers are interested in learning more about it, we recommend referring to business management textbooks.

The last planning timetable to be presented is the **critical path method** (CPM). Critical path method (CPM) charts are similar to PERT charts and are sometimes known as PERT/CPM (Modell, 1996). Like all the other planning timetables presented here, the CPM provides a graphical view of the project and predicts the time required to complete the project. But what is unique to CPM is that it focuses on time by showing which tasks are critical to maintaining the planning schedule and which are not (NetMBA, 2002–2007). Thus, the critical path is indicated and consists of the set of dependent tasks (each dependent on the preceding one) that together take the longest time to complete (Modell, 1996). The tasks on the path are critical because any delay in their completion will lengthen program implementation unless appropriate action is taken.

Phase 3: Establishing a System of Management

Once all the tasks have been identified and the timetable for completing them have been developed, planners need to turn their attention to how the program will be managed. "The efficient, satisfactory management of a health promotion program is vital to its long-term success" (Anspaugh et al., 2000, p. 124). **Management** has been defined as "the process of achieving results through controlling human, financial, and technical resources" (Johnson & Breckon, 2007, p. 293). Depending on the type of program being planned, the management process could range from consuming a small portion of a single planner's time and resources, such as when a smoking cessation program is being planned for 10 people, to needing several people working fulltime to manage a large community-wide program. Many of the tasks associated with the phase of implementation are presented later in this chapter. However, because of the complexity of principles associated with establishing a system of management we recommend readers refer to a management textbook (e.g., Johnson & Breckon, 2007) for more information on management techniques.

Phase 4: Putting the Plans into Action

Parkinson and Associates (1982) suggested three major ways of putting plans into action: by using a piloting process; by phasing it in, in small segments; and by initiating the total program all at once. These three strategies are best explained by using an inverted triangle, as shown in **Figure 12.3**. The triangle represents the number of people from the priority population who would be involved in the program based on the implementation strategy chosen. The wider portion of the triangle at the top would indicate offering the program to a larger number of people than is represented by the point of the triangle at the bottom.

These three different implementation strategies exist in a hierarchy. It is recommended that all programs go through all three of the strategies, starting with piloting, then phasing in, and finally implementing the total program. However, keep in mind that limited time and resources may not always allow planners to work through all three strategies.

Pilot Testing   Pilot testing (or piloting or field testing) the program is a crucial step. Even though planners work hard to bring a program to the point of putting it into action, it

Advantages

- More people involved
- Evaluation more meaningful with larger group

- Easier to cope with workload
- Gradual investment

- Opportunity to test program
- Close control of program

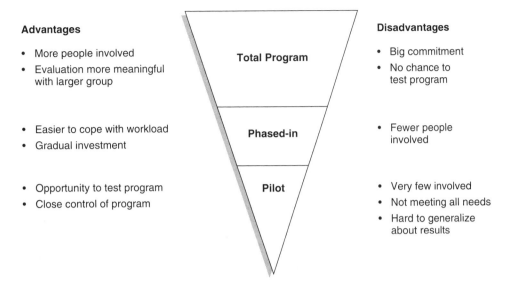

Disadvantages

- Big commitment
- No chance to test program

- Fewer people involved

- Very few involved
- Not meeting all needs
- Hard to generalize about results

Figure 12.3 Putting plans into action

is important to try to identify any problems with the program that might exist. Pilot testing allows planners to work out any bugs before the program is offered to a larger segment of the priority population, and also to validate the work that has been completed up to this point. For the most meaningful results, a newly developed program should be piloted in a similar setting and with people like those who will eventually use the program. Use of any other group may fail to identify problems or concerns that would be specific to the priority population. As an example of the piloting process, take the case of a hospital developing a worksite health promotion program that will be marketed to outside companies. It would be best if the program were piloted on a worksite group before it was marketed to worksites in the community. The hospital could look for a company that might want to serve as a pilot group, or it might use its own employees.

As part of piloting the program, planners should check on the following:

1. The intervention strategies were implemented as planned.

2. The intervention strategies worked as planned.

3. Adequate resources were available to carry out the program.

4. Participants in the pilot group had an opportunity to evaluate the program.

It is important to have the program participants critique such aspects of the program as content, approaches used, facilitator's effectiveness, space, accommodations, and other resources used. Such feedback will give planners insight into how to revise the program. If many changes are made in the program as a result of piloting, planners may want to pilot it again before moving ahead. This evaluation process during the piloting phase is part of process evaluation and will be discussed further in Chapter 13.

Phasing In Once a program has been piloted and revised, the program should, if applicable, be **phased in** rather than implemented in its entirety. This is especially true when there is a very large priority population. Phasing in allows the planners to have more control over the program and helps to protect planners and facilitators from getting in over their heads. There are several ways in which to phase in a program:

1. By different program offerings
2. By a limit on the number of participants
3. By choice of location
4. By participant ability

Say a comprehensive health promotion program was being planned for Blue Earth County, Minnesota. To phase in the program by different offerings, planners might offer stress-management classes the first six months. During the next six-month period, they could again offer stress management but also add smoking cessation programs. This process would continue until all offerings are included.

If the program were to be phased in by limiting the number of participants, planners might limit the first month's enrollment to 25 participants, expand it to 35 the second month, to 45 the third month, and so on, until all who wanted to participate were included. To phase in the program by location, it might initially be offered only to those living in the southwest portion of the county. The second year, it might expand to include those in the southeast, and continue in the same manner until all were included. A program planned for a college town might be offered first on campus, then off campus to the general public. A program phased in by participant ability might start with a beginning group of exercisers, then add an intermediate group, and finally include an advanced group.

Total Implementation Implementing the total program all at once, in most situations, would be a mistake. Rather, planners should work toward total implementation through the piloting and phasing-in processes. The only exceptions to this might be "one-shot" programs, such as programs designed around a single lecture, and possibly screening programs, but even then piloting would probably help.

First Day of Implementation No matter what program is being planned, there will be a "first day" for the program. The first day of the program, also referred to as the **program launch, program rollout,** or **program kick off,** is just an extension of the fourth P of marketing: Promotion (see Chapter 11). The focus of promotion is on creating and sustaining demand for the product (Weinreich, 1999). The creation of the demand for the product leads to the initiation of the program. As such, some special planning needs to take place for the first day of implementation. First, decide on a day when the program is to be rolled out. Consider launching the program to coincide with other already-occurring events or special days that can help promote the program. Examples include: starting a weight loss program at the beginning of the calendar year to coincide with New Year's resolutions, beginning a smoking cessation program on the third Thursday of November (the day each year for the American Cancer Society's Great American Smokeout), having immunization programs and physical examinations for children prior to the beginning of a new school year, launching a skin cancer prevention program on a college campus prior to the annual spring break, or rolling out the community-wide exercise program at the beginning of February, Heart Health month.

Second, kick off the program in style. This is important to bring attention to the program, and to create momentum and enthusiasm for the program (Chapman, 2006). Planners should consider having a first day that includes some special event such as a ribbon cutting, health screening, health fair, contest, appearance by a celebrity, or some other event that starts the program on a positive note. Celebrities need not be individuals with national or international recognition, but may be individuals such as an executive or supervisor of the organization for which the program is being planned (e.g., chief executive officer [CEO] or executive director), a visible or well-known person from the community (e.g., the mayor or a coach), or a common person who has been affected by the health problem on which the program will focus.

Third, consideration should be given to obtaining news coverage (print and/or broadcast) for the first day to further publicize the program. If it is decided to seek such coverage, you should (CDC, 2003):

- inform appropriate media representatives of your plans
- make arrangements to meet the media representatives at the designated time and place
- prepare the following and have them ready for the day:
  —press releases
  —video news releases
  —spokespersons trained to respond to inquires from media representatives

To get news coverage it might be useful to use a **news hook** to interest the media in the program being launched. By news hook, we mean something that would make the media want to cover the launch. The planners' organization may have newsworthy data or information related to the health problem being targeted by the program, or there may be a related news event that is receiving media attention that would help bring attention to the new program (CDC, 2003). For example, if the new program is aimed at reducing teen pregnancy and new state legislation has been proposed to assist in such efforts or an event related to teen pregnancy is currently an important news item, then linking the new program with those timely events can make it more newsworthy (CDC, 2003). Human interest stories also make for good news hooks. For example, if you are starting a smoking cessation program, getting former quitters to talk about how quitting changed their lives can be of interest to others. Or, if your program is aimed at teaching children what to do in an emergency situation, and you know of a child who has completed a similar program and was able to put the education to use in helping someone, many people would like to know about that. Planners should even consider linking the launch of the program with some important date in history to make it newsworthy. Linking the influenza epidemic of 1918 to launch the county-wide flu shot program may make it more newsworthy.

Phase 5: Ending or Sustaining a Program

The final phase of the implementation process is to determine how long to run a program. For some programs the answer will be simple; if the program met its goals and objectives and the priority population has been served to the fullest extent necessary, then the program can be ended. For example, a worksite health promotion may have a goal to certify 50% of the workforce in CPR. If that goal is reached, then the program's resources could be used on other health promotion programming. However, a greater concern facing most planners is how to sustain a needed program for a longer period of time when the goals and objectives have not been met (e.g., only half of those who were expected to get flu shots got them), or goals and objectives of the program are long-term in nature (e.g., providing food and shelter for the homeless). This is especially difficult when original program funding and other types of resources and support may end or be withdrawn. In Chapter 11, we presented information on how to maintain interest in program participants, but here we are referring to the maintenance and institutionalization of a program or its outcomes. Techniques that have been used by planners to sustain programs include: (1) working to institutionalize the program (see Chapter 3, Goodman & Steckler, 1989, and Goodman et al., 1993), (2) advocating for the program (see Chapter 8 for a discussion of advocacy), (3) partnering with other organizations/agencies with similar missions to share resources and responsibilities, and (4) by revisiting and revising the rationale used to create the program initially (see Chapter 3).

Concerns Associated with Implementation

Many matters of detail must be considered before and during the implementation process. Although we believe all the topics presented in this section are important, we feel that the topics of safety and medical concerns and ethical issues are the most important. That is why these topics are presented first.

Safety and Medical Concerns

The ultimate goal of most health promotion programs is to improve the health of its participants. As such, planners in no way want to put the health of participants in danger. Therefore, planners must give attention to the safety and medical concerns associated with health promotion programs. To insure the safety of participants, planners need to inform participants about the program they are considering joining. Only after they understand what the program is all about should they agree to participate. This concept is referred to as informed consent. More formally, **informed consent** has been defined as:

> the voluntary agreement of an individual, or his or her authorized representative, who has the legal capacity to give consent, and who exercises free power of choice, without undue inducement or any other form of constraint or coercion to participate in research [the program]. The individual must have sufficient knowledge and understanding of the nature of the proposed research [program], the anticipated risks and potential benefits, and the requirements of the research [program] to be able to make an informed decision (Levine, 1988, as stated in NIH, n.d., p. 1).

As a part of the process of obtaining informed consent from participants, program facilitators should:

1. Explain the nature and purpose(s) of the program.

2. Inform program participants of any inherent risks or dangers associated with participation and any possible discomfort they may experience.

3. Explain the expected benefits of participation.

4. Inform participants of alternative programs (procedures) that will accomplish the same thing.

5. Indicate to the participants that they are free to discontinue participation at any time.

In addition, planners must ask if the participants "have any questions, answer any such questions, and make it clear they should ask any questions they may have at any time during the program. Informed consent forms should be signed by participants before they enter the program" (Patton et al., 1986, p. 236).

Program planners must be aware that informed consent forms (sometimes called *waiver of liability* or *release of liability*) do not protect them from being sued. There is no such thing as a waiver of liability. If you are negligent, you can be found liable. However, informed consent forms do make participants aware of special concerns. Further, because people must sign the forms, they may not consider legal action even if they have a case, feeling that they were duly warned. **Box 12.2** presents a sample consent form.

Box 12.2 APPLICATION—EXAMPLE INFORMED CONSENT FORM

Consent to Perform Cholesterol Screening

I hereby grant permission to the Institute for Health Promotion personnel to perform a cholesterol screening on me. I am engaging in this screening voluntarily. I have been told this screening will provide an analysis of total blood cholesterol and that a trained employee will take my blood from a finger stick sample. This finger stick may be uncomfortable. I understand that the results of this screening are considered to be preliminary in nature and in no way conclusive. Results of a blood cholesterol screening like this can be affected by a number of factors including, but not limited to, smoking, stress level, amount of exercise, hormone levels, food eaten, heredity, and pregnancy. I also understand that my physician can perform a more complete blood lipid (fat) analysis for me, if I so desire.

Further, I have been told that all the information related to this screening is considered confidential.

I have read the above statement and understand what it means. I have also had an opportunity to ask questions about the screening, and all my questions have been answered to my satisfaction.

_____   _____   _____
Participant's signature   Date   Signature of Witness

NOTE TO PROGRAM PLANNERS: To ensure this form meets all related organizational policies and local and state laws, this form should be submitted to legal counsel before use.

Once participants have agreed to participate in a program, if the act of participating in the program puts anyone at medical risk (e.g., cardiovascular exercise programs), then these individuals need to obtain medical clearance before participating. Some organizations that conduct such programs on a regular basis will have a medical clearance form that will need to be completed. Typically, a physician who is familiar with the person's health history must sign the form. If such a form is not available, then steps need to be taken to create one and have it reviewed by a lawyer to make sure it includes all the necessary information.

After participants have medical clearance and are enrolled in a program, steps must be taken to ensure the safety and health of all associated with the program (i.e., participants and staff members). Providing a safe program includes: finding a safe program location (e.g., low-crime area), providing appropriate security at the location; ensuring that all building codes are met at the location, and ensuring that the classroom, locker rooms, laboratories, and any other facilities used are free of hazards. In addition to a safe environment, programs need qualified instructors (i.e., appropriately trained and certified), and planners need to be prepared for emergency situations by supplying the appropriate first-aid supplies and equipment, and developing an emergency care plan. **Box 12.3** provides a checklist of items that should be considered when creating an appropriate emergency care plan.

Box 12.3 CHECKLIST OF ITEMS TO CONSIDER WHEN DEVELOPING AN EMERGENCY CARE PLAN

1. Duties of program staff in an emergency situation are defined.
2. Program staff is trained (CPR and first aid) to handle emergencies.
3. Program participants are instructed what to do in an emergency situation (e.g., medical, natural disaster).
4. Participants with high-risk health problems are known to program staff.
5. Emergency care supplies and equipment are available.
6. Program staff has access to a telephone.
7. Standing orders are available for common emergency problems.
8. There is a plan for notifying those needed in emergency situations.
9. Responsibility for transportation of ill/injured is defined.
10. Injury (incident) report form procedures are defined.
11. Universal precautions are outlined and followed.
12. Responsibility for financial charges incurred in the emergency care process are defined.
13. The emergency care plan has been approved by the appropriate personnel.
14. The emergency care plan is reviewed and updated on a regular basis.

Ethical Issues

"Ethical issues permeate almost every decision and action undertaken in health education" (Goldsmith, 2006, p. 33), including many of the decisions associated with program planning. By **ethical issues** we mean situations where competing values are at play and program planners need to make a judgment about what is the most appropriate course of action. Here is an example of such an ethical issue. Planners may want to create an intervention that includes an economic incentive for a priority population that, for the most part, is composed of individuals with a low socioeconomic status. Because of the socioeconomic status of those in the priority population, the ethical issue that faces the planners is deciding at what dollar value does the incentive cross over from encouraging people to participate in a program to manipulating their participation in the program?

What guides ethical decision making? Most often, these decisions are compared to a standard of practice that has been defined by other professionals in the same field. For health promotion planners, the standard of practice is outlined in the *Code of Ethics for the Health Education Profession* developed by the Coalition of National Health Education Organizations (CNHEO, 1999) (see Appendix A for a copy of the Code). The preamble of the *Code* states: "The health educator is to aspire to the highest possible standards of conduct and to encourage the ethical behavior of those with whom they work" (CNHEO, 1999, p. 2). For program planners this means having integrity, and being honest, loyal, and accountable. Unethical practice leads to professional suicide; planners who act unethically damage their professional reputation and integrity (Bensley, 2003).

Many of the ethical issues that program planners will face revolve around the three fundamental principles of *The Belmont Report: Ethical Principles and Guidelines for the Protection of Human Subject Research* (National Commission, 1979). These principles include: (1) Respect for Persons, (2) Beneficence, and (3) Justice. Here are some examples of the application of these principles to program planning. The principle of *Respect for Persons* acknowledges the dignity and autonomy (i.e., freedom) of individuals, and requires that people with diminished autonomy (e.g., children, mentally disabled, and people with severe illnesses) be provided special protection (NIH, 2004). It is not unusual for health educators to be working with program participants who have values, behavior, including health behavior, and goals that are different than their own. Even though they are different, it is important to respect them. For example, health educators working in a family planning clinic may see clients choose a legal course of action that may be different than what they personally would select, but clients have the right to choose a course of action and it must be respected.

The principle of *Beneficence* requires program planners to protect participants by maximizing anticipated benefits and minimizing harms (NIH, 2004). This principle dates back to the Hippocratic Oath written by the famous Greek physician Hippocrates who lived from about 460 B.C. until 377 B.C. (Cottrell et al., 2009). The principle embodies two concepts doing good (i.e., **beneficence**) and not causing harm (i.e., **nonmaleficence**). "The Hippocratic maxim 'do no harm' has long been a fundamental principle of medical ethics" (NIH, 2004, p. 18), but also applies to the work of health educators. The concepts associated with this principle seem to be common sense, but yet well-intending health educators who may not be as well informed on best practices (see Chapter 8 for a discussion of best practices) could put participants at risk without knowing they are doing so. For example, in recent years much attention has been given to the public health issue of youth violence. Evidence shows that a number of well-meaning approaches to dealing with youth violence at all three levels of prevention—primary (i.e., holding youth back a grade in school), secondary (i.e., redirecting youth behavior or shifting peer group norm programs), and tertiary (i.e., "boot camps" for delinquent youths)—can bring harm to the youth (USDHHS, 2001c).

When dealing with the principle of beneficence, health educators may need to make ethical decisions revolving around the "benefit-harm ratio." For example, should a health educator be barred from releasing information about a person without his or her consent, even if it will benefit that person? Consider a high school sophomore who approaches the health teacher with confidential information that she is pregnant. Should the health teacher tell anyone else, such as the girl's parents?

The principle of *Justice* requires that program planners treat participants fairly (NIH, 2004). For example, the question of fairness may have ethical implications when it comes to charging a registration fee for a program. Because of the policies of the organization conducting the program, the program may need to turn a profit, but those in need of the program may not be able to afford the cost of registration. Other ethical issues of justice and fairness can arise from issues of sexism, racism, and other cultural biases.

The opportunities for dealing with ethical issues are many, and planners need to be prepared to handle them.

Legal Concerns

Legal liability is on the mind of many professionals today because of the concern over lawsuits. With this in mind, all personnel connected with the planned health promotion program, no matter how small the risk of injury to the participants (physical or mental), should make sure that they are adequately covered by liability insurance. In addition, program personnel should have an understanding of negligence and how to reduce one's risk of liability.

Negligence   Negligence is failing to act in a **prudent** (reasonable) manner. If there is a question whether someone should or should not do something, it is generally best to err on the side of caution. Negligence can arise from two types of **acts: omission** and **commission.** An act of *omission* is not doing something when you should, such as failing to warn program participants of the inherent danger in participation. An act of *commission* is doing something you should not be doing, such as leading an aerobic dance program when you are not trained to do so.

Reducing the Risk of Liability   The real key to avoiding liability is to reduce risk by planning ahead. Patton and colleagues (1986, p. 236) offer the following tips for reducing legal problems in exercise programs; however, similar advice would apply to all types of health promotion programs:

1. Be aware of legal liabilities (things you are legally responsible for).
2. Select certified instructors (in the activity and emergency care procedures) to lead classes and supervise exercise equipment (and for that matter all types of equipment).

3. Use good judgment in setting up programs and provide written guidelines for medical emergency procedures.

4. Inform participants about the risks and danger of exercise (or other activities) and require written informed consent.

5. Require that participants obtain medical clearance before entering an exercise program (or other strenuous programs).

6. Instruct staff members not to "practice medicine," but instead to limit their advice to their own area of expertise.

7. Provide a safe environment by following building codes and regular maintenance schedule for equipment.

8. Purchase adequate liability insurance for all staff.

With regard to item 8 in the preceding list, planners should check on the availability of liability insurance through (1) their employer or (2) special coverage from a professional organization.

Program Registration and Fee Collection

If the program you are planning requires people to sign up and/or pay fees, you will need to establish registration procedures. Program registration and fee collection may take place before the program (preregistration), by mail, in person, via an indirect method like payroll deduction, or at the first session. Planners should also give thought to the type of payment that will be accepted (cash, credit card, or check) and plan accordingly. Though it may seem obvious, some thought also must be given to the security of the money received. That is, how it will be handled, transported, and deposited or otherwise secured.

Procedures for Recordkeeping

Almost every program requires that some records be kept. Items such as information collected at registration, medical information, data on participant progress, and evaluations must be accounted for. The importance of privacy for those planners working in healthcare settings was further emphasized in 2003 with the enactment of the *Standards for Privacy of Individually Identifiable Health Information* section (The Privacy Rule) of the Health Insurance Portability and Accountability Act of 1996 (officially known as Public Law 104–191 and referred to as **HIPAA**). The Rule sets national standards that health plans, healthcare clearinghouses, and healthcare providers who conduct certain healthcare transactions electronically must implement to protect and guard against the misuse of individually identifiable health information. Failure to implement the standards can lead to civil and criminal penalties (USDHHS, 2007d).

The two techniques that are used to protect the privacy of participants are anonymity and confidentiality. **Anonymity** exists when no one, including the planners, can relate a participant's identity to any information pertaining to the program (Dane, 1990). Thus information associated with a participant may be considered anonymous when such information cannot be linked to the participant who provided it. In applying this concept, planners need to ensure that collected data had no identifying information attached to them such as the participant's name, social security number, or any other less common information.

Confidentiality exists when planners are aware of the participants' identities and have promised not to reveal those identities to others (Dane, 1990). When handling confidential data, planners need to take every precaution to protect the participants' information. Often this means keeping the information "under lock and key" while participants are active in a program, then destroying (i.e., shredding) the information when it is no longer needed.

Procedural Manual and/or Participants' Manual

Depending on the type and complexity of a program, there may be a need to develop a *program procedural manual* and/or *participants' manuals*. If a program is very involved (e.g., has several interventions or a very detailed curriculum) and/or may have a number of different people facilitating the program (i.e., one that will be used in a number of locations like an educational program of a voluntary health agency), there is probably a need to create a program procedural manual. The purposes of a program procedural manual (also sometimes referred to as a *training manual*) are to: (1) insure that all who are associated with the program understand the program and its parameters, (2) standardize the intervention so it can be replicated and to avoid what Basch and colleagues (1985) referred to as **Type III errors**—failure to implement the health education intervention properly (see Chapter 15 for a discussion of Type I and II errors), (3) provide ideas for facilitation, (4) provide additional background information on the topic, and (5) provide citations for additional resources.

Participant manuals may also be needed and/or useful for several reasons. First, they may be a good way of getting all program information into participants' hands at one time, including the educational materials and program procedures and guidelines. Second, they can help participants organize information they receive and keep it all in one place, especially if they are set up as loose-leaf notebooks or folders. Third, they can serve as a reference or resource for the participants. And fourth, if participants frequently use their manual as part of the program and become familiar with it, they may be more inclined to refer to it outside of the program sessions.

If a program is being developed in-house and manuals are needed, they will more than likely need to be developed in-house as well. Developing either type of manual—procedural or participant—in-house is a major task; therefore, adequate resources and time need to be given to developing the manuals. If a canned program is obtained from another organization (e.g., a voluntary health agency) or is being purchased from a vendor, it should more than likely include manuals.

Training for Facilitators

If a program that is being planned needs a specially qualified person (certified or licensed) to facilitate it, every effort must be made to secure such a person. This may mean having to hire a vendor to provide such a service. If funds to hire one are not available, others will need to be selected, trained, supported, and monitored appropriately. This may mean running your own training program or sending people to other training classes to become qualified facilitators.

Dealing with Problems

With the program up and running, the task of the planners is to anticipate and deal with problems that might arise and to do so in a constructive manner. Even if a program has been piloted, problems can still arise. Astute and effective planners must anticipate the possibility of things going wrong (Timmreck, 2003). "If problems are anticipated, they can be resolved more easily should they occur in the implementation process" (Timmreck, 2003, pp. 182–183). The problems that could be encountered can range from petty concerns to matters of life and death. Problems might involve logistics (room size, meeting time, or room temperature), participant dissatisfaction, or a personal or medical emergency. Whatever the problem, it should be worked out as much as possible to the satisfaction of all concerned. If there is a question of whether to accommodate a program participant or the program personnel, 99% of the time the participants should be satisfied. They are the lifeblood of all programs. As a part of this implementation concern, it might be a good idea to conduct a one-month evaluation asking questions similar to the ones asked in the piloting evaluation.

Reporting and Documenting

Planners need to give attention to reporting or documenting the ongoing progress of the program to interested others (Ross & Mico, 1980). Planners should keep others informed about the progress of the program for several different reasons, including (1) accountability, (2) public relations, (3) motivation of present participants, and (4) recruitment of new participants. The exact nature of the reporting or documenting will vary, but it is important for planners to keep all stakeholders informed.

SUMMARY

A great deal of work goes into developing a program before it is ready for implementation. The process used to implement a program may have much to say about its success. This chapter presents five phases planners can follow in implementing a program; (1) adoption of the program, (2) identifying and prioritizing the tasks to be completed: (3) establishing a system of management, (4) putting the plans into action, and (5) ending or sustaining a program. Also presented in this chapter are matters that need to be considered and planned for prior to and during implementation.

REVIEW QUESTIONS

1. What is meant by the term *implementation?*

2. Name and briefly describe the five phases of implementation presented in this chapter.

3. Briefly describe how each of the following planning timetables can be used:
   a. key activity chart
   b. Task Development Time Line
   c. Gantt chart
   d. PERT chart
   e. critical path method

4. What are three strategies from the modified model of Parkinson and Associates (1982) for implementing health promotion?

5. What are some techniques planners can use to enhance the first day of implementation? What does it mean to kick off a program?

6. What is meant by the term *informed consent*?

7. What can program planners do to ensure the health and safety of program participants?

8. What is an ethical issue? What are the three ethical principles associated with the *Belmont Report*?

9. Where can you find the *Code of Ethics for the Health Education Profession*?

10. What is negligence? What is the difference between an act of omission and an act of commission?

11. How can program planners reduce their risk of liability?

12. What implications does HIPAA have for planners?

13. What is the difference between anonymity and confidentiality?

14. What are procedural and participant manuals? When should they be used?

ACTIVITIES

1. Explain how you would implement a program you are planning, using a pilot study, phasing in, and total implementation. Also explain what you plan to do to "kick off" the program.

2. Develop an informed consent form that outlines the risks inherent in a program you are planning. Make sure the form includes a place for signatures of the participant and a witness and the date.

3. In a one-page paper, identify what you see as the biggest ethical concern of health promotion programming, and explain your choice.

4. Write a one-paragraph statement outlining the ethical stand your organization will take with regard to program implementation.

WEBLINKS

1. http://www.hhs.gov/ocr/hipaa/index.html

   United States Department of Health and Human Services (USDHHS)

   This is a page at the USDHHS website where you can get more information about the National Standards to Protect the Privacy of Personal Health Information.

2. http://www.history.com/tdih.do

   This Day in History

   This is a commercial web page. The site allows you to input a specific date to find out what historical events took place that day. It can be of use to planners when trying to make the kick off of the program "newsworthy" by linking it to a historical event.

3. http://www.cnheo.org

   Coalition for National Health Education Organizations (CNHEO)

   This is the home page of the CNHEO where you can find both the short and long versions of the *Code of Ethics for the Health Education Profession.*

4. http://www.asq.org/learn-about-quality/project-planning-tools/overview/gantt-chart.html

   American Society for Quality (ASQ)

   This is a web page from ASQ that provides information on how to create a Gantt chart.

5. http://www.nihtraining.com/ohsrsite/guidelines/belmont.html

   National Institutes for Health (NIH)

   This is a page at the NIH website that presents the *Belmont Report: Ethical Principles and Guidelines for the Protection of Human Subjects in Research.*

6. http://www.cancer.gov/clinicaltrials/understanding/simplification-of-informed-consent-docs

   National Cancer Institute (NCI)

   This is a page at the NCI website where you can get more information on informed consent forms. It includes a consent form template that was created to include all of the federally required elements for such a form for a research project.

7. http://cme.cancer.gov/clinicaltrials/learning/humanparticipant-protections.asp

   National Cancer Institute (NCI)

   This is a page at the NCI website that contains a free web-based course on the Human Participant Protections Education for Research Teams. This two-hour tutorial is designed for those involved in conducting research involving human participants, but it is also useful to program planners understanding the need for informed consent. Once completed, there is an option of printing a certificate of completion from your computer upon completing the course.

8. http://office.microsoft.com/en-us/excel/HA010346051033.aspx

Microsoft Office Online

This is a web page from Microsoft Office Online that shows how to create a Gantt chart using Microsoft Excel.

PART III

EVALUATING A HEALTH PROMOTION PROGRAM

The chapters in this section include an overview of the evaluation process, including how to plan an evaluation, analyze and interpret the data, and report the results. The chapters and topics presented in this section are:

CHAPTER 13
Evaluation: An Overview

CHAPTER 15
Data Analysis and Reporting

CHAPTER 14
Evaluation Approaches and Designs

Evaluation

An Overview

After reading this chapter and answering the questions at the end, you should be able to:

- Explain the two basic purposes for evaluation.
- Describe the process of conducting an evaluation.
- Compare and contrast the various types of evaluation.
- Identify some of the problems that may hinder an effective evaluation.
- List reasons why evaluation should be included in all programs.
- Explain the difference between internal and external evaluation.
- Describe several considerations in planning and conducting an evaluation.

KEY TERMS

baseline data	formative evaluation	process evaluation
effectiveness	impact evaluation	quality
evaluation	internal evaluation	standards of acceptability
evaluation consultant	institutional review boards	standards of evaluation
external evaluation	outcome evaluation	summative evaluation

Performing adequate and appropriate evaluation is necessary for any program regardless of size, nature, or duration. While it is true that program resources, namely the proportion of the budget that can be devoted to evaluation, as well as the evaluation expertise of the staff and partners, will influence the type and quality of the evaluation performed, every effort should be made to address the two most critical purposes of program evaluation: (1) assessing and improving **quality,** and (2) determining **effectiveness.** Planners who neglect evaluation do so at the peril of program funding and perhaps even professional reputation.

<table>
<tr><td>

Box 13.1   RESPONSIBILITIES AND COMPETENCIES
FOR HEALTH EDUCATORS

Responsibilities and competencies that are connected with the content in this chapter include:

Responsibility IV: Conduct Evaluation and Research Related to Health Education

                   Competency A: Develop plans for evaluation and research

                   Competency B: Review research and evaluation procedures

                   Competency D: Carry out evaluation and research plans

Source: NCHEC, SOPHE, & AAHE (2006)

</td></tr>
</table>

Evaluation is considered a major area of responsibility for certified health education specialists (NCHEC, SOPHE, & AAHE, 2006), and health educators or those employed in health promotion must understand: basic evaluation concepts and the sequence of evaluation, appropriate evaluation designs and methodology, and how to analyze and report evaluation data. Your credibility as a planner and health professional will often be linked directly to your ability to perform these important tasks.

This chapter presents an overview of evaluation. Specifically it introduces: evaluation terminology; the basic purposes of evaluation, including distinctions between formative (process) and summative (impact and outcome) evaluation; the process of conducting an evaluation; problems or barriers in program evaluation; and other issues to consider when conducting an evaluation. **Box 13.1** identifies the responsibilities and competencies for health educators that pertain to the material presented in this chapter.

Basic Terminology

In general terms, "evaluation is a process of reflection whereby the value of certain actions in relation to projects, programs, or policies are assessed" (Springett, 2003, p. 264). As it applies to health promotion, **evaluation** has been defined as "the comparison of an object of interest against a standard of acceptability" (Green & Lewis, 1986, p. 362). In this latter definition, the object of interest could be the entire health promotion program or any part of that program. The **standards of acceptability** are the minimum levels of performance, effectiveness, or benefits used to judge the value (Green & Lewis, 1986) and are typically expressed in the "outcome" and "criterion" components of a program's objectives (see Chapter 6 for information about objectives). **Box 13.2** lists a number of sources for standards of acceptability.

Several *types* of evaluation are used to address the two basic *purposes* of evaluation (i.e., assessing and improving quality and determining effectiveness). Process, or formative, evaluation relate to quality assessment and program improvement. Impact and outcome, or summative, evaluation measure program effectiveness.

In professional practice, the terms process evaluation and formative evaluation are used interchangeably and are usually synonymous. In theory, formative evaluation is somewhat more comprehensive and includes, in addition to process evaluation, such

---

Box 13.2   STANDARDS OF ACCEPTABILITY

Standard of Acceptability	Examples
Mandate (policies, statutes, laws) of regulating agencies	Percent of children immunized for school; percent of priority population wearing safety belts
Health status of the priority population	Rates of mortality and morbidity compared to state and national data
Values expressed in the local community	Type of school curriculum expected
Standards advocated by professional organizations	Passing scores, certification, or registration examinations
Norms established by research	Treadmill tests or percent body fat
Norms established by evaluation of previous programs	Smoking cessation rates or weight loss expectations
Comparison or control groups	Used in experimental or quasi-experimental studies

---

things as pre-testing certain program components (e.g., curriculum, video clips, public service announcements, language for potential legislation) with the priority population prior to implementation or pilot testing (testing the complete program with a small segment of the priority population before full-blown implementation). What is most important to remember is that both terms pertain to the process of quality, or program improvement. For example, assume a program is developed for women on breast cancer awareness consisting of three educational sessions: (1) cancer in general, (2) breast cancer specifically, and (3) self-breast examinations and mammography. Many factors could affect the quality of this program such as:

- Is the information accurate and current?
- Is the information and associated material appealing and interesting to participants?
- Are the most appropriate priority populations being addressed and reached with the program?
- Are behavior change strategies based on appropriate theory?
- Is the program being implemented as intended (as per protocol)?
- Is the facilitator (educator) qualified and knowledgeable?
- Do participants seem genuinely interested and engaged in the program?
- Are the physical surroundings (atmosphere of the room, heating/cooling, seating, etc.) of the educational sessions conducive to learning and behavior change?

Process evaluation addresses these and many other issues. But to expect our programs to be effective (i.e., women actually perform self-breast examinations and have mammograms conducted and, as a result, deaths due to breast cancer are ultimately decreased), planners and evaluators must ensure that the "process" of program delivery represents high quality and adherence to program protocols and guidelines.

With respect to the measurement of effectiveness, impact and outcome evaluation are generally synonymous with summative evaluation. Technically, impact evaluation relates to changes in behavior and, in some cases, changes in awareness, knowledge, attitudes, and skills, whereas outcome evaluation pertains to changes in health status such as mortality (death), morbidity (illness), or disability. In combination, attention to the quality and effectiveness of programs through proper evaluation helps ensure that program goals and objectives are accomplished. Ultimately, the true mark of program success should always be linked to the extent to which goals and objectives are achieved. Without evaluation, such claims can rarely, if ever, be made.

More formal definitions for *process, impact, outcome, formative*, and *summative evaluation* are presented below.

- **Process evaluation:** "Any combination of measurements obtained during the implementation of program activities to control, assure, or improve the quality of performance or delivery. Together with preprogram studies, makes up formative evaluation" (Green & Lewis, 1986, p. 364). Getting reactions from program participants about the times programs are offered or about program speakers are examples. Such measurements could be collected with a short questionnaire or focus group.

- **Impact evaluation:** Focuses on "the immediate observable effects of a program, leading to the intended outcomes of a program; intermediate outcomes" (Green & Lewis, 1986, p. 363). Measures of awareness, knowledge, attitudes, skills, and behaviors yield impact evaluation data.

- **Outcome evaluation:** Focuses on "an ultimate goal or product of a program or treatment, generally measured in the health field by mortality or morbidity data in a population, vital measures, symptoms, signs, or physiological indicators on individuals" (Green & Lewis, 1986, p. 364). Outcome evaluation is long-term in nature and takes more time and resources to conduct than impact evaluation.

- **Formative evaluation:** "Any combination of measurements obtained and judgments made before or during the implementation of materials, methods, activities or programs to control, assure or improve the quality of performance or delivery" (Green & Lewis, 1986, p. 362). Examples include, but are not limited to, pretesting, or pilot-testing a program.

- **Summative evaluation:** "Any combination of measurements and judgments that permit conclusions to be drawn about impact, outcome, or benefits of a program or method" (Green & Lewis, 1986, p. 366).

Even though the sets of terms are used to describe evaluation activities, there is some overlap among the terms as noted earlier (see **Figure 13.1**). Process evaluation occurs during the program and may be considered a form of formative evaluation. Impact and outcome evaluation occur at the completion of the program and are synonymous with summative evaluation. Both sets of evaluation terms (process, impact, and outcome; formative and summative) take into account the need to conduct evaluation before and/or during the program, and at the end of the program. Plans for all types of evaluation should be in place before or during program implementation.

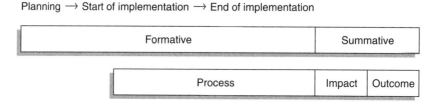

Figure 13.1 Comparison of evaluation terms

Purpose for Evaluation

In the most basic sense, programs are evaluated to gain information and make decisions. The types of evaluation are distinguished by how the information is going to be used. The information may be used by planners during the implementation of a program to make improvements in services (process evaluation). In other words, you do not want to continue indefinitely with a bad program. It may be used to see if certain immediate outcomes—such as knowledge, attitude, skills, and behavior change—have occurred (impact evaluation). It may also be used at the end of a program to determine whether long-term goals and objectives have been met (outcome evaluation). Capwell, Butterfoss, and Francisco (2000) identify six general reasons why stakeholders may want programs evaluated:

1. *To determine achievement of objectives related to improved health status:* Probably the most common reason for program evaluation is to determine if objectives of the program have been met. Evaluation for this reason may also be used to determine which of several programs was most effective in reaching a given objective.

2. *To improve program implementation:* Planners should always be interested in improving a program. Program evaluation can help planners understand why a par ticular intervention worked (Valente, 2002) or did not work, and thus, weak elements can be identified, removed, and replaced (Green & Lewis, 1986).

3. *To provide accountability to funders, community, and other stakeholders:* Many stakeholders are interested in the value of a program to a community, or if the program is worth its cost. Thus an evaluation may provide decision makers with the information to determine if the program funding should continue, discontinue, or expand.

4. *To increase community support for initiatives:* The results of an evaluation can increase the community awareness of a program. Positive evaluation information channeled through the media can help sell a program, which in turn may lead to additional funding.

5. *To contribute to the scientific base for community public health interventions:* Program evaluation can provide findings that can lead to new hypotheses about human behavior and community change, which in turn may lead to new and better programs.

6. *To inform policy decisions:* Program evaluation data can be used to impact policy within the community. For example, a number of communities have passed local ordinances based on the results of evaluative studies on secondhand smoke.

Framework for Program Evaluation

In 1999, the Centers for Disease Control and Prevention (CDC) (1999c) published an evaluation framework to be used for public health programs. The framework was developed by a working group that included evaluation experts, public health program managers and directors, state and local public health officials, teachers, researchers, U.S. Public Health Service agency representatives, and CDC staff members.

The framework (see **Figure 13.2**) is comprised of six steps that should be completed for any evaluation, regardless of the setting. They are not a prescription; rather, they are starting points for tailoring the evaluation. The early steps provide the foundation, and all steps should be finalized before moving to the next step:

- *Step 1—Engaging stakeholders:* This step begins the evaluation cycle. Stakeholders must be engaged to insure that their perspectives are understood. The three primary groups of stakeholders are (1) those involved in the program operations, (2) those served or affected by the program, and (3) the primary users of the evaluation results. Because stakeholders will decide the fate of the program based on the

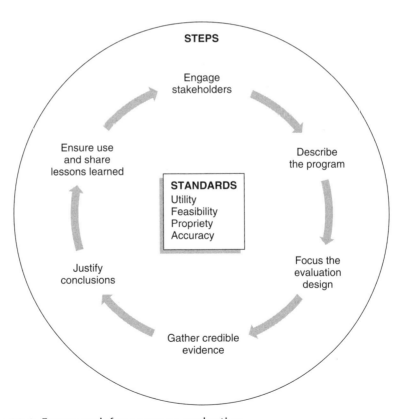

Figure 13.2 Framework for program evaluation

Source: Centers for Disease Control and Prevention (CDC) (1999c), p. 4.

evaluation results, it is important to understand their expectations up front. The scope and level of stakeholder involvement will vary with each program being evaluated.

- *Step 2—Describing the program:* This step sets the frame of reference for all subsequent decisions in the evaluation process. At a minimum, the program should be described in enough detail that the mission, goals, and objectives are known. Also, the program's capacity to effect change, its stage of development, and how it fits into the larger organization and community should be known. Usually, a logic model is used in this step to display a sequence of program events (see Chapter 1 for a discussion of logic models).

- *Step 3—Focusing the evaluation design:* This step entails making sure that the interests of the stakeholders are addressed while using time and resources efficiently. Among the items to consider at this step include articulating the purpose of the evaluation (i.e., gain insight, change practice, assess effects, affect participants' behavior), determining the users and uses of the evaluation results, formulating the questions to be asked, determining which specific evaluation design will be used, and finalizing any agreements about the process.

- *Step 4—Gathering credible evidence:* This step includes many of the items mentioned in Chapter 5. At this step, evaluators need to decide on the measurement indicators, sources of evidence, quality and quantity of evidence, and logistics for collecting the evidence.

- *Step 5—Justifying conclusions:* This step includes the comparison of the evidence against the standards of acceptability; interpreting those comparisons; judging the worth, merit, or significance of the program; and creating recommendations for actions based upon the results of the evaluation.

- *Step 6—Ensuring use and sharing lessons learned:* This step focuses on the use and dissemination of the evaluation results. When carrying out this final step, the needs of each group of stakeholders must be addressed.

In addition to the six steps of the framework, there are four **standards of evaluation**. These standards are noted in the box at the center of Figure 13.2. The standards provide practical guidelines for the evaluators to follow when having to decide among evaluation options. For example, these standards help evaluators avoid evaluations that may be accurate and feasible but not useful or those that would be useful and accurate but not feasible (CDC, 1999c). The four standards are:

- "Utility standards ensure that information needs of evaluation users are satisfied" (CDC, 1999c, p. 27).

- "Feasibility standards ensure that the evaluation is viable and pragmatic" (CDC, 1999c, p. 27). In other words, the evaluation is realistic and affordable.

- "Propriety standards ensure that the evaluation is ethical (i.e., conducted with regard for the rights and interests of those involved and effected)" (CDC, 1999c, p. 27).

- "Accuracy standards ensure that the evaluation produces findings that are considered correct" (CDC, 1999c, p. 29). This means findings are both valid and reliable.

Practical Problems or Barriers in Evaluation

Several authors (Solomon, 1987; Glasgow, Vogt, & Boles, 1999; Glasgow, 2002; NCI, 2002; Valente, 2002; Timmreck, 2003) have identified practical problems or barriers to effective evaluation. Some of the more common problems or barriers are presented below.

1. Planners either fail to build evaluation in the program planning process or do so too late (Solomon, 1987; Valente, 2002; Timmreck, 2003).

2. Resources (e.g., personnel, time, money) may not be available to conduct an appropriate evaluation (Solomon, 1987; NCI, 2002; Valente, 2002).

3. Organizational restrictions on hiring consultants and contractors (NCI, 2002).

4. Effects are often hard to detect because changes are sometimes small, come slowly, or do not last (Solomon, 1987; Glasgow, 2002; Valente, 2002).

5. Length of time allotted for the program and its evaluation (NCI, 2002).

6. Restrictions (i.e., policies, ethics, lack of trust in the evaluators) that limit the collection of data from those in the priority population (NCI, 2002).

7. It is sometimes difficult to distinguish between cause and effect (Solomon, 1987).

8. It is difficult to separate the effects of multistrategy interventions (Glasgow et al., 1999), or isolating program effects on the priority population from "real world" situations (NCI, 2002).

9. Conflicts can arise between professional standards and do-it-yourself attitudes (Solomon, 1987) with regard to appropriate evaluation design.

10. Sometimes people's motives get in the way (Solomon, 1987; Valente, 2002).

11. Stakeholders' perceptions of the evaluation's value (NCI, 2002).

12. Intervention strategies are sometimes not delivered as intended (i.e., type III error) (Glasgow, 2002), or are not culturally specific (NCI, 2002; Valente, 2002).

Examples of these problems in health promotion programs include not collecting initial information from participants because evaluation plans were not in place, failing to budget for the cost of the evaluation (e.g., printing questionnaires, additional staff, postage), or conducting the evaluation before a change can occur (e.g., changes in cholesterol level) or too long after program completion (e.g., long-term effects of a weight loss program). Those without evaluation expertise may conduct an evaluation without a sound design, such as not using appropriate sampling techniques or comparison groups. Program managers, who have a motivation to make their programs cost effective, may minimize costs and unwittingly exaggerate program benefits.

Awareness of these problems and development of strategies to deal with them may improve the accuracy of program evaluation. The remainder of this chapter discusses many approaches that can help minimize these problems, such as including evaluation in the early stages of program planning, accounting for ethical considerations, determining who will conduct the evaluation, carefully considering the evaluation design, increasing objectivity, and developing a plan to use the evaluation results.

Evaluation in the Program Planning Stages

As discussed in Chapter 6, the evaluation design must reflect the goals and objectives of the program. The results of the evaluation will determine whether the goals and objectives were met. To be most effective, the evaluation must be planned in the early stages of program development and should be in place before the program begins. Results from evaluations conducted early in the program planning process can assist in improving the program. Having a plan in place to conduct an evaluation before the end of a program will make collecting information regarding program outcomes much easier and more accurate.

Discussion on how evaluation plans can be included in program planning will focus on examples of formative and summative evaluations. The formative evaluation should provide feedback to the program administrator, with program monitoring beginning in the early stages. Collecting information and communicating it to the administrator quickly allows for the program to be modified and improved.

Data reflecting the initial status or interests of the participants (**baseline data**) or data from a needs assessment can be used to assess participant satisfaction. Additional information from the formative evaluation may indicate that the necessary staff have been hired, the program sites are available, brochures have been printed, participants are satisfied with the times the programs are offered, and classes are offered with the needs of the prospective participants in mind.

Initial data regarding the program should be analyzed quickly to make any necessary adjustments to the program. This type of evaluation can improve both new and existing programs. Information from the formative evaluation can be useful in answering questions, such as whether the programs are provided at convenient locations for the community members, whether the necessary materials arrived on time, and whether people are attending the workshops at all the various times they are offered.

By developing the summative evaluation plan at the beginning of the program, planners can ensure that the results will be less biased. Early development of the summative evaluation plan ensures that the questions answered reflect the original objectives and goals of the program. This type of evaluation can provide answers to many questions, such as whether the group approach or the individual approach was more effective in reducing tobacco use among the participants in a smoking cessation program, whether the participants in a weight loss program lost weight and kept the weight off, and how many people in the priority population increased their knowledge, changed their attitudes, or reduced their risks.

Ethical Considerations

Always remember that evaluation or research should never cause mental, emotional, or physical harm to those in the priority population. Evaluation participants should always be informed of the purpose and potential risks of any evaluation and should always give their consent before participating. Generally, evaluators assure the confidentiality and anonymity of evaluation responses. Although evaluation data are reported in the aggregate, no individual should ever have his or her personal information revealed in any setting or circumstance.

Because evaluations may have ethical considerations for the individuals involved, most colleges, universities, school systems, and large health organizations have boards to review the evaluation design and potential risk to participants. These groups are most often referred to as **institutional review boards** (IRBs) ["sometimes referred to as human subjects' committees, ethical review boards, research advisory committees" (Cottrell & McKenzie, 2005, p. 98)]. These boards serve to safeguard the rights, privacy, health, and well-being of those involved in the evaluation/research. Before conducting any evaluation or research involving human subjects, make sure to get IRB approval.

Who Will Conduct the Evaluation?

At the beginning of the program, planners must determine who will conduct the evaluation. The program evaluator must be as objective as possible and should have nothing to gain from the results of the evaluation. The evaluator may be someone associated with the program or someone from outside.

If an individual trained in evaluation and personally involved with the program conducts the evaluation, it is called an **internal evaluation.** For example, a local health department may use one of its own employees to serve as the evaluator of its programs. An internal evaluator would have the advantage of (1) being more familiar with the organization and the program history, (2) knowing the decision-making style of those in the organization, (3) being present to remind others of results now and in the future, and (4) being able to communicate technical results more frequently and clearly (Fitzpatrick et al., 2004). Conducting an internal evaluation is also less expensive than hiring additional personnel to conduct the evaluation. The major drawback, however, is the possibility of evaluator bias or conflict of interest. Someone closely involved with the program has an investment in the outcome of the evaluation and may not be completely objective. After all, a positive evaluation of the program may result in future funding that would enhance the positions of the staff members.

An **external evaluation** is one conducted by someone who is not connected with the program. Often an external evaluator is referred to as an **evaluation consultant.** Having someone from the state health department conduct evaluations for the local health department would be an example of an external evaluator. External evaluators are somewhat isolated, lacking the knowledge and experience of the program that the internal evaluator possesses. Evaluation of this nature is also more expensive, since an additional person must be hired to carry out the work. However, an external evaluator: (1) can often provide a more objective review and a fresh perspective, (2) can help to ensure an unbiased evaluation outcome, (3) brings a global knowledge of evaluation having worked in a variety of settings, and (4) "typically brings more breadth and depth of technical expertise" (Fitzpatrick et al., 2004, p. 23). **Box 13.3** presents a list of characteristics that program planners can use when selecting an external evaluator. In addition, when selecting an external evaluator, planners should look for someone with formal training in evaluation methods.

Whether an internal or external evaluator conducts the program evaluation, the main goal is to choose someone with credibility and objectivity. The evaluator must have a clear role in the evaluation design and accurately report the results regardless of the findings.

> **Box 13.3** CHARACTERISTICS OF A SUITABLE CONSULTANT
>
> - Is not directly involved in the development or administration of the program being evaluated
> - Is impartial about evaluation results (i.e., has nothing to gain by skewing the results in one direction or another)
> - Will not give in to any pressure by senior staff or program staff to produce particular findings
> - Will give the staff the full findings (i.e., will not gloss over or fail to report certain findings for any reason)
> - Has experience in the type of evaluation needed
> - Communicates well with key personnel
> - Considers programmatic realities (e.g., a small budget) when designing an evaluation
> - Delivers reports and protocols on time
> - Relates to the program
> - Sees beyond the evaluation to other programmatic activities
> - Explains both the benefits and risks of evaluation
> - Educates program personnel about conducting evaluation, thus allowing future evaluations to be done in house
> - Explains material clearly and patiently
> - Respects all levels of personnel
>
> *Source*: Thompson and McClintock (1998), p. 13

Evaluation Results

The question of who will receive the evaluation results is also an important consideration. The evaluation can be conducted from several vantage points, depending on whether the results will be presented to the program administrator, the funding source, the organization, or the public. These stakeholders may all have different sets of questions they would like answered. The evaluation results must be disseminated to groups interested in the program. Different aspects of the evaluation can be stressed, depending on the group's particular needs and interests. A program administrator may be interested in which approach was more successful, the funding source may want to know if all objectives were reached, and a community member may want to know if participants felt the program was beneficial.

The planning process of the evaluation should include a determination of how the results will be used. It is especially important in process and formative evaluation to implement the findings rapidly to improve the program. However, an action plan is needed in summative, impact, and outcome evaluation to ensure that the results are not filed away, but are used in the provision of future health promotion programs.

SUMMARY

Evaluation can be thought of as a way to make sound decisions regarding the worth or effectiveness of health promotion programs, to compare different types of programs, to eliminate weak program components, to meet requirements of funding sources, or to provide information about programs. The evaluation process takes place before, during, and after program implementation. If the evaluation is well designed and conducted, the findings can be extremely beneficial to the program stakeholders.

REVIEW QUESTIONS

1. What are the two basic purposes of program evaluation?

2. List and describe the six steps in CDC's framework for program evaluation.

3. List and describe the four standards in CDC's framework for program evaluation.

4. Give an example of a question that could be answered in a process evaluation, impact evaluation, and outcome evaluation.

5. What are some of the more common problems associated with or barriers to effective evaluation?

6. What different types of information could an evaluation provide for the various stakeholders (planners, funding source, administrators, and participants)?

7. Why is it important to begin the evaluation process in the program planning stages?

8. Explain how feedback from an evaluation can be used in program planning.

9. In what type of situation would an internal evaluation be more appropriate than an external evaluation?

10. What are the desirable characteristics of an external evaluator (evaluation consultant)?

ACTIVITIES

1. Describe how process, impact, and outcome evaluation could be used in a stress management program for college students.

2. Write a rationale to a funding source for hiring an external evaluator (evaluation consultant).

3. Review the evaluation component from a health promotion program in your community and/or discuss an evaluation plan with a planner or evaluator. Look for

the planning process used, the rationale for the data collection method, and how the findings were reported.

4. Assume you are responsible for selecting an evaluator for a health promotion program you are planning. Would you select an internal or an external evaluator? Explain your rationale. If you select an external evaluator (evaluation consultant), where do you think you could find such a person?

WEBLINKS

1. http://www.eval.org

   American Evaluation Association (AEA)

   This is the website for the AEA. The AEA is an international professional association of evaluators devoted to the application and exploration of program evaluation, personnel evaluation, technology, and many other forms of evaluation.

2. http://www.evaluationcanada.ca/site.cgi?s=1

   The Canadian Evaluation Society (CES)

   This is the website for the CES. The CES is a professional association of evaluators dedicated to the advancement of evaluation theory and practice. Information at this site is available in both English and French.

3. http://www.wkkf.org/Pubs/Tools/Evaluation/Pub770.pdf

   W.K. Kellogg Foundation (WKKF)

   This is the *WKKF Evaluation Handbook*. The handbook provides a framework for thinking about evaluation as a relevant and useful program tool. It was written primarily for project directors who have direct responsibility for the ongoing evaluation of W.K. Kellogg Foundation-funded projects.

4. http://www.cdc.gov/eval/index.htm

   Centers for Disease Control and Prevention (CDC)

   This is a page from the CDC website. This page is dedicated to the CDC Evaluation Working Group and its effort to promote program evaluation in public health. The site includes links to the CDC evaluation framework and additional resources that may help when applying the framework.

5. http://www.cdc.gov/mmwr/preview/mmwrhtml/rr4811a1.htm

   CDC Framework for Program Evaluation in Public Health

   This is CDC's framework described earlier in this chapter published in *Morbidity and Mortality Weekly Report*. This document describes in detail the six steps related to the framework.

6. http://www.rand.org/pubs/technical_reports/TR101/

   Getting to Outcomes: Promoting Accountability Through Methods and Tools for Planning, Implementation, and Evaluation

   An excellent evaluation resource related to establishing and measuring evidence-based program outcomes.

7. http://whqlibdoc.who.int/hq/2000/WHO_MSD_MSB_00.2e.pdf

   Process Evaluations

   This is a document on process evaluations from the World Health Organization. A good resource for designing and conducting process evaluations.

Evaluation Approaches and Designs

CHAPTER

CHAPTER OBJECTIVES

After reading this chapter and answering the questions at the end, you should be able to:
- Describe the difference between process and summative evaluation.
- Identify elements and strategies related to process evaluation.
- List some considerations in selecting an evaluation design.
- Compare and contrast quantitative and qualitative methods of evaluation.
- List the various qualitative methods that can be used in program evaluation.
- Differentiate among experimental, control, and comparison groups.
- Compare and contrast the major types of evaluation design.
- Identify the threats to internal and external validity and explain how evaluation design can increase control.

KEY TERMS

accountability
approaches
blind
capacity
comparison group
context
control group
cost-benefit analysis (CBA)
cost-effectiveness
    analysis (CEA)
cost-identification analysis
cost-utility analysis (CUA)

deductive
designs
dose
double blind
evidence
experimental design
experimental group
external validity
fidelity
generalizability
inclusion
inductive

interaction
internal validity
justification
measurement
multiplicity
nonexperimental design
orientation
pilot testing
posttest
pretest
pretesting
process evaluation

Key Terms, continued

qualitative method	recruitment	summative evaluation
quantitative method	resources	support
quasi-experimental design	response	triple blind
reach	satisfaction	

For the purpose of clarity, the term **process evaluation** will be used in this chapter synonymously with formative evaluation. As described in Chapter 13, there is little, if any, difference between process and formative evaluation among health promotion practitioners. Technically, formative evaluation is generally viewed as a more comprehensive approach and involves strategies such as pretesting and pilot testing—both addressed in this chapter. However, as evidenced by important writings in the field of health promotion (Steckler & Linnan, 2002; Saunders, Evans, & Joshi, 2005), the term process evaluation appears to be used more commonly. Summative evaluation will be used in this chapter to include any data collection related to changes in awareness knowledge, attitudes, skills, and more especially to improvements in health-enhancing behaviors (impact evaluation) as well as decreases in preventable death, disability, and injury (outcome evaluation).

As discussed in Chapter 13, program evaluation serves to: (1) assess and improve the quality of programs (process evaluation), and (2) assess effectiveness (summative evaluation). Based on stakeholder preferences, either process or summative evaluation may be performed independent of the other. As a general rule, however, it is recommended that both process and summative evaluation be performed, especially when a program is implemented for the first time.

This chapter focuses on evaluation approaches and designs. The term **approaches** refers to the use of either process or summative evaluation and suggests these two types of evaluation are clearly distinct. **Designs** relates to summative evaluation. Whereas process evaluation is typically defined with descriptions of associated elements and strategies, summative evaluations are generally associated with experimental, quasi-experimental, and nonexperimental designs. **Box 14.1** identifies the responsibilities and competencies for health educators that pertain to the material presented in this chapter.

Process Evaluation

At its core, process evaluation focuses on the quality of program content and program implementation. It quantifies what was done; when, where, and how it was done; who was reached; and how they participated (NCI, 2002). Process evaluation collects data and informs stakeholders of important findings that could improve a program or its delivery, and allows for appropriate changes before the program is fully implemented. Although a process evaluation can be performed to improve a program between implementation cycles (i.e., an evaluator identifies various issues that need to be addressed before the organization implements the program in the future), it is usually better to

Box 14.1 RESPONSIBILITIES AND COMPETENCIES FOR HEALTH EDUCATORS

Chapter 14 describes: evaluation approaches including process and summative evaluation, elements of formative evaluation, and evaluation designs. Responsibilities and competencies connected with this chapter include:

Responsibility IV: Conduct Evaluation and Research Related to Health Education

Competency A: Develop plans for evaluation and research

Competency B: Review research and evaluation procedures

Competency D: Carry out evaluation and research plans

Source: NCHEC, SOPHE, & AAHE (2006)

allow a process evaluation to inform and guide the development and implementation of a program as it actually unfolds. In cases where a program is implemented continuously, this distinction is not as clear or relevant.

Table 14.1 displays the elements of a comprehensive process evaluation. The degree to which these elements are used will be determined by many factors including the preferences of stakeholders. However, all 17 elements are important and have a bearing on program quality which, in turn, leads to program success.

Process evaluation occurs from the time of program inception through implementation. By nature, certain elements of the process evaluation are more applicable at the time of program inception. This is when planners either begin developing a new program or decide to use an existing program and tailor it to their priority population. For example, addressing the elements termed **justification** and **evidence** provide assurance that programs are supported by key stakeholders and that they are evidence-based. It is easy to make assumptions about these issues during a planning process. But addressing these key issues initially will orient and influence planners to make careful assessments about other program and evaluation components. In this regard, process evaluation can be beneficial before much, if any, time and effort are applied to the program.

Three additional elements displayed in Table 14.1 relate to issues that should be addressed early in the evaluation process. Assessing **capacity** requires evaluators to carefully examine the competency of those who are designing and implementing a program. This can be somewhat challenging if those performing the evaluation are the same professionals designing and implementing the program. Despite this inherent difficulty, planners and evaluators should identify the strengths and weaknesses of the internal staff and external partners and either invest in training or contract for external services as necessary. **Resources** relates to adequate funding and/or assistance from partner organizations. Although it is easy to underestimate program costs, evaluators performing a process evaluation should match the projected costs with the available resources to determine whether or not the program can be realistically implemented. Evaluators must also ensure that **orientation**, or the degree to which programs are adapted to the needs of the priority population, is adequately addressed. Professionals commonly assume that

Table 14.1 Elements of a comprehensive process evaluation

Justification	Degree to which a program, service, or activity is mandated or approved by relevant stakeholders and justified by needs assessment data and analysis.
Evidence	Degree to which the program, service, or activity is evidence-based (i.e., considered a best practice or promising approach or has otherwise been proven effective).
Capacity	Extent to which professionals have adequate knowledge, skills, and abilities to design and implement a program, service, or activity.
Resources	Adequacy of resources (e.g., budget, community resources or assistance, time).
Orientation	Degree to which the program, activity, or service is tailored to the priority population (i.e., culturally appropriate and consumer oriented).
Multiplicity	Degree to which multiple components are built into the program, service, or activity (e.g., education, communication, policy, environmental change).
Support	Degree to which a support component is built into a program, service, or activity (e.g., a hot line/quit line for a tobacco media campaign, development of walking paths for a community physical activity campaign).
Fidelity*	Extent to which the program, activity, or service was delivered as planned or as per protocol including the use of Gantt charts (i.e., timelines) and logic models.
Inclusion	Extent to which an adequate range and number of partners or organizations are involved with the program, service, or activity.
Accountability	Extent to which internal staff and external partners are fulfilling their responsibilities as planned, communicating needs, and making necessary adjustments.
Recruitment*	Quality and appropriateness of strategies used to promote a program, activity, or service and recruit participants.
Reach	Proportion of the priority population given the opportunity to participate in the program, activity, or service.
Response	Proportion of the priority population actually participating in the program, activity, or service.
Dose*	Number of program units delivered (e.g., presentations, products, services, messages).
Interaction	Quality of interactions (e.g., customer service; interpersonal, counseling, and presentation skills; clarity of instructions) between professionals and consumers.
Satisfaction	Degree to which consumers are satisfied with the program, service, or activity.
Context*	External factors that may influence program results (e.g., competing programs, conflicting messages, other confounders).

*Adapted from Steckler & Linnan, 2002 and Saunders, Evans, & Joshi, 2005

members of the priority population hold the same understanding and value for programs as those who design and implement the programs. Data from social marketing studies indicate this is not the case (Neiger & Thackeray, 2002). Assuring that programs are tailored to the values, wants, and needs of the priority population is an important component of a process evaluation and helps ensure that programs are more readily accepted by the priority population and that they result in the intended outcomes.

Two elements displayed in Table 14.1 relate to the development and content of a program. The term **multiplicity** relates to what is now generally viewed as a commonly held belief in health promotion that, compared with single-component programs, multiple-component programs are more effective. For example, the 5-a-Day program, as previously implemented at the national level, has included media components (public service announcements to increase fruit and vegetable consumption), supporting websites, educational curricula (including fruit and vegetable calculators, recipes, and food journals), environmental changes (ensuring that cafeterias provide appealing options for fruit and vegetables), and other activities such as grocery tours and collaborations with growers (CDC, 2007b). **Support,** a closely related concept to multiplicity, assures that programs have appropriate built-in reinforcement components to assist participants with the expected level of involvement and/or behavior change. For example, a well-baby program that promotes prenatal care through a media campaign cannot responsibly broadcast messages without an infrastructure that can support prenatal visits. In addition, a well-baby program of this nature should also be prepared to make referrals based on a variety of demographic variables within the priority population, including the ability to pay for services.

Certain elements in process evaluation such as *fidelity, inclusion,* and *accountability* relate to program implementation, including the development of appropriate and effective partnerships. **Fidelity** requires that programs are implemented either as intended or as per protocol. Because the results of effective programs are published in scientific journals or other reporting mechanisms, methods sections should provide a sequential order or step-by-step description of how the program was implemented. Practitioners should rely on this information to replicate the program. In addition, programs should routinely include some type of procedures outline or protocol that guides implementation. In this regard, process evaluation can assure that appropriate procedures are followed throughout implementation.

Oftentimes, the successful implementation of programs depends on the quality and quantity of partnerships. **Inclusion** assures that the right type and number of partners are involved with the program, and **accountability** ensures that both internal staff and partners are fulfilling their responsibilities as planned.

The natural inclination of most professionals or organizations is to include as many partners as possible to bear the burden of a program's cost and implementation. Care should be taken, however, to ensure that only those organizations that share the same values and commitment are included as program partners. This is not to suggest that organizations should not seek diverse or nontraditional partners. However, ideally, all partners should bring the same level of vision and energy to the program development and implementation process. Given these criteria, inclusion ensures that the right partners are involved with the program and accountability ensures that each partner organization performs its work.

Recruitment, reach, and **response** pertain to promoting the program and ensuring that people in the priority population are aware of the program, have the opportunity to participate in the program, and an adequate number actually participate in the program. Obviously, the budget, among other factors, influences the proportion of the priority population who has access to the program. Evaluators must develop projections for participation early, then match projections with actual participation. Furthermore, evaluators must determine whether methods for recruitment or promotion are appropriate based on communication capabilities and preferences of the priority population.

For example, newspaper advertisements will do little good if word of mouth communication (*viral marketing*) is a preferred channel within the priority population.

Dose is a measurement of how many units or program components were actually delivered to the priority population (e.g., number of educational sessions presented, number of nicotine devices distributed, number of car seats on loan, number of times a public service announcement was aired). Oftentimes, process evaluation is associated with dose. In other words, the practitioner tracks and reports how many products were distributed and equates this with the quality of a program. Although dose is an important element in process evaluation, it is only one element of a comprehensive approach. As an independent measurement, it cannot represent process evaluation nor should it serve as a proxy measure to describe the quality or value of a program. In addition, tracking and reporting dose should not be confused with program effectiveness that relates to changes in knowledge, attitudes, behaviors, and decreases in mortality, morbidity, and disability.

Interaction and **satisfaction** address the degree to which practitioners effectively work and communicate with program participants and how satisfied participants are with the program in general or with specific components. For example, a proven curriculum for weight loss among adults may be appealing to participants, theoretically grounded and technically sound in every way but not produce the expected results because of an ineffective instructor. A process evaluation can identify this problem and generate the necessary recommendations or adjustments. Likewise, data regarding participant satisfaction may produce important modifications during program implementation or in future applications of the program.

Finally, **context** assesses the presence of any confounding factors in the environment that may affect program participation or initial results. For example, participation in a school-based alcohol-free graduation celebration may be diminished by alternative venues that appeal more directly to the intended participants. Negative aspects of the physical environment or location of a program may have a harmful effect on program participation or retention. A television program showing disabling aspects of cancer aired at the same time a cancer screening program is initiated may scare potential program participants and dissuade their involvement. Because issues related to context may be the most difficult to modify, evaluators generally attempt to analyze context as part of the summative evaluation.

Strategies for conducting process evaluations are displayed and briefly described in **Table 14.2**. Although no single strategy is inherently superior to another, the element being evaluated (see Table 14.1) will largely influence the selection of the appropriate strategy. For example, a key informant interview would generally be appropriate if the evaluator is measuring *capacity* or *resources*. In this hypothetical situation, the key informant would probably be an administrator with adequate information about the skill sets of his/her staff and the type of budget that would be dedicated to the program. On the other hand, assessing *fidelity* can be accomplished with a protocol checklist. Certain elements can be addressed by one of many strategies or a combination of strategies. For example, assessing *interaction* or *satisfaction* can be accomplished by focus groups, in-depth interviews, or surveys.

Each of the strategies listed in Table 14.2 has a specific protocol for usage. Evaluators must ensure that these strategies are used appropriately and that data are not extrapolated or projected beyond their natural or appropriate use. For further explanation

Table 14.2 Procedures used in process evaluation

Focus Groups	Qualitative research wherein a trained moderator uses an interview guide or moderator's guide to ask questions about new programs, products, services, ideas, or topics to determine the attitudes, opinions, and preferences of a group of 6–12 individuals who are representative of the priority population.
Surveys	The collection of data, generally through questionnaires, from a representative sample of the priority population that allows evaluators to draw general conclusions about the entire priority population. May involve face-to-face interviews or written questionnaires, mailed questionnaires, telephone interviews, and electronic questionnaires, etc. An intercept survey attempts to approach consumers in their natural environments (e.g., grocery stores, malls, community events) for a brief face-to-face interview.
In-Depth Interviews	Formal interviews with program participants generally lasting a half hour or longer with the use of an interview guide and related probes. Allows evaluators to observe body language and facial expressions as prompts for additional questions and information.
Informal Interviews	Brief interviews with program participants that may take the form of a conversation rather than a formal interview.
Key Informant Interviews	Qualitative, in-depth interviews with individuals who understand the priority population and can represent their attitudes, values, and opinions to evaluators. Key informants are often people of influence within the priority population.
Direct Observation	A process wherein evaluators immerse themselves in the program as participants and assess the interactions between professionals and other participants, the general reactions and behaviors of the participants, and any problems or issues associated with program content and delivery. Use of this procedure sometimes involves concealing the observer from the program participants.
Expert Panel Reviews	A process wherein a small group of professionals, not associated with the program, but who have expertise related to the program, volunteer or are contracted to collect data, analyze the program, draw conclusions about its strengths and weaknesses, and make recommendations.
Quality Circles	A qualitative approach adapted from Japanese business practice whereby staff from the same program or work area meet regularly to discuss the strengths and weaknesses of a product, program, service, or activity and make recommendations for improvement. As an alternative to quality circles, evaluators may choose to interview program staff directly.
Protocol Checklist	A linear or sequential list of tasks or procedures that allows evaluators to compare how a program or policy is being implemented and compared with how it was originally intended to be implemented, or compared with what has been done elsewhere and reported in published studies or reports. Use of logic models may be used in lieu of the protocol checklist.
Gantt Chart	A type of bar chart that displays a program's timeline or project schedule. Whereas protocol checklists or logic models are not usually time phased, Gantt charts display the start and finish dates of key program elements (e.g., program objectives or key activities and tasks) (see Figure 12.2 for an example).
Program and Evaluation Forms	Program forms collected prior to program implementation may provide relevant information to evaluators (e.g., factors that have motivated participation, identification of goals, previous participation). Data from forms compiled during the program may reveal information helpful to program improvement (e.g., strengths, barriers, risks). Evaluation forms are generally administered at the conclusion of a program to measure the awareness, knowledge, attitudes, skills and behaviors and general levels of satisfaction as well as feedback on specific program components.

on specific strategies, see Chapter 4 for information on focus groups, survey methods, interviews, use of forms (existing records), and observations.

Two additional strategies, pretesting and pilot testing, though commonly associated with formative evaluation, are presented here as a way to assess the quality of distinct components associated with a program and to assess the overall quality of a program before full implementation occurs. Although the two terms are often used interchangeably, certain distinctions are important to make and understand.

Pretesting

Pretesting can be defined in at least two ways: (1) testing components of a program, service, or product with the priority population prior to implementation; and (2) collecting baseline data prior to program implementation that will be compared with posttest data to measure the effectiveness of programs. The type of pretesting that relates to formative or process evaluation pertains to the first definition—testing components of a program prior to program implementation. This type of pretesting is commonly associated with components of communication campaigns such as public service announcements, the content of media messages, and visual representations on posters or billboards. Accordingly, when pretesting is applied to health communications it has been defined as an evaluation that involves systematically collecting intended-audience reactions to messages and materials before the messages and materials are produced in final form (NCI, 2002). Pretesting, however, can be applied to any component of a program.

Pretesting assumes that program components have already been reviewed for evidence. That is, the component is demonstrated to be evidence-based in the literature or through some other reporting mechanism. Pretesting also assumes that practitioners have done their best to prepare program components in final form. In other words, it is not appropriate for practitioners to take short cuts and present materials with the mindset that members of the priority population will correct any flaws.

As stated, pretesting evaluates specific program components with members of the priority population. This may include specific sessions of an educational curriculum, a participant manual, draft language for a legislative bill, the visual presence and structural layout of a booth that will be used in a health fair, or messages and materials associated with a communication strategy. Many of the same strategies displayed in Table 14.2 are used to pretest program components. The most common strategies involve focus groups, in-depth interviews, and surveys (NCI, 2002). Practitioners would be well advised to receive training in these strategies before attempting to conduct them. Otherwise, it is wise to contract for services with professionals who do have experience and expertise.

Pilot Testing

Whereas pretesting focuses on specific program components, **pilot testing** (also referred to as field testing or alpha testing) generally assesses programs in limited areas and/or time periods (NCI, 2002). In other words, pilot testing generally presents the entire program to a limited and manageable number of members of the priority population so necessary modifications can be made before the program is implemented to the entire priority population. Pilot testing is also associated with testing the language and structure of questionnaires or other research instrumentation before a study is implemented (see Chapters 5 and 12 for more information on this application).

Pilot testing allows for "dry runs" to assess and measure the overall quality of the program. Occasionally, pilot testing may be associated with shorter durations of time compared with actual implementation time, but this is generally not advisable. Implementing the entire program to a limited number of people in the actual time frame is helpful for evaluators to discover important issues related to timing, spacing, and duration of interventions (see Chapter 12 for more information on this application). Pilot testing offers evaluators a wide angle or broad view of the program to assess how the entire program impacts participants.

Conducting a pilot test generally involves collecting data from participants. It is advisable to use the same data collection instruments that will be used in the actual implementation of the program to make adjustments to the instruments and program components simultaneously. The specific methodologies associated with summative evaluation are addressed later in this chapter and in Chapter 15. Chapter 5 also provides useful information on measurement, data collection, and sampling.

Summative Evaluation

If a program accounts for the elements displayed in Table 14.1 and passes all the tests of a comprehensive process evaluation, practitioners can assume that the collective efforts of stakeholders in designing and implementing a high-quality program will result in the expected outcomes stated in the program goals and objectives. These expected outcomes relate directly to **summative evaluation**, which, as defined in Chapter 13, is any combination of measurements that permit conclusions to be drawn about impact, outcome, or benefits of a program (Green & Lewis, 1986). Summative evaluation includes both impact evaluation, which focuses on intermediate indicators such as awareness, knowledge, attitudes, skills, and most importantly, behaviors. Outcome evaluation focuses on long-term program measures such as mortality, morbidity, or disability. A certain unwritten ethic associated with conducting a health promotion program suggests that although process evaluation is critical in the success of effective programs, practitioners should not be satisfied with this evaluation approach alone. Because health promotion programs are ultimately designed to enhance health and decrease or delay disease, evaluators must also measure indicators associated with summative evaluation. Although an element such as *dose* conducted in process evaluation provides important information, it does not account for meaningful change. For example, presenting and tracking, or measuring educational sessions about cholesterol reduction, is not the same process, nor nearly as valuable as actually helping clients decrease their cholesterol levels.

In addition to traditional measures in summative evaluation, outcomes can be determined by a number of factors, including years of life saved, number of smokers who quit, reduced absenteeism, number of pounds lost, and health care costs saved, due to health promotion programs.

Several different types of cost analysis can be used (McDermott & Sarvela, 1999; Levin & McEwan, 2001). **Cost-identification analysis** (or cost-feasibility analysis) is used to compare different interventions available for a program, often to determine which intervention would be the least expensive. With this type of analysis, evaluators identify the different items (i.e., personnel, facilities, curriculum, etc.) associated with a given intervention, determine a cost for each item, total the costs for that intervention, and then compare the total costs associated with each of several interventions. For example, if a health department was interested in providing a tobacco control program for a school district, it could conduct a cost-identification analysis on three different interventions: (1) teacher led, (2) peer education, and (3) voluntary agency provided. Costs for each of these interventions—such as staff time, staff benefits, curriculum materials, and volunteer training—would be identified, compared, and analyzed.

Cost-benefit analysis (CBA) looks at how resources can best be used. It will yield the dollar benefit received from the dollars invested in the program. **Cost-effectiveness analysis (CEA)** is used to quantify the effects of a program in monetary terms. It is more appropriate for health promotion programs than cost-benefit analysis, because a dollar value does not have to be placed on the outcomes of the program. Instead, a cost-effectiveness analysis will indicate how much it costs to produce a certain effect. For example, based on the cost of a program, the effect of years of life saved, number of smokers who stop smoking, or morbidity or mortality rates can be determined. A thorough explanation of both cost-benefit and cost-effectiveness analysis is presented in Appendix B in an article written by McKenzie (1986).

As noted in Appendix B, cost-benefit and cost-effectiveness analyses are not easy to perform. You are referred to two sources (CDC, 1999a; Goetzel et al., 1998) presented in Chapter 3 that should be useful in understanding more fully the complexities of these cost analyses.

A fourth type of cost analysis that is used with health promotion programs is **cost-utility analysis (CUA)**. This approach is different from the others in that the values of the outcomes of a program are determined by their subjective value to the stakeholders rather than their monetary cost. For example, an administrator may select a more expensive intervention for a program just because of the good public relations (i.e., the subjective value in the administrator's eye) for the organization. Or an administrator may survey those in the priority population to determine what outcomes they value from a program. Then, based on these data, the administrator selects the appropriate intervention.

Although many types of outcomes may be related to summative evaluation, the process itself is usually associated with the development of designs. This is particularly true of impact evaluation which requires a thoughtful design, including appropriate data collection procedures, valid and reliable questionnaires or other instruments, and proper analysis and data reporting. Outcome evaluation related to communities or large populations often involves analysis of vital statistics and trend data with the evaluator trying to account for *confounding variables* and determine what specific influence a certain program or combination of programs had in a community. In more controlled environments such as clinical or worksite settings, many of the same procedures related to designs used in impact evaluation can be applied to outcome evaluation.

An evaluation design is used to organize the summative evaluation and to provide for planned, systematic data collection, analysis, and reporting. A well-planned evaluation design helps ensure that the conclusions drawn about the program will be as accurate as possible. The design is developed during the early stages of program planning and has program goals and objectives as its focus. CDC's Framework for Program Evaluation (discussed in Chapter 13) suggests the study design should be addressed in *Step 3*, only after engaging stakeholders and describing the program. As designs are developed, evaluators must consider the audience and/or stakeholders who will read the results of the evaluation. In other words, the design must produce information that will answer the evaluation questions of stakeholders.

Selecting an Evaluation Design

There are few perfect evaluation designs, because no situation is ideal, and there are always constraining factors, such as limited resources. The challenge is to devise an *optimal* evaluation—as opposed to an *ideal* evaluation (CDC, 1999c). Planners should give much thought to selecting the best design for each situation. The following questions may be helpful in the selection of a design for summative evaluation:

- How much time do you have to conduct the evaluation?
- What financial resources are available?
- How many participants can be included in the evaluation?
- Are you more interested in qualitative or quantitative data?
- Do you have data analysis skills or access to statistical consultants?
- In what ways can validity be increased?
- Is it important to be able to generalize your findings to other populations?
- Are the stakeholders concerned with validity and reliability?
- Do you have the ability to randomize participants into experimental and control groups?
- Do you have access to a comparison group?

Dignan (1995) presents four steps in choosing an evaluation design. These four steps are outlined in **Figure 14.1**. The first step is to orient oneself to the situation. The evaluator must identify resources (time, personnel), constraints, and hidden agendas (unspoken goals). During this step, the evaluator must determine what is to be expected from the program and what can be observed.

The second step involves defining the problem—determining what is to be evaluated. During this step, definitions are needed for independent variables (what the sponsors think makes the difference), dependent variables (what will show the difference, e.g., awareness, knowledge, attitudes, skills, behaviors, disease prevalence), and confounding variables (what the evaluator thinks could explain additional differences).

The third step involves making a decision about the design—that is, whether to use qualitative or quantitative methods of data collection or both. The **quantitative method** is **deductive** in nature (applying a generally accepted principle to an individual case), so that the evaluation produces numeric (hard) data, such as counts, ratings, scores, or classifications. Examples of quantitative data include the posttest scores on a nutrition

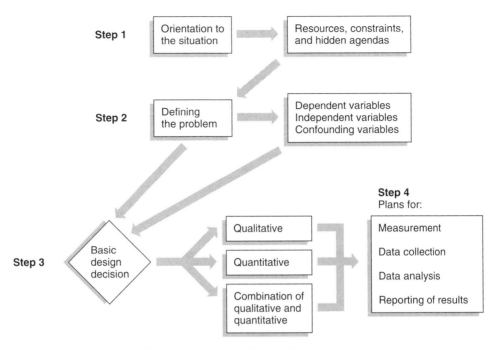

Figure 14.1 Steps in selecting an evaluation design

Source: From M. B. Dignan, *Measurement and Evaluation of Health Education*, 3/e, p. 151. Copyright © 1995. Reprinted by permission of Charles C. Thomas Publisher, Ltd., Springfield, Illinois.

knowledge test, a decrease in percent of body weight from pretest to posttest, and mortality rates related to cancer. This method is suited to programs that are well defined and compares outcomes of programs with those of other groups or the general population. It is the method most often used in evaluation designs.

The **qualitative method** is an **inductive** method (individual cases are studied to formulate a general principle) and produces narrative data, such as descriptions. This is a good method to use for programs that emphasize individual outcomes or in cases where other descriptive information from participants is needed. That is, qualitative data: provide depth of understanding, study motivation, enable discovery, are exploratory and interpretive, and allow insights into behavior and trends; quantitative data: measure level of occurrence, provide proof, and measure levels of actions and trends (NCI, 2002). **Box 14.2** provides a summary of the various qualitative methods presented by McDermott and Sarvela (1999).

Patton (1988) offers a checklist to determine whether qualitative data might be appropriate in a particular program evaluation. Collecting qualitative data may be a good strategy if there is a need to describe individual outcomes, to understand the dynamics and process of the programs, to obtain in-depth information on certain clients or sites, to focus on the diversity of program clients or sites, or to gather information to improve the program during process evaluation. Many of the strategies displayed in Table 14.2 use qualitative data.

Box 14.2 QUALITATIVE METHODS USED IN EVALUATION

Case studies: In-depth examinations of a social unit, such as an individual, family, household, worksite, community, or any type of institution as a whole

Content analysis: A systematic review identifying specific characteristics of messages

Delphi techniques: See Chapter 4 for an in-depth discussion of the Delphi technique

Elite interviewing: Interviewing that focuses on a certain type ("elite") of respondent

Ethnographic studies: A variety of techniques (participant-observer, observation, interviewing, and other interactions with people) used to study an individual or group

Films, photographs, and videotape recording (film ethnography): Includes the data collection and study of visual images

Focus group interviewing: See Chapter 4 for an in-depth discussion of focus group interviewing

Historical analysis: A review of historical accounts that may include an interpretation of the impact on current events

In-depth interviewing: A less structured, deeper interview in which the interviewees share their view of the world–See also Table 14.2

Kinesics: "The study of body communication" (p. 233)

Nominal group process: See Chapter 4 for an in-depth discussion of the nominal group process

Participant-observer studies: Those in which the observers (evaluators) also participate in what they are observing

Quality circle: "A group of people who meet at regular intervals to discuss problems and to identify possible solutions" (p. 236) – See also Table 14.2

Unobtrusive techniques: "Data collection techniques that do not require the direct participation or cooperation of human subjects" (p. 236) and include such things as unobtrusive observation, review of archival data, and study of physical traces

Source: Adapted from McDermott and Sarvela (1999)

Rather than choose one method, it may be advantageous to combine quantitative and qualitative methods. Steckler, McLeroy, and colleagues (1992) have discussed integrating qualitative and quantitative methods, since, to a certain extent, the weaknesses of one method is compensated for by the strengths of the other. **Figure 14.2** illustrates four ways that the qualitative and quantitative methods might be integrated. In Model 1, qualitative methods are used to help develop quantitative methods and instruments. For example, evaluators could use a focus group with stakeholders to determine what type of questions should be included on a data collection instrument. With Model 2, qualitative results are used to help interpret and explain findings from a quantitative evaluation. For example, evaluators could collect quantitative data from a large sample of people and more in-depth qualitative data from a few in the sample. Supplementing the hard data with anecdotal information further describes the findings. Model 3 is just the reverse of Model 2. In this

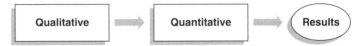

Model 1
Qualitative methods are used to help develop
quantitative measures and instruments.

Model 2
Qualitative methods are used to help explain quantitative findings.

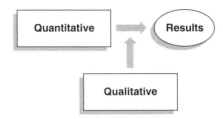

Model 3
Quantitative methods are used to embellish a primarily qualitative study.

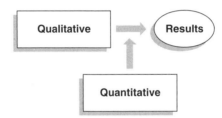

Model 4
Qualitative and quantitative methods are used equally and parallel.

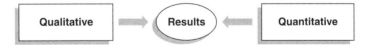

Figure 14.2 Four possible ways that qualitative and quantitative methods might be integrated

Source: A. Steckler et al., "Toward Integrating Qualitative and Quantitative Methods: An Introduction," *Health Education Quarterly*, 19(1), p. 5. Copyright © 1992. Reprinted by permission of Sage Publications.

model, quantitative results are used to help interpret predominately qualitative findings. For example, after observing a group of people for a period of time, evaluators may want to conduct a survey of the group. In the last model, Model 4, qualitative and quantitative data are used equally and parallel to cross-validate the findings.

The fourth step in selecting an evaluation design includes choosing how to measure the dependent variable, deciding how to collect the data (these components were discussed in Chapter 4) and how the data will be analyzed, and determining how the results will be reported. (These components are discussed in Chapter 15.)

Experimental, Control, and Comparison Groups

As in research studies, when evaluating a health promotion program, the group of individuals who receive the intervention is known as the **experimental group.** The evaluation is designed to determine what effects the program has on these individuals. To make sure that the effects are caused by the program and not by some other factor, a **control group** should be used. The control group should be as similar to the experimental group as possible, but the members of this group do not receive the program (intervention or treatment) that is to be evaluated.

Without the use of a properly selected control group, the apparent effect of the program could actually be due to a variety of factors (confounding variables), such as differences in participants' educational background, environment, or experience. By using a control group, the evaluator can show that the results or outcomes are due to the program and not to confounding variables. In an ideal situation, participants should be randomly selected, then randomly assigned to one of two groups, and finally it should be randomly determined which group would become the experimental group and which the control group. Theoretically, this would evenly distribute the characteristics of the participants. This technique increases the credibility of the evaluation by controlling for extraneous events and factors.

It is not always possible or ethical to assign participants to a control group, especially in population-based programs or if doing so would mean that they would be denied a necessary program or service. For example, a health promotion program could be designed for individuals with hypertension. Individuals diagnosed with hypertension could be referred by a physician into a health promotion class focused on reducing the risk factors associated with this disease. Denying some individuals access to the program in order to form a control group would clearly be unethical.

One way to deal with this problem is to provide the control group with an alternative program or to offer the regular program to the group at a later time (if a delay is not potentially harmful). Another alternative is to compare two programs: Offer an innovative program to some participants and continue the conventional program for others. Wagner and Guild (1989) see the advantage of this strategy as providing service to all participants (which fulfills a moral obligation) and still providing a comparison to assess the effectiveness of the innovative program.

Since the main purpose of social programs is to help clients, the client's viewpoint should be the primary concern. It is important to keep this in mind when considering ethical issues in the use of control groups. Conner (1980) identifies four underlying premises for the use of control groups in social program evaluation:

1. All individuals have a right to status quo services.
2. All individuals involved in the evaluation are informed about the purpose of the study and the use of a control group.

3. Individuals have a right to new services, and random selection gives everyone a chance to participate.

4. Individuals should not be subjected to ineffective or harmful programs.

The ethical issues that must be considered involve the potential denial of a service and allocation of scarce resources. When randomization is not feasible, planners should consider an equitable process of providing services for individuals while maintaining control over the evaluation design.

When participants cannot be randomly assigned to an experimental or control group, a nonequivalent group may be selected. This is known as a **comparison group.** It is important to find a group that is as similar as possible to the experimental group, such as two classrooms of students with similar characteristics or a group of residents in two comparable cities. Factors to consider include participants' age, gender, education, location, socioeconomic status, and experience, as well as any other variable that might impact program results.

Evaluation Designs

Measurements used in evaluation designs can be collected at three different times: after the program; both before and after the program; and several times before, during, and after the program. Remember from Chapter 5, **measurement** is defined by Green and Lewis (1986) as the method or procedure of assigning numbers to objects, events, and people.

Figure 14.3 presents evaluation designs commonly used in health promotion. In the figure, the letter O refers to measurement (or data collection), such as questionnaires, tests, interviews, observations, or other methods of gaining information. When multiple measurements are taken, the subscript number behind each O indicates the order in which the measurements are made. Measurement before the program begins is known as the **pretest,** and measurement after the completion of the program is known as the **posttest.** The letter X represents the program (intervention, or independent variable); the relative positions of the two letters in the table indicate when measurements are made in relation to when the program is provided. The figure also shows which groups receive the program and when participants are randomly assigned to groups [(R)].

Windsor and colleagues (2004) differentiate among three types of evaluation designs: experimental, quasi-experimental, and nonexperimental. **Experimental design** offers the greatest control over the various factors that may influence the results (confounding variables). It involves random assignment to experimental and control groups with measurement of both groups. This evaluation design produces the most interpretable and defensible evidence of effectiveness. **Quasi-experimental design** results in interpretable and supportive evidence of program effectiveness, but usually cannot control for all factors that affect the validity of the results. There is no random assignment to the groups, and comparisons are made on experimental and comparison groups. **Nonexperimental design,** without the use of a comparison or control group, has little control over the factors that affect the validity of the results.

Figure 14.3 Evaluation designs

I. Experimental design							
1. Pretest-posttest design							
— Experimental group	(R)	O_1	X	O_2			
— Control group	(R)	O_1		O_2			
2. Posttest-only design							
— Experimental group	(R)		X	O			
— Control group	(R)			O			
3. Time series design							
— Experimental group	(R)	O_1	O_2	O_3	X	O_4	O_5 O_6
— Control group	(R)	O_1	O_2	O_3		O_4	O_5 O_6
II. Quasi-experimental design							
1. Pretest-posttest design							
— Experimental group		O_1	X	O_2			
— Comparison group		O_1		O_2			
2. Time series design							
— Experimental group		O_1	O_2	O_3	X	O_4	O_5 O_6
— Comparison group		O_1	O_2	O_3		O_4	O_5 O_6
III. Nonexperimental design							
1. Pretest-posttest design							
— Experimental group		O_1	X	O_2			
2. Time series design							
— Experimental group		O_1	O_2	O_3	X	O_4	O_5 O_6

Key: (R) = Random assignment
O = Measurement/Observation
X = Program/Intervention

The most powerful design is the experimental design, in which participants are randomly assigned to the experimental and control groups. The difference between designs I.1 and I.2 in Figure 14.3 is the use of a pretest to measure the participants before the program begins. Use of a pretest would help assure that the groups are similar and provide baseline measurement. Random assignment should equally distribute any of the variables of the participants (such as age, gender, and race) between the different groups. Potential disadvantages of the experimental design are that it requires a relatively large group of participants and the intervention may be delayed for those in the control group.

A design more commonly found in evaluations of health promotion programs is the quasi-experimental pretest-posttest design using a comparison group (II.1 in Figure 14.3). This design is often used when a control group cannot be formed by random assignment. In such a case, a comparison group (a nonequivalent control group) is identified, and both groups are measured before and after the program. For example, a program on fire safety for two fifth-grade classrooms could be evaluated by using pre- and post-knowledge tests. Two other fifth-grade classrooms not receiving the program could serve as the comparison group. Similar pretest scores between the comparison and experimental groups would indicate that the groups were equal at the beginning of the program. However, without random assignment, it would be impossible to be sure that other variables (a unit on fire safety in a 4-H group, distribution of smoke detectors, information from parents) did not influence the results.

Sometimes participants cannot be assigned to a control group and no comparison group can be identified. In such cases, a nonexperimental pretest-posttest design (III.1 in Figure 14.3) can be used, but the results are of limited significance, because changes could be due to the program or to some other event. An example of this type of nonexperimental design would be the measurement of safety belt use after a community program on that topic. An increase in use might mean that the program successfully motivated individuals to use safety belts; however, it could also reveal the impact of increased enforcement of the mandatory safety belt law, of a traffic fatality in the community, or a safety article in the local newspaper.

A time series evaluation design (I.3, II.2, III.2 in Figure 14.3) can be used to examine differences in program effects over time. Random assignment to groups (I.3) offers the most control over factors influencing the validity of the results. The use of a comparison group (II.2) offers some control; without a control group or comparison group (III.2), it is possible to determine changes in the participants over time, but one cannot be sure that the changes were due only to the program.

In the time series design, several measurements are taken over time both before and after the program is implemented. This process helps to identify other factors that may account for a change between the pretest and posttest measurements and is especially appropriate for measuring delayed effects of a program. A time series design could be used in a weight loss program to indicate the amount of weight loss over time and the ability to maintain a desired weight.

When more than one experimental group is part of the evaluation, they can be included in the designs that have been discussed. These designs could be used to evaluate several types of programs—for example, to compare the effect of lectures, workshop, and self-study. Measurements could be collected from all groups at the same points in time, and programs could occur simultaneously.

Another design that may be used is the staggered treatment design (see **Figure 14.4**), which is used to determine the effects of a program over time by including several measurements after the end of the program. It also indicates the effects of testing, since not all groups in this design receive a pretest. The staggered treatment design can also be used in quasi-experimental and nonexperimental designs, although with the limitations of not using a control group or comparison group.

Figure 14.4 Staggered treatment design

Experimental group 1	(R)	X	O_1		O_2		O_3		O_4
Experimental group 2	(R)		O_1	X	O_2		O_3		O_4
Experimental group 3	(R)				O_1	X	O_2		O_3
Experimental group 4	(R)							X	O_1

Key: (R) = Random assignment
    O = Measurement/Observation
    X = Program/Intervention

Internal Validity

The **internal validity** of evaluation is the degree to which change that was measured can be attributed to the program. Many factors can threaten internal validity, either singly or in combination, making it difficult to determine if the outcome was brought about by the program or some other cause. Cook and Campbell (1979) have identified some of the threats to internal validity, summarized as follows:

- *History* occurs when an event happens between the pretest and posttest that is not part of the health promotion program. An example of history as a threat to internal validity is having a national antismoking campaign coincide with a local smoking cessation program.

- *Maturation* occurs when the participants in the program show pretest-to-posttest differences due to growing older, wiser, or stronger. For example, in tests of muscular strength in an exercise program for junior high students, an increase in strength could be the result of muscular development and not the effect of the program.

- *Testing* occurs when the participants become familiar with the test format due to repeated testing. This is why it is helpful to use a different form of the same test for pretest and posttest comparisons.

- *Instrumentation* occurs when there is a change in measurement between pretest and posttest, such as the observers becoming more familiar with or skilled in the use of the testing format over time.

- *Statistical regression* is when extremely high or low scores (which are not necessarily accurate) on the pretest are closer to the mean or average scores on the posttest.

- *Selection* reflects differences in the experimental and comparison groups, generally due to lack of randomization. Selection can also interact with other threats to validity, such as history, maturation, or instrumentation, which may appear to be program effects.

- *Mortality* refers to participants who drop out of the program between the pretest and posttest. For example, if most of the participants who drop out of a weight loss program are those with the least (or the most) weight to lose, the group composition is different at the posttest.

- *Diffusion or imitation of treatments* results when participants in the control group interact and learn from the experimental group. Students randomly assigned to an innovative drug prevention program in their school (experimental group) may discuss the program with students who are not in the program (control group), biasing the results.

- *Compensatory equalization of treatments* occurs when the program or services are not available to the control group and there is an unwillingness to tolerate the inequality. For instance, the control group from the previous example (students not enrolled in the innovative drug prevention program) may complain, since they are not able to participate.

- *Compensatory rivalry* is when the control group is seen as the underdog and is motivated to work harder.

- *Resentful demoralization of respondents receiving less desirable treatments* occurs among participants receiving the less desirable treatments compared to other groups, and the resentment may affect the outcome. For example, an evaluation to compare two different smoking cessation programs may assign one group (control) to the regular smoking cessation program and another group (experimental) to the regular program plus an exercise class. If the participants in the control group become aware that they are not receiving the additional exercise class, they may resent the omission, and this may be reflected in their smoking behavior and attitude toward the regular program.

The most significant way in which threats to internal validity can be controlled is through randomization. By random selection of participants, random assignment to groups, and random assignment of types of intervention or no intervention to groups, any differences between pretest and posttest can be interpreted as a result of the program. When random assignment to groups is not possible and quasi-experimental or nonexperimental designs are used, the evaluator must make all threats to internal validity explicit and then rule them out one by one.

External Validity

The other type of validity that should be considered is **external validity,** or the extent to which the program can be expected to produce similar effects in other populations. This is also known as **generalizability.** The more a program is tailored to a particular population, the greater the threat to external validity, and the less likely it is that the program can be generalized to another group.

As with internal validity, several factors can threaten external validity. They are sometimes known as *reactive effects*, since they cause individuals to react in a certain way. The following are several types of threats to external validity:

- *Social desirability* occurs when individuals give a particular response to try to please or impress the evaluator. An example would be children who tell the teacher they brush their teeth every day, regardless of their actual behavior.

- *Expectancy effect* is when attitudes projected onto individuals cause them to act in a certain way. For example, in a drug abuse treatment program, the facilitator may feel that a certain individual will not benefit from the treatment; projecting this attitude may cause the individual to behave in self-defeating ways.

- *Hawthorne effect* refers to a behavior change because of the special status of those being tested. This effect was first identified in an evaluation of lighting conditions at an electric plant; workers increased their productivity when the level of lighting was raised as well as when it was lowered. The change in behavior seemed to be due to the attention given to them during the evaluation process.

- *Placebo effect* causes a change in behavior due to the participants' belief in the treatment.

Cook and Campbell (1979) discuss the threats to external validity in terms of statistical interaction effects. These include interaction of selection and treatment (the findings from a program requiring a large time commitment may not be generalizable to individuals who do not have much free time); interaction of setting and treatment (evaluation results from a program conducted on campus may not be generalizable to the worksite); and interaction of history and treatment (results from a program conducted on a historically significant day may not be generalizable to other days).

Conducting the program several times in a variety of settings, with a variety of participants, can reduce the threats to external validity. Threats to external validity can also be counteracted by making a greater effort to treat all subjects identically. In a **blind** study, the participants do not know what group (control or experimental group) they are in. In a **double blind** study, the type of group participants are in is not known by either the participants or the planners. In a **triple blind** study, this information is not available to the participants, planners, or evaluators.

It is important to select an evaluation design that provides both internal and external validity. This may be difficult, because lowering the threat to one type of validity may increase the threat to the other. For example, tighter evaluation controls make it more difficult to generalize the results to other situations. There must be enough control over the evaluation to allow evaluators to interpret the findings while sufficient flexibility in the program is maintained to permit the results to be generalized to similar settings.

SUMMARY

This chapter focused on evaluation approaches and design elements and strategies for conducting a comprehensive process evaluation were presented. Distinctions between process and summative evaluations were made and key issues related to summative evaluation were outlined.

The steps for selecting an evaluation design were also presented with a discussion about quantitative and qualitative methods. Evaluation design should be considered early in the planning process. Evaluators need to identify what measurements will be taken as well as when and how. In doing so, a design should be selected that controls for both internal and external validity.

REVIEW QUESTIONS

1. List the elements of a comprehensive process evaluation and describe when in the design and implementation process they are most appropriately applied.

2. Match the strategies for process evaluation with the appropriate elements.

3. What is the difference between cost-benefit analysis and cost-effectiveness analysis? Which is more appropriate for use in health promotion programs?

4. What is the difference between quantitative and qualitative evaluation? When would one method be more appropriate than the other? How could they be combined in an evaluation design?

5. Name at least five different qualitative methods of evaluation and describe each.

6. What are the advantages of using a control group? What types of evaluation design do not use control groups? What is the difference between a control group and a comparison group?

7. What is the difference between experimental, quasi-experimental, and nonexperimental designs? What are the strengths and weaknesses of each?

8. What is the difference between internal validity and external validity?

9. What are some considerations in the selection of an evaluation design presented in this chapter? What considerations can you add to this list?

ACTIVITIES

1. Interview the manager of a health promotion program of your choice about how he/she measures quality. How many elements of process evaluation can you detect?

2. Look at an evaluation of a health promotion program that has been conducted in your community. Identify the evaluation approach that it most closely follows. Discuss your view with the program evaluator.

3. Develop an evaluation design for a program you are planning. Explain why you chose this design, and list the strengths and weaknesses of the design.

4. If you were hired to evaluate a safety belt program in a community, what evaluation design would you use and why? Assume you have all the resources you need to conduct the evaluation.

5. Explain what evaluation design you would use in evaluating the difference between two teaching techniques. Why would you choose this design?

WEBLINKS

1. http://www.wmich.edu/evalctr/checklists/

   The Evaluation Center at Western Michigan University (WMU)

   This is a page from the Evaluation Center at WMU website. This site provides evaluation specialists and users with refereed checklists. The site's purpose is to improve the quality and consistency of evaluations and enhance evaluation capacity through the promotion and use of high-quality checklists targeted to specific evaluation tasks and approaches. Visitors to this site can download a number of checklists and information on how to create them.

2. http://oerl.sri.com/

   Online Evaluation Resource Library (OERL)

   This is the website for the OERL. This library, funded by the National Science Foundation (NSF), was developed for professionals seeking to design, conduct, document, or review project evaluations. OERL's resources include instruments, plans, and reports from evaluations that have proven to be sound and representative of current evaluation practices.

3. http://www.ericae.net/main.htm

   Educational Resources Information Center (ERIC)

   This is a page from the ERIC Clearinghouse on Assessment and Evaluation website. The site offers a variety of resources and seeks to provide balanced information concerning educational assessment, and resources to encourage responsible test use.

4. http://national.unitedway.org/outcomes/

   United Way of America (UWA)

   This is a page from UWA's website. This page is titled *Outcome Measurement Resource Network*. The *Resource Network* offers information, downloadable documents, and links to resources related to the identification and measurement of program- and community-level outcomes.

5. http://whqlibdoc.who.int/hq/2000/WHO_MSD_MSB_00.2e.pdf

   World Health Organization

   A helpful PDF document on process evaluation that supplements material in this chapter. Describes why a process evaluation should be performed and how to do a process evaluation.

6. http://www.rand.org/pubs/technical_reports/TR101/

   Rand Organization—Getting to Outcomes

   This document, which focuses on substance abuse, provides an excellent explanation of promoting accountability through methods and tools for planning, implementation, and evaluation. One focus of the document is how to get to outcomes that justify prevention programs in general.

CHAPTER 15

Data Analysis and Reporting

CHAPTER

CHAPTER OBJECTIVES

After reading this chapter and answering the questions at the end, you should be able to:

- Define *data management*.
- List examples of univariate, bivariate, and multivariate analysis and explain how they could be used in evaluation.
- Differentiate between descriptive and inferential statistics.
- Explain the difference between the null hypothesis and the alternative hypothesis in significance testing.
- Define *level of significance, Type I error,* and *Type II error.*
- Define *independent variable* and *dependent variable*.
- Describe how statistical results can be interpreted.
- Describe the format for the evaluation report, guidelines for presenting data, and ways to enhance the report.
- Discuss ways to increase the utilization of the evaluation findings.

KEY TERMS

alpha level
alternative hypothesis
analysis of variance
  (ANOVA)
bivariate data analysis
chi-square
correlations
data management
dependent variables
descriptive statistics
independent variables

inferential statistics
level of significance
mean
measures of central tendency
measures of spread or
  variation
median
missing data
mode
multiple regression
multivariate data analysis

null hypothesis
practical significance
program significance
range
statistical significance
t-tests
Type I error
Type II error
univariate data analysis
variable

Like all other aspects of evaluation, the types of data analysis to be used in the evaluation should be determined in the program-planning stage. Basically, the analysis determines whether the outcome was different from what was expected. The evaluator then draws conclusions and prepares reports and/or presentations. The types of analysis to be used and how the information is presented are determined by the evaluation questions and the needs of the stakeholders.

This chapter describes different types of analyses commonly used in evaluating health promotion programs. To present them in detail or to include all possible techniques is beyond the scope of this text. If you need more information, refer to statistics textbooks, research methods and statistics courses, or statistical consultants. **Box 15.1** identifies the responsibilities and competencies for health educators that pertain to the material presented in this chapter.

Evaluations that suffer from major methodological problems are not likely to inspire confidence. A common problem is inadequate documentation of methods, results, and data analysis. The evaluation itself should be well designed; the report should contain a complete description of the program, objective interpretation of facts, information about the evaluation design and statistical analysis, and a discussion of features of the study that may have influenced the findings. In order to add accurate findings to the knowledge base of the profession, appropriate evaluation standards should be adopted to serve as guidelines for reporting and reviewing evaluation research (Moskowitz, 1989).

Data Management

Once the data have been collected (see Chapter 4 for data collection methods), they must be organized in such a manner that they can be analyzed in order to interpret the findings. To do this, the data, no matter if they are quantitative or qualitative, must be coded, cleaned, and organized into a usable format. These steps are collectively referred to as **data management**. By coded, we mean that the data are assigned labels so that they

---

Box 15.1	RESPONSIBILITIES AND COMPETENCIES FOR HEALTH EDUCATORS

Chapter 15 describes: managing data collected in evaluations or other research; types of data analysis; applications of data analyses; interpreting data; reporting the results of evaluation, including designing written reports and how and when to present evaluation reports; and increasing the use of evaluation results. Responsibilities and competencies that are connected with the content in this chapter include:

Responsibility IV: Conduct Evaluation and Research Related to Health Education

Competency A: Develop plans for evaluation and research

Competency E: Interpret results from evaluation and research

Competency F: Infer implications from findings for future health-related activities

Source: NCHEC, SOPHE, & AAHE (2006)

can be read and understood by a computer. To code data, a coding system must be established. The coding system outlines the process "through which raw data become translated for various forms of analysis (such as frequency counts, descriptive statistics, cross tabulations and other statistical procedures)" (McDermott & Sarvela, 1999, p. 77). For example, if the answer to a question on an instrument is yes, "yes" answers may be coded as the number "1" when entered into the computer, while "no" answers may be coded as a number "2." In addition to creating the coding scheme for raw data, a coding system also establishes rules for dealing with coding problems such as when respondents circle both "yes" and "no" for their answer to a question, or when neither "yes" nor "no" is circled but rather the space between the "yes" and "no" is circled.

Once the data have been coded and prior to being entered into a computer system, they must be cleaned. "Data cleaning entails checking that the values are valid and consistent; i.e., all values correspond to valid question responses" (Valente, 2002, p.136). For example, if the possible range of answers for a particular question is 1 to 3 and the frequency distribution identifies some 4s, those instruments with the 4s on them must be identified and checked to determine if the person completing the instrument made an error or if there was an error made by the person coding the data. If it was a data coding error, it should be corrected. If the person completing the data collection instrument made an error, it would be treated as no response to that question or as **missing data** (Cottrell & McKenzie, 2005). Once the cleaning of the data has been completed, the appropriate data analysis can begin.

Data Analysis

The goal of data analysis is to reduce, organize, synthesize, and summarize information in order to make sense of it and to be able to make inferences about the priority population (Fitzpatrick et al., 2004; McDermott & Sarvela, 1999). Regardless of the type of data analysis to be used, the analysis begins with the identification of the variables of interest. A **variable** is a characteristic or attribute that can be measured or observed (Creswell, 2002). In program evaluation, the variables are divided into independent and dependent variables. **Independent variables** are those that are either controlled by the evaluator or cause or exert some influence, whereas the **dependent variables** are the outcome variables being studied. In other words "Independent variables influence dependent variables" (Valente, 2002, p. 165). Examples of independent variables include exposure to an intervention, gender, race, age, education, and income, while dependent variables may include awareness, knowledge, attitudes, skills, and behaviors.

Statistics are used to analyze the variables. **Descriptive statistics** are used to organize, summarize, and describe characteristics of a group, while **inferential statistics** are concerned with relationships and causality in order to make generalizations (or inferences) about a population based upon findings from a sample. Statistical analyses also allow evaluators to measure the association and relationships between and among variables. When one variable is analyzed, it is called **univariate data analysis**. Analysis of two variables is called **bivariate** and analysis of more than two variables is referred to as **multivariate data analysis**.

The choice of a type of analysis is based on the evaluation questions, the type of data collected, and the audience who will receive the results (Newcomer & Wirtz, 2004). For some types of evaluation, descriptive data are all that is needed, and techniques are chosen to determine frequencies, counts, or other univariate procedures. Other evaluation questions focus on testing a hypothesis about relationships between variables; in such cases, more elaborate statistical techniques are needed. **Box 15.2** contains examples of the types of evaluation questions that can be answered by using different types of data analyses.

The level of measurement (i.e., nominal, ordinal, interval, or ratio, discussed in Chapter 5) is an important factor in selecting the type of data analysis. For the most part, analytical techniques have been developed for use with selected levels of measurement. In other words, not all analytical techniques can be used with all levels of measurement. For example, multiple regression analysis is a technique that has been reserved for use with interval and ratio data. Newcomer and Wirtz (2004) have created a very useful summary (see **Table 15.1**) to assist evaluators in selecting appropriate statistical techniques.

The issue of who will be the recipients of the final evaluation report should also be considered when selecting the type of analysis. Evaluators want to be able to present the evaluation results in a form that can be understood by the stakeholders. With regard to this issue, it is probably best to err on the side of too simple an analysis rather than one that is too complex.

Finally, regardless of the type of analysis selected for an evaluation, the method should be chosen early in the evaluation process and in place before the data are collected.

Univariate Data Analyses

Univariate data analyses examine one variable at a time. It is common for univariate analyses to be descriptive in nature. As noted earlier, descriptive statistics are used to

---

Box 15.2 EXAMPLES OF EVALUATION QUESTIONS ANSWERED USING UNIVARIATE, BIVARIATE, AND MULTIVARIATE DATA ANALYSIS

Univariate Analysis	Bivariate Analysis	Multivariate Analysis
What was the average score on the cholesterol knowledge test?	Is there a difference in smoking behavior between the individuals in the experimental and control groups after the healthy lifestyle program?	Can the risk of heart disease be predicted using smoking, exercise, diet, and heredity?
How many participants at the worksite attended the healthy lifestyle presentation?	Is peer education or classroom instruction more effective in increasing knowledge about the effects of drug abuse?	Can mortality risk among motorcycle drivers be predicted from helmet use, time of day, weather conditions, and speed?
What percentage of the participants in the corporate fitness program met their target goal?	Do students' attitudes about bicycle helmets differ in rural and urban settings?	

Table 15.1   Selecting statistical techniques

Purpose of the Analysis	How the Variables Are Measured	Appropriate Technique	Appropriate Test for Statistical Significance	Appropriate Measure of Magnitude
To compare a sample distribution to a population distribution	Nominal/ordinal	Frequency counts	Chi-square	NA
	Interval	Means and medians Standard deviations/interquartile range	Chi-square	NA
To analyze the relationship between two variables	Nominal/ordinal	Contingency tables	Chi-square	Difference in column percentages
	Interval	Contingency tables/test of differences of means of proportions	Chi-square or t-test	Difference in column percentages or in means
To reduce the number of variables through identifying factors that explain variation in a larger set of variables	Interval	Factor analysis	NA	Pearson's correlations; Eigenvalues
To sort units into similar clusters or groupings	Nominal/ordinal/interval	Cluster analysis; discriminant functions analysis	F; Wilk's Lambda	Cannonical/correlation coefficient[2]
To predict or estimate program impact	Nominal/ordinal dependent variable	Log linear regression	t and F	Odds estimates
	Interval dependent variable	Regression	t and F	R^2, beta weights
To describe or predict a trend in a series of data collected over time	Nominal, ordinal, or interval independent variables but interval dependent variable	Regression	t and F	R^2, beta weights

Note: NA = not applicable

Source: J. S. Wholey et al., *Handbook of Practical Program Evaluation*, p. 397. Copyright © 1994 by John Wiley and Sons. Used with permission.

describe, classify, and summarize data. Summary counts (frequencies) are totals, and they are the easiest type of data to collect and report. Summary counts could be used in process evaluation—for example, to count the number of participants in blood pressure screening programs at various sites. The information would assist the planners in publicizing sites with low attendance or adding additional personnel to busy sites. Other examples of frequencies, or summary counts, are, for instance, the number of participants in a workshop, those who scored over 80% on a knowledge posttest, or the number of individuals wearing a safety belt.

Measures of central tendency are other forms of univariate data analyses. The **mean** is the arithmetic average of all the scores. The **median** is the midpoint of all the scores, dividing scores ranked by size into equal halves. The **mode** is the score that occurs most frequently. These are all useful in describing the results, and reporting all three measures of central tendency will be especially helpful if extreme scores are found.

Measures of spread or variation refers to how spread out the scores are. **Range** is the difference between the highest and lowest scores. For example, if the high score is 100 and the low score is 60, the range is 40. Measures of spread or variation—such as range, standard deviation, or variance—can be used to determine whether scores from groups are similar or spread apart.

Bivariate Data Analyses

Bivariate data analyses are used to study two variables simultaneously. Such analyses "are usually used to determine the presence of relationships or differences between groups" (McDermott & Sarvela, 1999, p. 300). When using bivariate analyses, it is common to state evaluation questions in the form of hypotheses. The **null hypothesis** holds that there is no observed difference between the groups. The **alternative hypothesis** says that there is a difference between the groups. For example, a null hypothesis might state that there is no difference between the two groups, say men and women, in knowledge about cancer risk factors, while the alternative hypothesis states that there is a difference.

Statistical tests are used to determine if the relationships or differences between groups are statistically significant. **Statistical significance** "refers to whether the observed differences between the two or more groups are real or not, or whether they are chance occurrences" (McDermott & Sarvela, 1999, p. 300). In other words, statistical tests are used to determine whether the null hypothesis is rejected (meaning a relationship between the groups probably does exist) or whether it is failed to be rejected (indicating that any apparent relationship between groups is due to chance).

There is the possibility that the null hypotheseis can be rejected when it is, in fact, true; this is known as **Type I error**. There is also the possibility of failing to reject the null hypothesis when it is, in fact, not true; this a **Type II error**. The probability of making a Type I error is reflected in the alpha level. The **alpha level,** or **level of significance,** is established before the statistical tests are run and is generally set at .05 or .01. This indicates that the decision to reject the null hypothesis is incorrect 5% (or 1%) of the time; that is, there is a 5% probability (or 1% probability) that the outcome occurred by chance alone.

When a smaller alpha level is used (.01 or .001), the possibility of making a Type I error is reduced; at the same time, however, the possibility of a Type II error increases. An example of a Type I error is the adoption of a new program due to higher scores on a knowledge test, when, in reality, increases in knowledge occurred by chance and the new program is not more effective than the existing program. An example of a Type II error is not adopting the new program when it is, in reality, more effective.

Bivariate analyses that are commonly used in program evaluation include chi-square, *t*-tests, analysis of variance, and correlations. **Chi-square** is a statistical test "that measures the association between two nominal and/or ordinal variables" (Valente, 2002, p. 170). An example of this type of analysis would be measuring the association of grade levels (e.g., third and fifth grades) with the attitudes of children toward the use of bicycle helmets (i.e., strongly agree, agree, disagree, and strongly disagree).

While chi-square is used to study nominal and/or ordinal variables, *t*-**tests** and **analysis of variance (ANOVA)** are statistical tests used to study group differences when the dependent variables involve interval or ratio data (e.g., scores on a test). There are several situations in which a *t*-test could be used. The most common use of a *t*-test is to determine whether a variable changed significantly in one group at two different points in time, such as between baseline before the intervention (pretest) and at follow-up after the intervention (posttest). This type of *t*-test is called a dependent *t*-test. A second common use of a *t*-test is to study the differences between two groups at a single point in time. An example of such a situation is the comparison of nutrition knowledge test scores after two groups have been exposed to different nutrition education interventions. This type of *t*-test is called an independent *t*-test.

ANOVA is a statistical test that could be used to study differences between two groups just like a *t*-test, but is more commonly used to study differences between more than two groups. For example, an ANOVA could be used to determine if there was a difference in the test scores of three groups (i.e., different age groups like 15–24, 25–45, and 46–65 year olds) on a physical activity knowledge test following exposure to a single health promotion intervention.

While the bivariate analyses discussed so far are used to determine if differences exist between groups, **correlations** are used to study the strength and direction of relationships between two variables (McDermott & Sarvela, 1999). Correlations are expressed as values between +1 (a positive correlation) and −1 (a negative correlation), with a 0 indicating no relationship between the variables. "The higher the value of the correlation coefficient is (regardless of direction) the stronger the relationship between the two variables" (McDermott & Sarvela, 1999, p. 304).

Correlation between variables indicates only a relationship; this technique does not establish cause and effect. An example of the use of correlation would be to determine the relationship between safety belt use and age of the driver. If older people were found to wear their safety belts more often than younger people, that would constitute a positive correlation between age and belt use. If younger people wore their safety belts more often, it would be a negative correlation. If age made no difference in who wore the belts more often, the correlation would be 0.

Multivariate Data Analyses

Multivariate data analyses are used to study three or more variables simultaneously. Typically, such analyses are used in more advanced evaluation designs, and thus will not be discussed in detail here because of the scope of this text. Examples of multivariate analyses include multiple regression, discriminant analysis, and factor analysis. Of these, the one most commonly used in health promotion evaluation is **multiple regression**. "There are many different types of multiple regression, including stepwise regression, logistic regression, and general linear regression" (McDermott & Sarvela, 1999, p. 305). Though the procedures and applications for various types of regression differ, they are "useful in exploring relationships among variables or in exploring the independent effects of many variables on one dependent variable" (Fitzpatrick et al., 2004, p. 359). An example of the latter would be trying to predict the risk of heart disease (the dependent variable) using the independent variables of smoking, exercise, diet, and family history.

Applications of Data Analyses

Many evaluation concepts have been presented—so many, in fact, that you might find it difficult to keep them all clear in your mind or to apply them. Therefore a few examples here will help you see how to move from a program goal to an intervention to an evaluation design to data analysis. To illustrate these concepts, a couple of statistics have been selected that are commonly used with health promotion programs: chi-square and *t*-tests.

Case #1

Program goal: Reduce the prevalence of smoking in the priority population
Priority population: The 70 employees of The Mitchell Company who smoke
Intervention (independent variable): Two different smoking cessation programs
Variable of interest (dependent variable): Smoking cessation after one year
Evaluation design: R   A X_1 O_1
                        R   B X_2 O_1

where:

R = random assignment
A = group A
B = group B
X_1 = method 1
X_2 = method 2
O_1 = self-reported smoking behavior

Data collected: Nominal data; quit yes or no

| | *Smoking Employees* | |
	Group A **Method 1**	**Group B** **Method 2**
Quit	24%	33%
Did not quit	76%	67%

Data analysis: A chi-square test of statistical significance can be used to test the null hypothesis that there is no difference in the success of the two groups.

Case #2

Program goal: Increase the AIDS knowledge of the priority population
Priority population: The 1,200 new freshmen at Julia University
Intervention (independent variable): A two-hour lecture-discussion program given during the freshmen orientation program
Variable of interest (dependent variable): AIDS knowledge
Evaluation design: O_1 X O_2

where:

$$O_1 = \text{pretest scores}$$
$$X = \text{two-hour program at freshman orientation}$$
$$O_2 = \text{posttest scores}$$

Data collection: Ratio data; scores on 100-point-scale test

	Test Results	
	Pretest	**Posttest**
Number of students	1,200	1,200
Mean score	69.0	78.5

Data analysis: A dependent *t*-test of statistical significance can be used to test the null hypothesis that there is no difference between the pre- and posttest means on the knowledge test.

Case #3

Program goal. To improve the testicular self-examination skills of the priority population
Priority population: All boys enrolled in the eighth grade at Jones Junior High School
Intervention (independent variable): Two-week unit on testicular cancer
Variable of interest (dependent variable): Score on testicular self-exam skills test
Evaluation design: A O_1 X O_2
                        B O_1 O_2

where:

$$A = \text{eighth-grade boys at Jones Junior High School}$$
$$B = \text{eighth-grade boys at Hastings Junior High School}$$
$$O_1 = \text{pretest scores}$$
$$X = \text{two-week unit on testicular cancer}$$
$$O_2 = \text{posttest scores}$$

	Test Results	
	Jones Junior High ($n = 142$)	**Hastings Junior High ($n = 131$)**
Pre	62	63
Post	79	65

Data collected: Ratio data; scores on 100-point skills test

Data analysis: An independent *t*-test of statistical significance can be used to (1) test the null hypothesis that there is no difference in the pretest scores of the two groups because the groups were not randomly assigned, and (2) test the null hypothesis that there is no differences in the posttest scores of the two groups.

Interpreting the Data

With the data analyses completed, attention must turn to interpreting the data. By interpretation we mean attaching meaning to the analyzed data and drawing conclusions (Fitzpatrick et al., 2004). "Interpretation should be characterized by careful, fair, open methods of inquiry."

To insure that the interpretation is fair and as objective as possible, it is recommended that the interpretation not be the sole responsibility of the evaluator or, for that matter, any other single person. At the beginning of Chapter 13 when we began our discussion of evaluation, we spoke of the importance of making sure that the evaluation process is a collaborative process that includes representation from all of the stakeholders. That principle applies not only to the planning of the evaluation, but also to the interpretation of the data. Several authors (Fitzpatrick et al., 2004; Patton, 1986; Solomon, 1987; Weiss, 1984) have recommended bringing the stakeholders and evaluator together in one or more meetings to systematically review the findings. Such meetings take advantage of the diverse perspectives of the stakeholders, as well as allow for a discussion of the implications of various interpretative conclusions.

There is no single method used to interpret data. In fact, a number of different methods could be used. Fitzpatrick and colleagues (2004) have identified eight methods that have served well in the past. They include:

1. Determining whether objectives have been achieved;

2. Determining whether laws, democratic ideals, regulations, or ethical principles have been violated;

3. Determining whether assessed needs have been reduced;

4. Determining the value of accomplishments;

5. Asking critical reference groups to review the data and to provide their judgments of successes and failures, strengths, and weaknesses;

6. Comparing results with those reported by similar entities or endeavors;

7. Comparing assessed performance levels on critical variables to expectations of performance or standards;

8. Interpreting results in light of evaluation procedures that generated them (p. 364)

Finally, the interpretation of the results must distinguish between **program significance (practical significance)** and statistical significance. Programmatic significance measures the meaningfulness of a program regardless of statistical significance. Statistical significance is determined by statistical testing. It is possible—especially when a large number of people are included in the data collection—to have statistically significant results that indicate gains in performance but are not meaningful in terms of program goals. For example, say the mean scores on a knowledge test of two groups are 70 and 69 (out of 100 points). If the groups are large enough, it would be possible that the difference in the scores (i.e., 1 point) could be statistically significant. But in practical terms, does the group with a mean score of 70 have more knowledge that will translate to more informed consumers? Probably not! Thus spending extra dollars on the program that generated the mean score of 70 versus the less expensive program that generated a mean score of 69 would really not be cost-effective. Statistical significance is similar to reliability in that they are both measures of precision. It is important to consider whether statistical significance justifies the development, implementation, and costs of a program (Fink & Kosecoff, 1978).

Evaluation Reporting

The results and interpretation of the data analyses, as well as a description of the evaluation process, are incorporated into the final report to be presented to the stakeholders. The report itself generally follows the format of a research report, including an introduction, methodology, results, conclusions, and discussion.

Some may see the creation of an evaluation report as a waste of time or a nonessential step in the larger process of evaluation; however, an evaluation report is essential for several reasons (Wurzbach, 2002). An evaluation report can provide:

- the discipline to help you critically analyze the results of the evaluation and think about any changes you should make as a result
- a tangible product for your agency
- evidence that your program or materials have been carefully developed—to be used as a sales tool with gatekeepers (e.g., television station public service directors)
- a record of your activities for use in planning future programs
- assistance to others who may be interested in developing similar programs or materials
- a foundation for evaluation activities in the future (e.g., it is easier to design a new questionnaire based on one you have previously used than to start anew) (p. 590)

The number and type of reports needed are determined at the beginning of the evaluation based on the needs of the stakeholders. For a process evaluation, reports are needed early and may be provided on a weekly or monthly basis. The process evaluations may be formal or informal, ranging from scheduled presentations to informal telephone calls. They must be submitted on time in order to provide immediate feedback so that program modifications can be made. Generally, a report is submitted at the end of an evaluation and may be written and/or oral.

Evaluators must be able to communicate to all audiences when presenting the results of the evaluation. The reaction of each audience—participants, media, administrators, funding source—must be anticipated in order to prepare the necessary information. In some cases, technical information must be included; in other cases, anecdotal information may be appropriate. The evaluator must fit the report to the audience as well as prepare for a negative response if the results of the evaluation are not favorable. This involves looking critically at the results and developing responses to anticipated reactions.

The format for communicating the evaluation results may include several methods, such as a technical report, journal article, news release, meeting, presentation, press conference, letter, or workshop. Generally, more than one method is selected in order to meet the needs of all stakeholders. For example, following an innovative worksite health promotion program, the evaluator might prepare a news release for the community, a letter to all staff who participated, a technical report for the funding source, and an executive summary for the administrators.

Designing the Written Report

As previously mentioned, the evaluation report follows a similar format to that used in a research report. The evaluation report generally includes the following sections:

- *Abstract or executive summary:* This is a summary of the total evaluation including goals and objectives, methods, results, conclusions, and recommendations. It is a concise presentation of the evaluation since it may be the only portion of the report that some of the stakeholders may read. Most abstracts/executive summaries range in length from 150 to 600 words.

- *Introduction:* This section of the report includes a complete description of the program and the evaluation, including the rationale or justification for the program and evaluation. Goals and objectives of the program are listed, as are the evaluation questions to be answered.

- *Methods/procedures:* The methods/procedures section includes information on the evaluation design, priority populations, instruments used, and how the data were collected and analyzed.

- *Results:* This section is the main part of the report. It includes the findings from the evaluation, summarizing and simplifying the data and presenting them in a clear, concise format. Data are presented for every evaluation question.

- *Conclusions/recommendations:* This section uses the findings (presented in the previous section) to answer the evaluation questions. The results are interpreted to determine significance and explanations. Judgments and recommendations are included in this section; they may have been made by the evaluator and/or the administrator, depending on the evaluation model used.

Box 15.3 summarizes what is included in the evaluation report.

Presenting Data

The data that have been collected and analyzed are presented in the evaluation report. The presentation of the data should be simple and straightforward. Graphic displays and tables may be used to illustrate certain findings; in fact, they are often a central part of the report. They also often make it easier for the readers of a written report or the audience for an oral report to understand the findings of an evaluation. Graphic displays should be self-explanatory. In fact, it is usually ill-advised to describe in the text too much of what is already displayed in a table or figure. When presenting the data in graphic form it is often helpful to include a frame of reference—such as a comparison

Box 15.3 WHAT TO INCLUDE IN THE EVALUATION REPORT	
Abstract/executive summary	Overview of the program and evaluation
	General results, conclusions, and recommendations
Introduction	Purpose of the evaluation
	Rationale or justification for the evaluation
	Program and participant description (including staff, materials, activities, procedures, etc.)
	Goals and objectives
	Evaluation questions
Methods/procedures	Design of the evaluation
	Priority population
	Instrumentation, including information on validity and reliability
	Sampling procedures
	Data collection procedures
	Pilot study results
	Data analyses procedures
Results	Description of findings from data analyses
	Answers to evaluation questions
	Addresses any special concerns
	Explanation of findings
	Charts and graphs of findings
Conclusions/recommend-ations	Interpretation of results
	Conclusions about program effectiveness
	Limitations
	Program recommendations
	Determining if additional information is needed

with national, state, local, or other data—and explain any limitations of the data. If graphic displays are used in a report, it is recommended (USDHHS, CDC, no date) that such displays are appropriate for the results:

1. Use horizontal bar charts to focus attention on how one category differs from another.

2. Use vertical bar charts to focus attention on a change in a variable over time.

3. Use cluster bar charts to contrast one variable among multiple subgroups.

4. Use line graphs to plot data for several periods and show a trend over time.

5. Use pie charts to show the distribution of a set of events or a total quantity.

If many tables are included, the main ones can be placed in the text of the report and the rest relegated to an appendix. **Box 15.4** lists guidelines to follow when presenting data in the evaluation report and/or presentation.

Box 15.4	GUIDELINES FOR PRESENTING DATA

1. Use graphic methods of presenting numerical data whenever possible.

2. Build the results and discussion section of the evaluation report—and perhaps other sections as well—around tables and figures. Prepare the tables and graphs first; then write text to explain them.

3. Make each table and figure self-explanatory. Use a clear, complete title, a key, label, footnotes, and so forth.

4. Discuss in the text the major information to be found in each table and figure.

5. Experiment with, and consider using, as many graphs as you have the time and ingenuity to prepare. Not only do they communicate clearly to your audiences, they also help you to see what is happening.

6. Because graphs tend to convey fewer details than numerical tables, consider providing both tables and graphs for the same data, where appropriate.

7. If you have used a mixed evaluation design with both quantitative and qualitative data collection procedures, use the direct quotations and descriptions from the qualitative results to add depth and clarity to information reported graphically.

8. When presenting complicated graphs to a live audience, give some instruction about how to read the graph and a few sample interpretations of simpler versions, then present the real data.

9. When a complete draft of the report has been completed, ask yourself the following questions:
   a. Do the figure titles give a comprehensive description of the figures? Could someone browsing through the report understand the graphs?
   b. Are both axes of every graph clearly labeled with a name?
   c. Is the interval size marked on all axes of graphs?
   d. Is the number of cases on which each summary statistic has been based indicated in each table or on each graph?
   e. Are the tables and figures labeled and numbered throughout the report?
   f. If the report is a lengthy one, does it include a list of tables and figures at the front following the table of contents?

Source: L. L. Morris et al., *How to Communicate Evaluation Findings.* Copyright © 1987. Reprinted by permission of Sage Publications.

How and When to Present the Report

Evaluators must consider carefully the logistics of presenting the evaluation findings. They should discuss this with the decision makers involved in the evaluation. An evaluator may be in the position of presenting negative results, encountering distrust among staff members, or submitting a report that will never be read. Following are several suggestions for enhancing the evaluation report:

• Give key decision makers advance information on the findings; this increases the likelihood that the information will actually be used and prevents the decision makers from learning about the results from the media or another source.

- Maintain anonymity of individuals, institutions, and organizations; use sensitivity to avoid judging or labeling people in negative ways; maintain confidentiality of the final report according to the wishes of the administrators; maintain objectivity throughout the report (Windsor et al., 2004).
- Choose ways to report the evaluation findings so as to meet the needs of the stakeholders, and include information that is relevant to each group.

Increasing Utilization of the Results

Far too often an evaluation will be conducted and a report submitted to the decision makers, but the recommendations will not be implemented. This occurs for a variety of reasons. Decision makers may not use findings because they are conducting the evaluation only to fulfill the requirements of the funding source, to serve their own self-interest, or to gain recognition for a successful program. Even decision makers who plan to use the evaluation results in their health promotion program may find that they are unable to state the evaluation question or that the final report contains language and concepts that are unfamiliar to them. Weiss (1984) developed the following guidelines to increase the chances that evaluation results will actually be used:

1. Plan the study with program stakeholders in mind and involve them in the planning process.

2. Continue to gather information about the program after the planning stage; a change in the program should result in a change in the evaluation.

3. Focus the evaluation on conditions about the program that the decision makers can change.

4. Write reports in a clear, simple manner and submit them on time. Use graphs and charts within the text, and include complicated statistical information in an appendix.

5. Base the decision on whether to make recommendations on how specific and clear the data are, how much is known about the program, and whether differences between programs are obvious. A joint interpretation between evaluator and stakeholders may be best.

6. Disseminate the results to all stakeholders, using a variety of methods.

7. Integrate evaluation findings with other research and evaluation about the program area.

8. Provide high-quality research.

SUMMARY

Evaluation questions developed in the early program-planning stages can be answered once the data have been analyzed. Descriptive statistics can be used to summarize or describe the data, and inferential statistics can be used to generate or test hypotheses.

These statistics are generated by applying the appropriate univariate, bivariate, and/or multivariate analysis. Evaluators then interpret the data and present the results to the stakeholders via a formal or informal report.

REVIEW QUESTIONS

1. What are some common problems with evaluations, and how can these problems be reduced or overcome?

2. What is meant by the term *data management*?

3. What is the difference between descriptive and inferential statistics?

4. What are some types of univariate data analyses used in evaluation? When would these be used?

5. How are bivariate and multivariate data analyses used in evaluation?

6. Explain the concepts of hypothesis testing, level of significance, Type I error, and Type II error.

7. What is the role of evaluators and decision makers in interpreting the results and making recommendations?

8. What is the difference between statistical significance and program significance?

9. What information is included in the written evaluation report? How is the information modified for various audiences?

10. What are some guidelines for presenting data in an evaluation report?

11. How can the evaluation report be enhanced?

12. How can the evaluator increase the likelihood of utilization of the evaluation findings?

ACTIVITIES

1. Obtain an actual report from a program evaluation. Look for the type of statistical tests used, level of significance, independent and dependent variables, interpretation of the findings, recommendations, and format for the report.

2. Discuss evaluation with a decision maker from a health agency. Find out what types of evaluation have been conducted, who has conducted them, what the findings have been, whether the findings were implemented, and how the information was reported.

3. Compare an evaluation report with a research report. What are the similarities and differences? How could you improve the report?

4. Using data that you have generated or data presented by your instructor, create one table and one graph.

WEBLINKS

1. http://www.astho.org/

   Association of State and Territorial Health Officials (ASTHO)

   This is the website for the ASTHO. The ASTHO is the national nonprofit organization representing the state and territorial public health agencies of the United States, the U.S. Territories, and the District of Columbia. ASTHO's members are the chief health officials of these jurisdictions. At this site you can link to all the state and territorial public health agencies where you can find various examples of the presentation of health data using charts, graphs, and tables.

2. http://www.cancercontrol.cancer.gov/index.html

   National Cancer Institute (NCI)

   This is a web page from the NCI website. This is the page that provides information on cancer control and population sciences. This site includes evaluation reports on a number of cancer education programs including the well-known 5-a-Day program.

3. http://www.adb.org/Evaluation/reports/

   Asian Development Bank (ADB)

   This is a web page from the ADB website. The ADB, established 1966, is a multilateral development finance institution dedicated to reducing poverty in Asia and the Pacific. At this web page you can find a number of the final evaluation reports created by the ADB. These reports provide good examples of how final evaluation reports are formatted. Some of the reports deal with health-related topics.

4. http://www.cdc.gov/phtrain/

   Centers for Disease Control and Prevention (CDC)

   This is a web page from the CDC website that lists public health training and employment opportunities. Several of the training opportunities relate to statistical data analysis and reporting.

5. http://www.cdc.gov/nchs/

   National Center for Health Statistics (NCHS)

   This is the website for the NCHS. It is a rich source of information about America's health and provides many examples of the presentation of health data.

6. http://www.nhtsa.dot.gov/stsi/

   State Traffic Safety Information (STSI)

   This is a web page from the National Center for Statistical Analysis of the National Highway Traffic Safety Administration website. STSI presents a by-state profile of traffic safety data and information including: crash statistics, economic costs, legislation status, funding programs, and more. It provides a lot of examples of the presentation of health data using charts, graphs, and tables.

Appendixes

Code of Ethics for the Health Education Profession

Unabridged Version

Preamble

The Health Education profession is dedicated to excellence in the practice of promoting individual, family, organizational, and community health. Guided by common ideals, Health Educators are responsible for upholding the integrity and ethics of the profession as they face the daily challenges of making decisions. By acknowledging the value of diversity in society and embracing a cross-cultural approach, Health Educators support the worth, dignity, potential, and uniqueness of all people.

The Code of Ethics provides a framework of shared values within which Health Education is practiced. The Code of Ethics is grounded in fundamental ethical principles that underlie all health care services: respect for autonomy, promotion of social justice, active promotion of good, and avoidance of harm. The responsibility of each health educator is to aspire to the highest possible standards of conduct and to encourage the ethical behavior of all those with whom they work.

Regardless of job title, professional affiliation, work setting, or population served, Health Educators abide by these guidelines when making professional decisions.

Article I: Responsibility to the Public

A Health Educator's ultimate responsibility is to educate people for the purpose of promoting, maintaining, and improving individual, family, and community health. When a conflict of issues arises among individuals, groups, organizations, agencies, or institutions, health educators must consider all issues and give priority to those that promote wellness and quality of living through principles of self-determination and freedom of choice for the individual.

Section 1

Health Educators support the right of individuals to make informed decisions regarding health, as long as such decisions pose no threat to the health of others.

Section 2

Health Educators encourage actions and social policies that support and facilitate the best balance of benefits over harm for all affected parties.

Section 3

Health Educators accurately communicate the potential benefits and consequences of the services and programs with which they are associated.

Source: The Coalition of National Health Education Organizations, Ethics Task Force, November 9, 1999 <www.cnheo.org/>. Reprinted by permission.

Section 4

Health Educators accept the responsibility to act on issues that can adversely affect the health of individuals, families, and communities.

Section 5

Health Educators are truthful about their qualifications and the limitations of their expertise and provide services consistent with their competencies.

Section 6

Health Educators protect the privacy and dignity of individuals.

Section 7

Health Educators actively involve individuals, groups, and communities in the entire educational process so that all aspects of the process are clearly understood by those who may be affected.

Section 8

Health Educators respect and acknowledge the rights of others to hold diverse values, attitudes, and opinions.

Section 9

Health Educators provide services equitably to all people.

Article II: Responsibility to the Profession

Health Educators are responsible for their professional behavior, for the reputation of their profession, and for promoting ethical conduct among their colleagues.

Section 1

Health Educators maintain, improve, and expand their professional competence through continued study and education; membership, participation, and leadership in professional organizations; and involvement in issues related to the health of the public.

Section 2

Health Educators model and encourage nondiscriminatory standards of behavior in their interactions with others.

Section 3

Health Educators encourage and accept responsible critical discourse to protect and enhance the profession.

Section 4

Health Educators contribute to the development of the profession by sharing the processes and outcomes of their work.

Section 5

Health Educators are aware of possible professional conflicts of interest, exercise integrity in conflict situations, and do not manipulate or violate the rights of others.

Section 6

Health Educators give appropriate recognition to others for their professional contributions and achievements.

Article III: Responsibility to Employers

Health Educators recognize the boundaries of their professional competence and are accountable for their professional activities and actions.

Section 1

Health Educators accurately represent their qualifications and the qualifications of others whom they recommend.

Section 2

Health Educators use appropriate standards, theories, and guidelines as criteria when carrying out their professional responsibilities.

Section 3

Health Educators accurately represent potential service and program outcomes to employers.

Section 4

Health Educators anticipate and disclose competing commitments, conflicts of interest, and endorsement of products.

Section 5

Health Educators openly communicate to employers expectations of job-related assignments that conflict with their professional ethics.

Section 6

Health Educators maintain competence in their areas of professional practice.

Article IV: Responsibility in the Delivery of Health Education

Health Educators promote integrity in the delivery of health education. They respect the rights, dignity, confidentiality, and worth of all people by adapting strategies and methods to meet the needs of diverse populations and communities.

Section 1

Health Educators are sensitive to social and cultural diversity and are in accord with the law when planning and implementing programs.

Section 2

Health Educators are informed of the latest advances in theory, research, and practice, and use strategies and methods that are grounded in and contribute to the development of professional standards, theories, guidelines, statistics, and experience.

Section 3

Health Educators are committed to rigorous evaluation of both program effectiveness and the methods used to achieve results.

Section 4

Health Educators empower individuals to adopt healthy lifestyles through informed choice rather than by coercion or intimidation.

Section 5

Health Educators communicate the potential outcomes of proposed services, strategies, and pending decisions to all individuals who will be affected.

Article V: Responsibility in Research and Evaluation

Health Educators contribute to the health of the population and to the profession through research and evaluation activities. When planning and conducting research or evaluation, health educators do so in accordance with federal and state laws and regulations, organizational and institutional policies, and professional standards.

Section 1

Health Educators support principles and practices of research and evaluation that do no harm to individuals, groups, society, or the environment.

Section 2

Health Educators ensure that participation in research is voluntary and based on the informed consent of the participants.

Section 3

Health Educators respect the privacy, rights, and dignity of research participants, and honor commitments made to those participants.

Section 4

Health Educators treat all information obtained from participants as confidential unless otherwise required by law.

Section 5

Health Educators take credit, including authorship, only for work they have actually performed and give credit to the contributions of others.

Section 6

Health Educators who serve as research or evaluation consultants discuss their results only with those to whom they are providing service, unless maintaining such confidentiality would jeopardize the health or safety of others.

Section 7

Health Educators report the results of their research and evaluation objectively, accurately, and in a timely fashion.

Article VI: Responsibility in Professional Preparation

Those involved in the preparation and training of Health Educators have an obligation to accord learners the same respect and treatment given other groups by providing quality education that benefits the profession and the public.

Section 1

Health Educators select students for professional preparation programs based upon equal opportunity for all, and the individual's academic performance, abilities, and potential contribution to the profession and the public's health.

Section 2

Health Educators strive to make the educational environment and culture conducive to

the health of all involved, and free from sexual harassment and all forms of discrimination.

Section 3

Health Educators involved in professional preparation and professional development engage in careful preparation; present material that is accurate, up-to-date, and timely; provide reasonable and timely feedback; state clear and reasonable expectations; and conduct fair assessments and evaluations of learners.

Section 4

Health Educators provide objective and accurate counseling to learners about career opportunities, development, and advancement, and assist learners to secure professional employment.

Section 5

Health Educators provide adequate supervision and meaningful opportunities for the professional development of learners.

Abridged Version

Preamble

The Health Education profession is dedicated to excellence in the practice of promoting individual, family, organizational, and community health. The Code of Ethics provides a framework of shared values within which Health Education is practiced. The responsibility of each Health Educator is to aspire to the highest possible standards of conduct and to encourage the ethical behavior of all those with whom they work.

Article I: Responsibility to the Public

A Health Educator's ultimate responsibility is to educate people for the purpose of promoting, maintaining, and improving individual, family, and community health. When a conflict of issues arises among individuals, groups, organizations, agencies, or institutions, health educators must consider all issues and give priority to those that promote wellness and quality of living through principles of self-determination and freedom of choice for the individual.

Article II: Responsibility to the Profession

Health Educators are responsible for their professional behavior, for the reputation of their profession, and for promoting ethical conduct among their colleagues.

Article III: Responsibility to Employers

Health Educators recognize the boundaries of their professional competence and are accountable for their professional activities and actions.

Article IV: Responsibility in the Delivery of Health Education

Health Educators promote integrity in the delivery of health education. They respect the rights, dignity, confidentiality, and worth of all people by adapting strategies and methods to meet the needs of diverse populations and communities.

Article V: Responsibility in Research and Evaluation

Health Educators contribute to the health of the population and to the profession through research and evaluation activities. When planning and conducting research or evaluation, health educators do so in accordance with federal and state laws and regulations, organizational and institutional policies, and professional standards.

Article VI: Responsibility in Professional Preparation

Those involved in the preparation and training of Health Educators have an obligation to accord learners the same respect and treatment given other groups by providing quality education that benefits the profession and the public.

Cost-Benefit and Cost-Effectiveness as a Part of the Evaluation of Health Promotion Programs

Abstract

Economic evaluation should be a component of program evaluation. To encourage and help with this process, definitions of common economic terms, a review of the literature, steps for conducting an economic evaluation, and the use of economic evaluation with health promotion program is presented.

Introduction

The idea of promoting good health practices is not new in the United States. However, it is only in recent years that the concept of health promotion has grown in popularity and that the number of health promotion programs has flourished. The growth has occurred because of the ". . .increasing evidence of an association between patterns of lifestyle and health status of individuals and population groups, and associations between environmental and workplace hazards and the health and well-being of communities and workers" (Work Group on Health Promotion/Disease Prevention, 1987).

Though the number of health promotion programs continues to increase, the evaluation of said programs lags behind. There are several reasons for this. First, many of the first generation health promotion programs were developed without regard to an appropriate plan of evaluation. Thus data were not and could not be collected. Second, the very nature of health promotion programs, that of being "in the field" and being geared toward the long-term outcome of "improved health," makes them difficult to evaluate. Concerns such as evaluation expertise, confidentiality of participants, and resources of time, money, and personnel have proven to be stumbling blocks in collecting the needed data.

If health promotion programs are to prosper and grow, empirical evidence of their worth should be provided. This can be done only through appropriate evaluation of the programs, evaluation that pays considerable attention to problems of design and measurement, and that can be reproducible. Green (1979) stated that "Evaluation of a health promotion plan certifies its appropriateness and its effectiveness and ensures that the practitioner is accountable to the patient (consumer), the community, and the hospital administrator." Though Green's comments were directed toward hospital health promotion programs, these same ideas can be transferred

Source: J. F. McKenzie "Cost-Benefit and Cost-Effectiveness as a Part of the Evaluation of Health Promotion Programs," *The Eta Sigma Gamman, 18*(2) (1986): 10–16. Reprinted by permission from *Journal of Eta Sigma Gamma: The Health Educator,* formerly *The Eta Sigma Gamman.*

to any health promotion setting because all program planners need to be accountable to the consumer (Work Group on Health Promotion/Disease Prevention, 1987).

The question now is not whether or not health promotion programs should be evaluated but how should it be done? Green (1979) has defined three different levels of evaluation—process, impact, and outcome. Process evaluation deals with the professional practice of those presenting the health promotion program. Impact evaluation is concerned with the immediate difference that the health promotion program has on the knowledge, attitude, behavior, and environment. Outcome evaluation focuses on long-term concerns such as morbidity, mortality, and years of survival following the health promotion program. There are many strategies for evaluating health promotion programs within each of these levels, and they have been thoroughly covered in the works of Windsor, Baranowski, Clark, and Cutter (1984) and Green and Lewis (1986). However, there is one evaluation strategy that these authors have addressed that merits further discussion because of the importance being placed on it in today's practice: the economic evaluation of health promotion programs. In the business world the economic evaluation of a program is often referred to as the "bottom line."

In writing about corporate health promotion programs, Fielding (1982, p. 85) has stated:

> Although current evidence suggests a very favorable return on investment for disease prevention and health promotion programs, much more information is needed to quantify costs and benefits and to suggest which models work best in different corporate settings. Therefore, it is imperative that all efforts include long-term evaluation of effects of programs on both direct and indirect costs.

The remaining portion of this paper will focus on the economic evaluation of health promotion programs. This refers to the cost-benefit and cost-effectiveness analysis (CBA and CEA, respectively) of the programs.

Definitions of CBA and CEA

Simply stated, CBA and CEA are formal analytical techniques used for comparing the negative and positive consequences of alternative uses of resources. They are not formulas for making decisions, but rather are tools to help individuals make decisions (Warner & Luce, 1982). More specifically, Green and Lewis (1986, p. 361) have defined cost-benefit as "a measure of the cost of an intervention relative to the benefits it yields, usually expressed as a ratio of dollars saved or gained for every dollar spent on the program," and cost-effectiveness as "a measure of the cost of an intervention relative to its impact, usually expressed in dollars per unit of effect." Common CEA measures may include years of life saved, days of morbidity and disability avoided, number of smokers who quit, and number of pounds lost.

When first reading these definitions, they appear to be very much alike. The basic technical distinction between CBA and CEA lies in the process of valuing the desirable consequences of health promotion programs (Warner & Luce, 1982). CBA requires that all desirable consequences be expressed in monetary (dollar) terms. For many of the consequences this is a manageable task, but there are some desirable consequences that researchers have found most difficult to quantify in dollars—the value of human life may be the most notable. Several researchers (Rice, 1966; Cooper and Rice, 1976; Acton, 1976) have offered means of dealing with the problem.

More recently the difference between CBA and CEA seems to be fading. Warner and Luce have pointed out that as they have reviewed the literature on CBA and CEA, the two techniques are becoming more alike in the way analysts are applying the concepts. They have indicated that "recent sophisticated health care CEAs are incorporating some dollar-valued benefits into the cost side of the equation (as negative costs), and increasing recognition of the meaning of CBA in health care is bringing it closer to CEA. The human capital approach to measuring indirect benefits in CBA values livelihood, not life itself; thus a CBA is really a net dollar benefit for some nonmonetized health outcomes. The newer, more sophisticated CEA seems to be a significant step forward in that it combines the best of both CBA and CEA" (Warner & Luce, 1982, p. 213).

The Popularity of CBA and CEA

The evaluation techniques of CEA and CBA are by no means new concepts, for they can be traced back hundreds of years. However, there has been a tremendous growth in their use and interest in the health professions in the past fifteen years. Much of this growth has paralleled the increase of health care costs during the same period of time. Many feel that this burgeoning interest of CEA and CBA in the health professions has resulted from health professionals seeking to identify and convey the meaning of cost-beneficial and cost-effective health care interventions. It is now quite common to find CBA and CEA citations on most all health care topics.

Review of Literature

As Warner and Hutton (1980) have pointed out, the contributions to the health care CBA and CEA literature have grown exponentially in recent years. Over the years the majority of the literature has dealt with medical interventions. Since this paper is focused on nonmedical interventions—health promotion activities—the medical intervention CBA and CEA literature is not reviewed here. However, it is well presented in Warner and Luce (1982).

The references to the nonmedical CBA and CEA literature are much more limited. The nonmedical literature falls into three major areas—public health measures (i.e., water fluoridation, food inspection, etc.), identification of health risks via screenings (for hypertension, cancer, and other diseases), and personal health lifestyle (i.e., exercise, smoking, nutrition, stress, etc.). Public health measures have generally not been considered a part of health promotion activities. And even though screenings have been a portion of a number of health promotion programs, it is the category of personal health lifestyle on which most health promotion programs are planned. It is this literature that is reviewed below.

A number of reviews of the CBA and CEA of health promotion type activities have been found in the literature (Fielding, 1982; Rogers, Eaton, & Bruhn, 1981; Scheffler & Paringer, 1980; and Warner, 1979). These reviews report on basically two types of studies. One group includes studies that have calculated a CBA or CEA on a specific health problem in terms of what the costs and benefits would be for the entire United States if a health promotion program were implemented. One such paper is presented by Kristein (1977). In his paper, Kristein examines several different health concerns such as hypertension, cancer of the colon, heavy cigarette smoking, alcohol abuse, and breast cancer. A summary of his heavy cigarette smoking calculations provides a good example of this approach. He calculated that the costs of heavy cigarette smoking were approximately $20.3 billion (in 1975 dollars). This includes the cost of hospital care, medical care, absenteeism, and premature deaths. If a smoking cessation program were implemented for the 22 million heavy smokers in the United States (a 1975 estimate) at $125 per person and there was a 25% success rate, Kristein estimated a cost-benefit ratio of 1.8 to 1.0.

This means that for every dollar put into such a program a $1.80 could be saved. This type of CBA is useful in showing that smoking cessation programs can provide financial benefits, but the exactness of the figures must be put into perspective because of the lack of detail in the analysis.

The other major group of studies that appear in the reviews are those that report on the results of a CBA or CEA calculated on a specific health promotion activity offered by a specific organization. For example, Fielding (1982) has reviewed the results of a number of employee health promotion programs. His findings show that a number of different techniques have been used to calculate CBAs and CEAs, and that calculations are based on a number of assumptions and thus the results are difficult to compare. In another paper, Fielding (1984) offers the following example:

> Campbell's analysis of the savings attributable to their colorectal cancer screening programs hinges on assumptions regarding the number of cases of colorectal cancer that would have occurred in the absence of screening, and the direct and indirect costs associated with each case. It also assumes that all cases prevented were due to on-site screening rather than screening that occurred in another setting (e.g., doctor's office or HMO) at the encouragement of an outside health professional. While these estimates of savings due to health promotion measures are useful in showing the value companies themselves have placed in the savings, it is difficult to know if their assertions can be applied to other companies. (p. 259)

Further indication of the inconsistency in the way CBA and CEA for health promotion activities have been calculated was noted by Rogers et al. (1981, p. 333)—". . .carefully designed cost analyses have not been conducted so that various approaches can be compared as to the expense, as well as to short-term

impact and long-term outcome." There is clearly a need for authors to describe in detail all the steps they follow in calculating their CBA or CEA so that other evaluators can use the same steps and thus be able to compare results.

The health promotion literature includes more reports of CBAs and CEAs on identification of health risks than in personal health lifestyle change, with more reports dealing with hypertension screening programs than any other (Alderman, Madhavan, & Davis, 1983; Erfurt & Foote, 1984; Foote & Erfurt, 1977; Ruchlin & Alderman, 1980; and Ruchlin, Melcher, & Alderman, 1984). Only two recent reports on personal health lifestyle change could be found. One dealt with weight loss (Seidman, Sevelius, & Ewald, 1984) and the other with smoking cessation (Weiss, Jurs, Lesage, & Iverson, 1984). Scheffler and Paringer (1980) have pointed out the need for empirical evidence of the economic soundness of other lifestyle change programs such as physical exercise and dietary changes.

Finally, there are many more reports using CEA than CBA in the health promotion literature. Only two reports of CBA (Alderman et al., 1983; and Weiss et al., 1984) could be found. All others were CEAs. The reasons for this will become clear from subsequent discussion.

Calculating CBAs and CEAs

As suggested in preceding portions of this paper, the calculation of CBAs and CEAs for health promotion activities is no easy task. In most cases they will be difficult and in some cases impossible to calculate. However, if evaluations of health promotion activities are going to be complete, they should be attempted.

Though there are certain processes that must be included in calculating CBAs and CEAs, the exact steps one could use may vary. The important point to remember is that whatever steps are used, they should be reported accurately and in detail so others can replicate and compare results. The steps presented below are a combination of techniques suggested by a governmental agency and several different individuals (OTA, 1978; OTA, 1980; Rogers et al., 1981; Shepard & Thompson, 1979; and Warner & Luce, 1982).

Step 1: Defining the Problem

The initial step in calculating a CBA or CEA is defining the problem to be analyzed. The problem should be stated as clearly and explicitly as possible. Seemingly small differences in the definition of the problem could have a large impact on the calculated costs, benefits, and effects. The statement of the problem should also clearly specify for whom the analysis is going to be calculated. For example, a cost-analysis of a health promotion program would differ greatly if it were being calculated from the employer's point of view as opposed to the costs, benefits, and effects experienced by the employee.

Commonly defined problems for which health promotion programs are usually designed deal with either a specific health concern or an economic issue. An example of a problem that deals with a health concern might be to reduce the risk of cardiovascular disease in white collar employees, while a problem revolving around an economic issue may be to reduce the amount of money the company spends on health insurance claims per year. Both of these problems would be appropriate for calculating a CBA or CEA; however, for the purposes of this paper, the cardiovascular disease problem will be used as an example through the remaining steps in the process.

Step 2: Specifying the Objectives

Closely related to defining the problem is setting one or more objectives against which programmatic alternatives are to be evaluated. If the defined problem is not readily measurable, further specification may help qualify it. For example, the problem of reducing cardiovascular disease in white collar employees is too broad to be readily quantified.

A possible specification of an appropriate objective would be to reduce the risk of cardiovascular disease in this employee group by getting 50% of the high-risk employees in an appropriate exercise program. It is known that the high-risk group includes individuals who have hypertension and are overweight. These individuals cost a company more money in medical care, accidents, etc. than individuals without them. Exercise has been shown to help both of these health concerns.

Step 3: Identifying Alternatives

To determine if a specific approach to a problem is cost-effective or cost-beneficial, it needs to be compared to other approaches that could also be used to achieve the stated objectives. Again using the problem of cardiovascular disease as an example, an alternative approach may be to reduce disease via a nutrition and weight control program as opposed to the exercise program.

When identifying alternatives for health promotion programs, it should be noted that the alternatives do not need to attack the problem using similar approaches. For example, if the problem is to reduce health costs due to cigarette smoking within an organization, one cost analysis may be completed on an educational smoking cessation approach. Another analysis of costs could be calculated on the alternative which mandates, via a company policy, that there be no smoking in the workplace.

It is helpful to keep the following concerns in mind when identifying appropriate alternatives: (1) select only alternatives that are believed to be potentially quite cost-effective, (2) select alternatives that offer variety in their approach, and (3) select alternatives that would be appropriate for comparison—do not select an alternative that is obviously an inappropriate approach for solving the problem (i.e., getting *every* employee to adopt a specific exercise program).

Step 4: Describing Production Relationships

The first three steps of this process set the conceptual framework for calculating a CBA or CEA. When one describes the production relationships, he/she is creating the technical framework for the quantitative assessment and comparison of costs and benefits of the alternatives. This may be the most important step in the CBA and CEA processes. To set up the technical framework, the evaluator must identify the resources necessary to carry out the alternative, explain how the resources are combined, and then predict the outcome(s). As Warner and Luce (1982) have pointed out, this can be completed in several different ways ranging from a simple flow chart to a sophisticated, multi-equation computer simulation.

In the cardiovascular disease problem, the resources would include personnel time—of both the high-risk employees participating in this program and the program leaders, educational materials (i.e., booklets, films, handouts, etc.), supplies (i.e., exercise clothing, laundry expenses, etc.), pre- and postprogram exercise testings, preprogram medical examinations, fee for facility use, and any other preparticipant program expenses. The outcomes of the program may include 50% of the participants getting involved in a lifelong exercise program, 50% reducing their weight, and 75% getting their blood pressure under control. These in turn may result in fewer health insurance claims because of reduced illness, less absenteeism, and fewer accidents, thus increasing productivity. In the long run it is hoped these programs will decrease both morbidity and premature mortality.

As one can see from this example, this step can become quite involved. One may need to examine previous programs—conducted either in house or in another setting—or obtain the services of a technical consultant to try to adequately identify all resources and outcomes. However, the evaluator of the health promotion programs should be aware that even this additional work may not ensure the identification of all health outcomes. It is because of this inability to identify specific health outcomes that the use of CBA with health promotion programs has been limited. If the health benefits of a program cannot be identified, then one cannot put a dollar value on them and thus the cost of the benefit cannot be analyzed. For example, what are the health benefits of a nutrition education program? Unless these benefits can be identified,* CBA would be an inappropriate cost analysis technique to use with health promotion programs.

On the other hand, CEA can be applied very well to some health promotion programs. For the outcomes of concern are not benefits but effects, and with a CEA the evaluator is not required to put a dollar value on the effects. Thus when analyzing the nutrition education program, one can identify effects such as the reduction of calorie intake or the reduction of serum fat levels without trying to identify the health benefit of such. It should be noted that these effects are immediate (i.e., reduction in calories) or intermediate (i.e., decrease in serum fat levels) outcomes only and not long-term (i.e., decreased premature mortality) like some financiers of health promotion programs want to see.

Whether one is using CBA or CEA, the more completely the production relationships have been described, the easier it will be to

---

*See the related literature section of this paper for examples of where evaluators have been able to apply CBA to health promotion programs.

complete steps 5 and 6 in the process—analyzing costs, benefits, and effectiveness.

Step 5: Analyzing the Costs

Costs should be defined as those resources that one must give up to gain some benefit or effect (Warner & Luce, 1982). This would include not only those direct controllable costs but also overhead uncontrollable costs.

The cost of some resources may be obvious. Using the cardiovascular disease example, it may be very easy to determine the cost of the educational materials because they can be purchased at a cost of Y per set. The cost of the group leader may be obvious, too, but how about the cost of the four volunteers who are helping conduct the program? Since the program could not be run without the four volunteers, this is a cost to the program. In this situation the economic concept of "opportunity cost" would be used. "The opportunity cost is its value in another use" (Warner & Luce, 1982, p. 77). So if these volunteers were not helping in this program, how much would they be worth in another setting? It may be found that they would be worth $7.50 per hour working in a similar capacity at a local health agency. Therefore their cost could be determined with this figure.

Since one of the major reasons for calculating CBA and CEA is to be able to compare alternatives, it is important that costs (and for that matter benefits and effects) of the different alternatives are calculated in a similar manner. For example, if one is comparing different cardiovascular exercise programs and both programs include the help of volunteers, the same opportunity costs should be used in determining the total cost of volunteers.

Step 6: Analyzing Benefits and Effectiveness

There are usually numerous desired outcomes (benefits) that result from health promotion programs. Some are obvious while others are much more difficult to identify. For this reason, it may help the evaluator to try to categorize the different outcomes. Warner and Luce (1982) have identified the following classification scheme for outcomes associated with health care activities: (1) personal health benefits—improvements in health such as increased life expectancy, decreased morbidity, and reduced disability; (2) health care resource benefits—the saving of unused resources resulting from the implementation of an activity (for example, an exercise program could reduce the resources put into cardiac surgery); (3) other economic benefits—desired outcomes that are not identified as either health or health care benefits, such as work productivity; (4) other social benefits—desired outcomes that have positive social effects like increased access to health services or compassion; and (5) intermediate outcomes—benefits that occur prior to a final outcome. Because it is sometimes difficult to measure final outcomes, one often must use the intermediate outcome. For example, the long-term impact of an exercise program on one's health would be difficult to determine, but one could measure the intermediate outcome of weight loss.

It should be noted that not all outcomes are benefits. The best example of this appears in screening programs when false positive outcomes appear. If such outcomes do exist, they need to be treated as costs.

The measurement of benefits and effectiveness is very much like the measurement of costs in that some aspects are straightforward while others are very difficult. For example, not all social benefits can be quantified, such as compassion. There is no standard unit of compassion on which one could attach a dollar value.

It is at this point in the calculations of CBA and CEA that the differences in the two analyses can be seen. The CEA ends with the measurement of effectiveness. No dollar value is placed on the outcomes. Thus, the number of lives saved, trips to the health clinic, or persons involved in the exercise program are all that are needed. However, in order to calculate a CBA, monetary units must be attached to each outcome. This is not too difficult when market prices are available. But they are not always available, and the one area that has caused considerable discussion is trying to put a monetary label on the "value of life." Techniques that have been used include (1) human capital—value of being productively employed in the labor market plus the direct benefit of health care resource savings, (2) willingness to pay—value that individuals place on reducing risks of death and illness, (3) court awards in civil cases—value of productive life and emotional costs, and (4) life insurance holdings—value of one's life insurance.

Step 7: Discounting

A necessary step in calculating an accurate CBA or CEA is that of discounting. Since the costs and benefits of some programs do not occur entirely in the present, for comparison purposes all future costs and monetary values of future benefits should be discounted to their present value. In other words, a dollar today is worth more to an individual than the promise of having the dollar tomorrow and more still than having the dollar the day after tomorrow. "The discount rate attempts to adjust for what a dollar invested today would earn in interest" (Collen & Goodman, 1985). ". . .Discounting is particularly important in the case of preventive activities since so many of the benefits occur well into the future. In

addition, discounting helps to explain how 'postponing' illness costs can have the effect of 'containing them'" (Warner, 1979).

To carry out the discounting process, one must first decide on a discount rate. The discount rate expresses the degree to which tomorrow's dollar loses value relative to today's dollar. Since there is little consensus on what discount rate should be used and because the particular discount rate chosen can have a substantial impact on the outcome of the analysis [In relative terms, low discount rates tend to favor projects whose benefits occur in the distant future (OTA, 1980)], CBAs and CEAs are usually calculated using several different rates, usually ranging from 3–10%. This process of using several different rates is called sensitivity analysis.

For example, if one wanted to spend $1,000 today on an exercise program expecting to save $2,000 in medical costs in five years, there would be a need to discount the benefit ($2,000) to its estimated present value. For the sake of the example the discount rate will be set at 5%. The present discounted value today of the net benefit would be $567 ($1,567–$1,000) and not $1,000 ($2,000–$1,000).

Both time (in years) and the discount rate impact the discounted value. Tables 1 and 2 illustrate the effect of each. Table 1 shows how an expected $2,000 benefit decreases in value over time when the discount rate stays constant (5% in this example).

Table 1   Effect of time on discounted value

Discount Rate	Time (in years)	Present Value of Cost	Present Value of Benefit	Present Value of Net Benefit
.05	0	$1,000	$2,000	$1,000
.05	1	$1,000	$1,905	$905
.05	2	$1,000	$1,814	$814
.05	5	$1,000	$1,567	$567
.05	10	$1,000	$1,228	$228
.05	20	$1,000	$754	$-246

Table 2 illustrates how again a $2,000 benefit decreases in value as the discount rate increases and the time stays constant (5 years in this example).

It is obvious from these tables that given a large enough discount rate and/or a substantial number of years, the net benefit could be a negative number. Such a number would indicate that the costs would outweigh the benefits and the cost-benefits ratio would be less than 1.0 to 1.0. In other words, it would cost more than one dollar to get a dollar worth of benefit.

For those interested in other examples of the discounting process, see Collen and Goodman (1985) and Warner and Luce (1982).

Step 8: Analyzing Uncertainties

As has been demonstrated throughout this discussion of calculating a CBA or CEA, there will be times when the evaluator will be uncertain of some data that need to be included. In such cases several alternatives are available to the evaluator. As with discounting, the evaluator could use a sensitivity analysis. For example, if the evaluator were figuring a CEA on a smoking cessation program and was not sure of the cost of an instructor for the program, he/she could make several different estimates of the cost. Each of these estimates could then be "plugged into" the analysis to give the evaluator a range for the CEA.

Another approach to dealing with uncertainties would be to elicit the help of a group of experts in the field. Such a technique is called consensus development. With this technique a group of experts is brought together to listen to a presentation of uncertain areas. Following the presentation, the group is then isolated to discuss the presentation and to reach a consensus as to what should be used in place of the uncertain data.

Step 9: Interpreting the Results

Because of all the concerns noted in calculating a CBA or CEA, one needs to be careful in interpreting the results of an analysis. There are many assumptions and uncertainties that both the evaluator and/or the interpreter of the results could overlook. Thus, one needs to proceed with caution when reading the analysis reports.

Assuming all steps have been carried out properly and appropriate CBA and CEA data have been calculated, the decision maker must not forget that the economic evaluation is only one piece of the data needed to make decisions about programs. Most programs have important ethical, legal, and/or societal issues that must be identified and discussed before final program decisions can be made.

Using CBAs and CEAs with Health Promotion Programs

The need for incorporating an economic component in the evaluation of a health promotion program should be obvious. The question that remains is, what specific technique would be

Table 2   Effect of discount rate on discounted value

Discount Rate	Time (in years)	Present Value of Cost	Present Value of Benefit	Present Value of Net Benefit
0	5	$1,000	$2,000	$1,000
3	5	$1,000	$1,725	$725
5	5	$1,000	$1,567	$567
7	5	$1,000	$1,426	$426
10	5	$1,000	$1,242	$242
15	5	$1,000	$994	$−6

most appropriate? In most situations the answer would be CEA. The reasons for using CEA as opposed to CBA with health promotion programs are: (1) the inability to determine and then measure all the effects of a program, and (2) the inability to put a monetary value on the measured effect. These inabilities of not being able to identify the effects and then in turn being able to determine the value (in dollars) of these effects are critical steps in the CBA process. Without them an evaluator could not calculate an accurate CBA. It would probably be a rare situation in which a CBA would be an appropriate technique to use in an evaluation of a health promotion program. Even if an evaluator were able to determine these values, there are some (Fielding, 1979; Kristein, 1983) who believe the cost-benefit ratio would not favor the health promotion programs. These individuals have indicated that there are several cost issues that evaluators to date have not considered when calculating a CBA. One of these issues revolves around the additional costs of human longevity. When an individual lives longer, he/she is more likely to have incurred additional medical costs and an employer will have to pay pensions for a longer period of time.

Conclusion

Many of the early health promotion programs planned in this country were implemented on the premise that it was more economically sound to spend healthcare dollars on prevention activities than on curing disease. At the present time, there is little empirical data to prove such economic evaluation—even though CBA and CEA have been used in many other areas of the health care system. As one looks to the future, it seems reasonable that if health promotion program planners are going to convince policy makers that such programs are an effective means of improving health status, then economic evaluation must be a part of the total evaluation process.

References

Acton, J. (1976). Measuring the monetary value of lifesaving programs. *Law and Contemporary Problems, 40,* 46.

Alderman, M. H., Madhavan, S., & Davis, T. (1983). Reduction of cardiovascular disease events by worksite hypertension treatment. *Hypertension, 5* (supplement V). V138–V143.

Collen, M., & Goodman, C. (1985). Cost-effectiveness and cost-benefit analysis. In Institute of Medicine, *Assessing Medical Technologies* (pp. 136–144, 160–164). Washington, D.C.: National Medical Press.

Cooper, B., & Rice, D. (1976). The economic cost of illness revisited. *Social Security Bulletin, 39,* 21.

Erfurt, J. C., & Foote, A. (1984). Cost-effectiveness of work-site blood pressure control programs. *Journal of Occupational Medicine, 26,* 892–900.

Fielding, J. E. (1982). Effectiveness of employee health improvement programs. *Journal of Occupational Medicine, 24,* 907–916.

Fielding, J. E. (1984). Health promotion and disease prevention at the worksite. In L. Breslow (Ed.), *Annual Review in Public Health* (pp. 237–265). Palo Alto, California: Annual Reviews, Inc.

Fielding, J. E. (1979). Preventive medicine and the bottom line. *Journal of Occupational Medicine, 21,* 79–88.

Foote, A., & Erfurt, J. C. (1977). Controlling hypertension: A cost-effective model. *Preventive Medicine, 6,* 319–343.

Green, L. W. (1979). How to evaluate health promotion. *Hospitals, 53,* 106–108.

Green, L. W., & Lewis, F. M. (1986). *Measurement and evaluation in health education and health promotion.* Palo Alto, California: Mayfield Publishing Company

Kristein, M. M. (1977). Economic issues in prevention. *Preventive Medicine, 6,* 252–264.

Kristein, M. M. (1983). How much can business expect to profit from smoking cessation? *Preventive Medicine, 12,* 358–381.

Office of Technology Assessment, U.S. Congress. (1978). *Assessing the efficacy and safety of medical technologies.* Washington, D.C.: U.S. Government Printing Office.

Office of Technology Assessment, U.S. Congress (1980). *The implications of cost-effectiveness analysis of medical technology/ background paper #1: Methodological issues and literature review.* Washington, D.C.: U.S. Government Printing Office.

Rogers, P. J., Eaton, E. K., & Bruhn, J. G. (1981). Is health promotion cost effective? *Preventive Medicine, 10,* 324–339.

Rice, D. (1966). *Estimating the cost of illness.* U.S. Department of Health, Education and Welfare, PHS, Health Economic Series No. 6.

Ruchlin, H. S., & Alderman, M. H. (1980). Cost of hypertension control at the workplace. *Journal of Occupational Medicine, 22,* 795–800.

Ruchlin, H. S., Melcher, L. A., & Alderman, M.H. (1984). A comparative economic analysis of work-related hypertension care programs. *Journal of Occupational Medicine, 26,* 45–49.

Scheffler, R. M., & Paringer, L. (1980). A review of the economic evidence on prevention. *Medical Care, 18,* 473–484.

Schwartz, R. M., & Rollins, P. L. (1985). Measuring the cost benefit of wellness strategies. *Business and Health, 2,* 10, 24–26.

Seidman, L. S., Sevelius, G. G., & Ewald, P. (1984). A cost-effective weight loss program at the worksite. *Journal of Occupational Medicine, 26,* 725–730.

Shepard, D. S., & Thompson, M. S. (1979). First principles of cost-effectiveness analysis in health. *Public Health Reports, 94,* 535–543.

Warner, K. E., & Hutton, R. C. (1980). Cost-benefit and cost-effective analysis in health care. *Medical Care, 18,* 1069–1084.

Warner, K. E., & Luce, B. R. (1982). *Cost-benefit and cost-effectiveness in health care: Principles, practice, and potential.* Ann Arbor, Michigan: Health Administration Press.

Warner, K. E. (1979). The economic implications of preventive health care. *Social Science and Medicine, 13C,* 227–237.

Weiss, S. J., Jurs, S., Lesage, J. P., & Iverson, D. C. (1984). A cost-benefit analysis of a smoking cessation program. *Evaluation and Program Planning, 7,* 337–346.

Windsor, R. A., Baranowski, T., Clark, N., & Cutter, G. (1984). *Evaluation of health promotion and education programs.* Palo Alto, California: Mayfield Publishing Company.

Work Group on Health Promotion/Disease Prevention. (1987). Criteria for the development of health promotion and education programs. *American Journal of Public Health, 77,* 89–92.

Glossary

action objective type of impact objective that describes the action or behavior in which the priority population will engage

action research see *participatory research*

action stage a stage of change in which a person has changed overt behavior for less than six months

active participants those who take part in most group activities

act of commission doing something you should not be doing

act of omission not doing something you should be doing

Administrative and Policy Assessment part of the fourth phase of PRECEDE-PROCEED, "an analysis of the policies, resources, and circumstances prevailing in an organizational situation to facilitate or hinder the development of the health program" (Green & Kreuter, 2005, p. G–1)

administrative objective see *process objective*

Advanced level 1 health educator "the level of a health educator with a baccalaureate or master's degree and five years' experience or more in the field of health education" (NCHEC, SOPHE, & AAHE, 2006, p. 56)

Advanced level 2 health educator "the level of a health educator with a doctoral degree and five years' experience or more in the field of health education" (NCHEC, SOPHE, & AAHE, 2006, p. 56)

advisory board see *planning committee*

alpha level the level of statistical significance (usually set at .01 or .05)

alternative hypothesis the hypothesis that holds there is a difference between two groups, treatments, or interventions

analysis of variance (ANOVA) a statistical test used to study group differences when the dependent variables involved represent interval or ratio data

anonymity exists when there is no link between personal information and the person's identity

APEX-PH Assessment Protocol for Excellence in Public Health—a planning model developed by the National Association of County and City Health Officials in 1991 for city and county health departments

assessment the "estimation of the relative magnitude, importance, or values of objects observed" (Cottrell et al., 2009, p. 361)

attitude objective those that describe the desired attitude of those in the priority population

attitude toward the behavior "the degree to which performance of the behavior is positively or negatively valued" (Ajzen, 2006)

aversive stimulus unpleasant consequence of a behavior

awareness objective those that describe of what those in the priority population will become aware

barriers things that keep people from obtaining the product or adopting a behavior

baseline data data collected prior to program implementation to serve as a comparison with data collected during the program, or more typically, with data collected at the completion of a program

basic priority rating (BPR) a process used to prioritize needs assessment data

behavioral capability knowledge and skills necessary to perform a behavior

behavioral change theories "specify the relationships among causal processes operating both within and across levels of analysis" (McLeroy, Steckler et al., 1992, p. 3)

behavioral objectives see *action objective*

beneficence doing good

benefits value or outcome the priority population receives as a result of obtaining the product

best experiences interventions from prior or existing programs of others that have not gone through the critical research and evaluation studies and thus fall short of best practice criteria but nonetheless show promise in being effective

best practices "recommendations for an intervention, based on critical review of multiple research and evaluation studies that substantiate the efficacy of the intervention in the populations and circumstances in which the studies were done, if not its effectiveness in other populations and situations where it might be implemented" (Green & Kreuter, 2005, p. G–1)

best processes original intervention strategies that the planners create on their own based on their knowledge and skills of good planning processes

bias a preference that inhibits impartiality

bias data those data that have been distorted because of the way they have been collected

bivariate data analysis analysis of two variables

blind study an evaluation wherein participants do not know if they belong to the experimental group or control group

bottom up see *grassroots*

brand "name, term, design, symbol, or any other feature that identifies one seller's good or service as distinct from those of other sellers" (American Marketing Association, 2007)

budget a "formal statement of the estimated revenues and expeditures" (Johnson & Breckon, 2007, p. 170)

canned program one that has been developed by an outside group and includes the basic components and materials necessary to implement a program

categorical funding funds that are earmarked or dedicated to support programs aimed at a specific health problem or determinant (i.e., risk factor)

CDCynergy a six-phase social marketing planning model developed by the Centers for Disease Control and Prevention in the mid-1990s

census everyone in a population

chi-square a statistical test that measures the association between two nominal and/or ordinal variables

citizen initiated see *grassroots*

cluster sampling a type of probability sample that selects participants from a sampling frame as groups not individuals

coalition a "formal, long-term alliance among a group of individuals representing diverse organizations, factors, or constituencies within the community who agree to work together to achieve a common goal" (Butterfoss & Whitt, 2003, p. 354)

codes of practice guidelines or criteria for offering a certain type of program

communication channel route through which a message is delivered to the priority population

community a "group of people who have common characteristics" (Turnock, 2004, p. 383)

community advocacy a process in which the people of the community become involved in the institutions and decisions that will impact their lives

community building an "orientation to community that is strength based rather than need based and stresses the identification, nurturing, and celebration of community assets" (Minkler, 2005a, p. 4)

community capacity the "characteristics of communities that affect their ability to identify, mobilize, and address social and public health problems" (Goodman et al., 1999, p. 259)

community development a "process designed to create conditions of economic and social progress for the whole community with its active participation and fullest possible reliance on the community's initiative" (United Nations, 1955, p. 6)

community empowerment where community members control decision making

community forum a process that brings people from the priority population to discuss problems and needs

community organization the "process by which community groups are helped to identify common problems or goals, mobilize resources, and in other ways develop and implement strategies for reaching the goals they have collectively set" (Minkler & Wallerstein, 2005, p. 26)

community organizing the process of community organization

comparison group as part of a summative evaluation or research study, a nonequivalent group (not randomly selected) that does not receive the treatment or program but is compared with the experimental group

Competency Update Project (CUP) a six-year, multiphase process carried out by the health education profession in order to reverify the role of the entry-level health educator and to distinguish it from the role of the advanced-level health educator

concepts primary elements or the building blocks of a theory (Glanz et al., 2002b)

concurrent validity a form of criterion validity in which a new instrument and an established valid instrument that measure the same characteristics are given to the same population and the new instrument correlates positively with the established instrument

conditions a major component of an objective that describes when or how the outcome will be observed

confidentiality exists when there is a link between personal information and the person's identity but that information is protected from others

construct a concept developed, created, or adopted for use with a specific theory (Kerlinger, 1986)

construct validity "the degree to which a measure correlates with other measures it is theoretically expected to correlate with" (Valente, 2002, p. 161)

consumer-based planning a planning process that incorporates the wants, needs, and preferences of the priority population directly into interventions and implementation

contemplation stage a stage of change in which a person intends to take action in the next six months

content validity the "assessment of the correspondence between the items composing the instrument and the content domain from which the items were selected" (DiIorio, 2005, p. 213)

contingencies what happens if the objectives in a behavior change contract are either met or not met

continuum theories those that identify variables that influence action and combine them into a prediction equation (Weinstein et al., 1998)

control group as part of a summative evaluation or research study, a randomly selected group of individuals, similar to the experimental group

that does not receive the treatment or program but is compared with the experimental group

convergent validity "the extent to which two measures which purport to be measuring the same topic correlate (that is, converge)" (Bowling, 2005, p. 12)

correlation represents the strength and direction of relationships between two variables

cost-benefit analysis (CBA) measures dollars spent on a program versus dollars saved or gained

cost-effectiveness analysis (CEA) measures dollars spent on a program versus the impact achieved

cost-identification analysis compares interventions to determine which is least expensive in the context of impact achieved

cost-utility analysis values of the outcomes of a program are determined by their subjective value to the stakeholders rather than monetary cost

criterion a major component of an objective that describes how much change will occur

criterion-related validity the "extent to which data generated from a measurement instrument are correlated with the data generated from a measure (criterion) of the phenomenon being studied, usually an individual's behavior or performance" (Cottrell & McKenzie, 2005, p. 307)

critical path method (CPM) similar to PERT (see *PERT*) but focuses on total time to complete the tasks and the critical dependent tasks

culture the "patterned ways of thought and behavior that characterize a social group, which are learned through socialization processes and persist through time" (Coreil, Bryant, & Henderson, 2001, p. 29)

cultural competent the ability "to understand and respect values, attitudes, beliefs, and mores that differ across cultures, and to consider and respond appropriately to these differences in planning, implementing, and evaluating health education and health promotion programs and interventions" (Joint Committee, 2001, p. 99)

cultural sensitivity implies knowledge that cultural differences exist and does not assign values to those differences (Anderson & Fenichel, 1989)

curriculum a "written plan outlining what students will be taught (a course of study)" (ASCD, 2007, ¶. 3)

data management the process of organizing, coding, and cleaning data in a useable format for the purpose of analysis and reporting

decisional balance refers to the pros and cons of behavioral change

Delphi technique a "group process that generates a consensus through a series of questionnaires" (Gilmore & Campbell, 2005, p. 67)

dependent variable an outcome variable or end result indicator in an evaluation or study

descriptive statistics data used to organize, summarize, and describe characteristics of a group

Diffusion of Innovations theory explains a pattern for how innovations (e.g., products) are adopted in a population

direct reinforcement consequence given in a specific situation to increase a behavior

discriminant validity "requires that the construct should not correlate with dissimilar (discriminant) variables" (Bowling, 2005, p. 12)

disincentive consequence for not acting in a certain way; also used as a means to discourage the consumer from purchasing a product or behaving in a certain way.

doers those who are willing to take on work to complete a task

dose the number of program units delivered

double blind study an evaluation wherein neither participants nor those implementing the program know which group is experimental and which group is the control

early adopters in the Diffusion of Innovations theory, the second group of people to adopt the innovation; often comprised of opinion leaders

early majority in the Diffusion of Innovations theory, the people who are interested in the innovation, but will need external motivation to become involved

ecological perspective a view that there are a number of different sized populations (i.e., individuals, families, schools, employers, social networks, organizations, communities) within the environment

educational and ecological assessment the third phase of PRECEDE-PROCEED wherein planners identify predisposing, reinforcing, and enabling factors that contribute to problems identified in earlier phases of the model

effectiveness in evaluation, a measure usually associated with the outcomes of a program—that is,

did the program result in changes in awareness, knowledge, attitudes, skills, or especially behavior, and did the program result in improved health status (i.e., less mortality, morbidity, and disability).

efficacy expectations people's competency feelings

elaboration amount of effortful processing people put into receiving messages

emotional-coping responses dealing with sources of anxiety that surround a behavior

empowered community "one in which individuals and organizations apply their skills and resources in collective efforts to meet their respective needs" (Israel et al., 1994)

enabling factor "any characteristic of the environment that facilitates action and any skill or resource required to attain a specific behavior" (Green & Kreuter, 2005, p. G–3)

entry-level health educator those who are taking their first professional position in health education and possess a baccalaureate or master's degree and less than five years' experience

environmental objective type of impact objective that describes how the environments (i.e., emotional, physical, social) around the priority population will change

epidemiological assessment the second phase of PRECEDE-PROCEED, wherein planners identify specific health goals or problems that contribute to the social goals or problems identified in Phase 1; and "the identification of etiological factors, or determinants of health in the genetics, behavioral patterns, and environment of the population" (Green & Kreuter, 2005, pp. 11–12)

epidemiology "the study of the distribution and determinants of health-related states or events in specific populations, and the application of this study to control health problems" (Last, 2007, p. 111)

ethical issues situations where competing values are at play and program planners need to make a judgment about what is the most appropriate course of action

evaluation the "comparison of an object of interest against a standard of acceptability" (Green & Lewis, 1986, p. 362)—may be formative (including process evaluation) or summative in nature

evaluation approach refers to the use of either process or summative evaluation and suggests these two types of evaluation are clearly distinct

evaluation consultant an external evaluator

evaluation design used to organize the summative evaluation and to provide for planned, systematic data collection, analysis, and reporting

evaluation standards practical guidelines for evaluators to follow

evidence a body of data that can be used to make decisions about planning

evidence-based practice process of systematically finding, appraising, and using evidence as the basis for decision making when planning a health promotion program (Cottrell & McKenzie, 2005)

exchange process of the marketer providing a product and its benefits to the consumer in trade for the consumer paying a price

executive participants core group who are committed to resolution of the concern

expectancies values people place on an expected outcome

expectations anticipation of certain outcomes from a certain behavior

experimental design random assignment to experimental and control groups with measurement of both groups

experimental group as part of a summative evaluation or research study, a group of individuals that receives the treatment or program

external evaluation evaluation conducted by an individual or organization not affiliated with the organization conducting the program

external personnel individuals from outside the planning agency/organization or people from within the priority population

external validity extent to which the program can be expected to produce similar effects in other populations

face validity if, on the face, the measure appears to measure what it is supposed to measure (McDermott & Sarvela, 1999)

fairness whether a measure is "appropriate for the individuals of various ethnic groups with different backgrounds, gender, educational levels, etc." (Torabi, 1994, p. 56)

field study the most strenuous form of pilot testing in which people from the priority population assess the process being tested in a setting that is just like or closely represents the setting in which the program will be implemented

flexibility as related to program planning, a process that is adapted to the needs of stakeholders

flex time a system in which employees can vary their work schedule to meet their personal needs

fluidity as related to program planning, a process that is sequential and logical in nature

focus group an "exploratory process that is used for generating hypotheses, uncovering attitudes and opinions, and acquiring and testing new ideas" (Gilmore & Campbell, 2005, p. 98)

formative evaluation "any combination of measurements obtained and judgments made before or during the implementation of materials, methods, activities, or programs to control, assure or improve the quality of performance or delivery" (Green & Lewis, 1986, p. 362)

formative objective see *process objective*

functionality as related to program planning, an assurance that the outcome of planning is improved health conditions, not just the production of a program plan

Gantt chart a program management charting method that provides a graphical illustration of the time frame for tasks to be completed and what has been completed to date

gatekeepers those who control, both formally and informally, the political climate of a community

goal general statement of intent (Neiger & Thackeray, 1998)

grant money money that is received from a funded grant proposal

grantsmanship the ability to write grant proposals that are funded

grassroots a step of community organizing in which those within the community recognize the issue of concern

Guide to Community Preventive Services (Community Guide) the "body of evidence and recommendations approved by the Task Force on Community Preventive Services" (Zara et al., 2005, p. 479)

hard money an ongoing source of funding that is part of the operating budget

health advocacy the "processes by which the actions of individuals or groups attempt to bring about social and/or organizational change on behalf of a particular health goal, program, interest, or population" (Joint Committee on Terminology, 2001, p. 7)

health assessments include instruments known as health risk appraisals/assessments (HRAs), health status assessments (HSAs), various lifestyle-specific assessment instruments, and wellness and behavioral/habit inventories (SPM Board of Directors, 1999)

health behavior behaviors that impact a person's health

Health Belief Model a behavior change model that hypothesizes that health-related action is based on the interaction of motivation, perceived threat of a health problem, and reduction of the threat at an acceptable cost

health communication the use of strategies to inform and influence individual and community decisions to enhance health (NCI, 2002)

Health Communication Model a four-phase program planning model for health communication developed by the National Cancer Institute

health education "any combination of planned learning experiences based on sound theories that provide individuals, groups, and communities the opportunity to acquire information and the skills needed to make quality health decisions" (Joint Committee on Terminology, 2001, p. 99)

health educator a "professionally prepared individual who serves in a variety of roles and is specifically trained to use appropriate educational strategies and methods to facilitate the development of policies, procedures, interventions, and systems conducive to the health of individuals, groups, and communities" (Joint Committee on Terminology, 2001, p. 100)

Health Insurance Portability and Accountability Act of 1996 (HIPAA) (Public Law 104–191) sets national standards that health plans, healthcare clearinghouses, and healthcare providers who conduct certain healthcare transactions electronically must implement to protect and guard against the misuse of individually identifiable health information

health promotion "any planned combination of educational, political, environmental, regulatory or organizational mechanisms that support actions and conditions of living conducive to the health of individuals, groups, and communities" (Joint Committee on Terminology, 2001, p. 101)

Healthy Communities a movement that began in the 1980s with assistance from the World Health Organization to mobilize and empower partnerships within cities and communities to enhance health and well-being

Healthy People U.S. government publication that brought together much of what was known about the relationship of personal health behavior and health status

Healthy Plan-It a six-phase planning model developed by the Centers for Disease Control and Prevention in 2000 to strengthen in-country management training capacity in the health sector of developing countries

impact evaluation evaluation that focuses on the immediate observable effects of a program (e.g., awareness, knowledge, attitudes, skills, environment, and behaviors) leading to the intended outcomes of a program (Green & Lewis, 1986)

impact objectives a category of objectives comprised of the four types of learning objectives (i.e., awareness, knowledge, attitudes, and skills), action or behavioral, and environmental objectives

implementation the "act of converting planning, goals, and objectives into action through administrative structure, management activities, policies, procedures, regulations, and organizational actions of new programs" (Timmreck, 1997, p. 328)

incentives reward for achieving a goal; also used as a means to entice the consumer to purchase the product or adopt a behavior

independent variable a variable that is manipulated, selected, or measured by the evaluator which causes or exerts some influence on the dependent variable

inferential statistics data used to determine relationships and causality in order to make generalizations or inferences about a population based on findings from a sample

influencers those who control resources to facilitate the planning and implementation of a program

informed consent agreeing to participate after knowing the full implications of what they are agreeing to

in-house materials educational materials developed by the program planners

in-kind support nonfinancial support of a program such as free materials or volunteer time

innovators in the Diffusion of Innovations theory, the very first people to adopt the innovation

institutional review board (IRB) a group of individuals with authority to grant or deny permission to conduct evaluation or research. These boards serve to safeguard the rights, privacy, health, and well-being of those involved in the research.

instrumentation a "collective term that describes all measurement instruments used" (Cottrell & McKenzie, 2005, p. 311)

intention an "indication of a person's readiness to perform a given behavior, and it is considered to be the immediate antecedent of behavior" (Ajzen, 2006)

interactive contact methods data collection methods wherein those collecting the data interact with those from whom the data are being collected

internal consistency reliability the intercorrelations among individual items on the instrument, that is, whether all items on the instrument are measuring part of the total area

internal evaluation evaluation conducted by one or more individuals employed by, or in some other way affiliated with, the organization conducting the program

internal personnel individuals from within the planning agency/organization or from within the priority population

internal validity degree to which change that was measured can be attributed to the program under investigation

interrater reliability rater reliability using two or more raters

interval level measures a measurement form that put data into categories that are mutually exclusive, exhaustive, and rank ordered; furthermore, the distance between categories can be measured and there is no absolute zero

intervention "to come or occur between two things, events, or points in time; to come in or between so as to hinder or alter an action" (Anderson et al., 2002, p. 447)

intervention alignment part of the fourth phase of PRECEDE-PROCEDE wherein planners match appropriate strategies and interventions with projected changes and outcomes identified in earlier phases (Green & Kreuter, 2005)

Intervention Mapping a six-phase program planning model guided by diagrams and matrices that incorporate outputs of the assessment process with relevant theory to help develop appropriate interventions for priority populations

intrarater reliability rater reliability that is established by a single rater

key activity chart a program management charting method that presents the key activities or tasks, an estimate of when they will take place, and the time needed to complete them

key informants strategically placed individuals in a community who have the knowledge and ability to report on the needs of those in the priority population

knowledge objective type of impact objective that describes the information those in the priority population will learn

laggards in the Diffusion of Innovations theory, people who are not very interested in innovation and would be the last to adopt it

lapse a single slip back to an old behavior while attempting a behavior change

late majority in the Diffusion of Innovations theory, the people who are interested in the innovation but are more skeptical and need external motivation to become involved

learning objectives a category of objectives comprised of four levels of objectives (i.e., awareness, knowledge, attitudes, and skills)

lesson the amount of material that can be presented during a single educational encounter

lesson plan the written outline of a lesson

levels of measurement a hierarchy of four measurement levels (nominal, ordinal, interval, and ratio)

likelihood of action weighing the threat of disease against the difference between benefits and barriers

literature the articles, books, and other documents that explain the past and current knowledge about a particular topic

locality development a form of community organizing that is "heavily process oriented, stressing consensus, and cooperation and aimed at building group identity and a sense of community" (Minkler & Wallerstein, 2005, p. 30)

locus of control perception of the center of control over reinforcement

logic model "a simplified picture of a program, initiative, or intervention" (UW-Ex, 2002a, p. 2) that "shows the logical relationships among the resources that are invested, the activities that take place, and the benefits or changes that result" (UW-Ex, 2002a, p. 2)

macro practice methods of professional change that deal with issues beyond the individual, family, and small group level

maintenance stage a stage of change in which a person has changed overt behavior for more than six months

management the "process of achieving results through controlling human, financial, and technical resources" (Johnson & Breckon, 2007, p. 293)

MAPP Mobilizing for Action through Planning and Partnerships—a six-phase program planning model developed by the National Association of County and City Health Officials in 2001

mapping the visual representation of data by geography or location, linking information to a place (Kirschenbaum & Russ, 2005)

mapping community capacity a process of mapping community assests

market the buyer, consumer, or priority population who has an interest in the product

marketing a "set of processes for creating, communicating, and delivering value to customers" (American Marketing Association, 2007)

marketing mix combination of the product, price, place, and promotion.

MATCH Multilevel Approach to Community Health—a five-phase program planning model developed in the late 1980s

mean the arithmetic average of all scores in data analysis

measurement the method or procedure of assigning numbers to objects, events, and people (Green & Lewis, 1986)

measurement instrument the item used to measure the variables

measures of central tendency forms of univariate data analysis involving the mean, median, and mode

median the midpoint of all scores in data analysis

mission statement a short narrative that describes the general focus or purpose of a program

mode the score or response that occurs most frequently in data analysis

model generalized, hypothetical description, often based on an analogy, used to analyze or explain something (Glanz et al., 2002b)

multiple regression a statistical test that explores the relationships between multiple independent variables and one dependent variable

multiplicity refers to the number of components or activities that make up an intervention

multivariate data analysis analysis of more than two variables

need the "difference between the present situation and a more desirable one" (Gilmore & Campbell, 2005, p. 6)

needs assessment the process of identifying, analyzing, and prioritizing the needs of a priority population

negative punishment removing a positive reinforcer to decrease a behavior

negative reinforcement removing a negative reinforcer or aversive stimulus to increase a behavior

negligence failing to act as a reasonable (prudent) person would

networking interaction among professionals in order to share information

news hook news that the media would want to cover

no contact methods data collection methods wherein those collecting the data had no contact with those from whom the data were collected

nominal group process a highly structured process in which a few knowledgeable representatives (five to seven) are asked to qualify and quantify specific needs

nominal level measures a measurement form that put data into categories that are mutually exclusive and exhaustive

nonexperimental design use of pretest and posttest comparisons, or posttest analysis only, without a control group or comparison group

nonmaleficence not causing harm

nonprobability sample type of sample in which all in the survey population do not have an equal and known probability of being selected

nonproportional stratified random sample a form of stratified random sample in which the sampling units are selected so that there is equal representation from the strata

null hypothesis the hypothesis that holds there is no difference between two groups, treatments, or interventions

objectives statements that specify intermediate accomplishments or benchmarks

observation "notice taken of an indicator" (Green & Lewis, 1986, p. 363)

obtrusive observation when people are aware they are being measured, assessed, or tested

occasional participants those who become involved on an irregular basis and usually only when major decisions are made

opinion leaders those who are well respected in a community and can accurately represent the views of the priority population

ordinal level measures a measurement form that put data into categories that are mutually exclusive, exhaustive, and rank ordered

organizational culture the norms and traditions of an organization

outcome a major component of an objective that describes what will change as a result of the program

outcome evaluation evaluation that focuses on the end result of a program generally measured by improvements in mortality, morbidity, or vital measures of symptoms, signs, or physiological indicators (Green & Lewis, 1986)

outcome expectations value placed on expected outcomes

outcome objective a type of objective that describes the change in health status, social benefits, risk factors, or quality of life of the priority population

ownership a feeling that is derived from participating in the development of a program

PACE-EH Assessment Protocol for Excellence in Public Health—a three-phase program planning model and the forerunner to the MAPP model, developed in 1991, by the National Association of County and City Health Officials

parallel (or equivalent or alternate) **forms reliability** focuses on whether different forms of the same instrument when measuring the same participants will produce similar results

participation and relevance "community organizing that 'starts where the people are' and engages community members as equals" (Minkler & Wallerstein, 2005, p. 35)

participatory data collection where those in the priority population participate in the data collection

participatory research research characterized by community empowerment, collaboration, acquisition of knowledge through hands-on participation, and a focus on social change

PATCH an acronym for a planning process called Planned Approach to Community Health

peer education a process wherein individuals are educated by others who have similar characteristics or standing as themselves

penetration rate number in the priority population exposed or reached

perceived barriers costs that must be overcome in order to follow a health recommendation

perceived behavioral control perceived ease or difficulty of performing the behavior

perceived benefits belief that a certain action could improve one's health

perceived seriousness/severity belief that if a disease or condition were contracted it could be serious

perceived susceptibility belief that one is vulnerable to a certain disease or condition

perceived threat belief that one is vulnerable to a serious health problem or to the sequelae of that illness or condition

PERT acronym for Program Evaluation and Review Technique; a program management charting method that provides a graphical illustration of the time frame for tasks to be completed that includes three estimates of time—optimistic, pessimistic, and probabilistic

phased in implementation of a program by limiting the number of people able to start the program at any given time

photovoice those in the priority population are provided with cameras and skills training, then use the cameras to convey their own images of the community's problems and strengths

pilot testing a set of procedures used to try out various processes during program development using a small group of participants prior to implementation

place where the priority population has access to the product or where they may engage in the desired behavior

planning committee the collective group of individuals who have the responsibility of creating a program and then overseeing its implementation and evaluation

planning models those used for planning, implementing, and evaluating programs

planning parameters the boundaries in which the planning committee must work when planning, implementing, and evaluating the program

population as it relates to sampling, those in the universe specified by time or place

population-based approach planning processes used with large populations

positive punishment adding something to a situation that decreases a behavior

positive reinforcement a consequence of a behavior that is enjoyable or makes a person feel good

posttest testing components of a program, service, or product with the priority population after the completion of a program

potential building blocks located resources originating outside the neighborhood and controlled by people outside

PRECEDE-PROCEED Predisposing, Reinforcing, Enabling Constructs in Ecological Diagnosis and Evaluation—Policy, Regulatory, and Organizational Constructs in Educational and Environmental Development—a widely known and robust eight-phase program planning model

precontemplation stage a stage of change in which a person has no intentions to take action in the next six months

predictive validity a form of criterion validity in which the measurement used will be correlated with another measurement of the same phenomenon at another time

predisposing factor "any characteristic of a person or population that motivates behavior prior to the occurrence of the behavior" (Green & Kreuter, 2005, p. G–6)

preliminary review a form of pilot testing in which colleagues of planners review a process being tested

preparation a stage of change in which a person intends to take action in the next 30 days and has taken some behavioral steps in this decision

prepilot a form of pilot testing in which five or six people from the priority population assess the process being tested

pretest testing components of a program, service, or product with the priority population prior to implementation

pretesting can be defined in one of two ways: (1) testing components of a program, service, or product with the priority population prior to implementation; and (2) collecting baseline data prior to program implementation that will be compared with posttest data to measure the effectiveness of programs

price what the priority population gives up to obtain the product and its associated benefits

primary building blocks assets located in the neighborhood and largely under the control of those who live in the neighborhood

primary data original data collected by the planners

priority population the people for whom the program is intended

probability sample type of sample in which all in the survey population have an equal and known probability of being selected

process evaluation "any combination of measurements obtained during the implementation of program activities to control, assure, or improve the quality of performance or delivery" (Green & Lewis, 1986, p. 364)

process objective a type of objective that expresses the tasks or activities to be carried out by the program planners

processes of change a construct of the transtheoretical model that describes the covert and overt activities that people use to progress through the stages of change (Prochaska et al., 1998)

product something (i.e., goods, services, events, experiences, information, ideas, or behaviors) that fulfills a need customers have and provides a benefit they value; obtained for a price in the exchange

profit margin the percent of financial gain after all the expenses are paid

program kick off see *program launch*

program launch the first day of program implementation

program objective see *outcome objective*

program ownership a feeling by those in the priority population that the program in part belongs to them

program rollout see *program launch*

promotion marketing communication strategy for letting the priority population know about the product and how to obtain or purchase it

proportional stratified random sample a form of stratified random sample in which the sampling units are selected in the same proportion that the strata exist in the survey population

proposal a formal written request for funding

proxy measure an outcome measure that provides evidence that a behavior has occurred

prudent acting as a reasonable person would act in a given situation

psychometric qualities an instrument's validity, reliability, and fairness

public domain available for anyone to use without permission

punishment any event that follows a behavior which decreases the probability that the same behavior will be repeated in the future

qualitative data information presented in narrative form used in evaluation to provide detailed summaries or descriptions of observations, interactions, or verbal accounts (e.g., data from focus groups, in-depth interviews)

qualitative measure "tend to produce data in the language of the subjects, rarely with numerical values attached to observations" (Green & Lewis, 1986, p. 151)

quality in evaluation, a measure usually associated with how a program is implemented and what can be done to improve program delivery

quantitative data information expressed in numerical terms that can be compared on scales

quantitative measure "rely on more standardized data collection and reduction techniques, using predetermined questions or observational indicators and established response items" (Green & Lewis, 1986, p. 151)

quasi-experimental design use of a treatment group and a nonequivalent (nonrandomized) comparison group with measurement of both groups

random-digit-dialing a method of selecting participants using random combinations of numbers to create telephone numbers

random selection a method of selecting participants in which all in the survey population have an equal chance or known probability of being selected

randomized controlled trial research designs that include randomization, control groups, and experimental groups

range the difference between the highest and lowest scores in data analysis

rater (or observer) **reliability** associated with the consistent measurement (or rating) of an observed event by the same or different individuals (or judges or raters) (McDermott & Sarvela, 1999)

ratio level measure a measurement form that puts data into categories that are mutually exclusive, exhaustive, and rank ordered; furthermore, the distance between categories can be measured and there is an absolute zero

recidivism slipping back to an old behavior after attempting a behavior change

reciprocal determinism behavior changes that result from the interaction between the person and the environment

reinforcement any event that follows a behavior which increases the probability that the same behavior will be repeated in the future (Skinner, 1953)

reinforcing factor "any reward or punishment following or anticipated as a consequence of a behavior, serving to strengthen the motivation for the behavior after it occurs" (Green & Kreuter, 2005, p. G–7)

relapse breakdown or failure in a person's attempt to change or modify a behavior (Marlatt & George, 1998)

relapse prevention a self-control program to help individuals to anticipate and cope with the problem of relapse in the behavior change process (Marlatt & George, 1998)

reliability "an empirical estimate of the extent to which an instrument produces the same result (measure or score), applied once or two or more times" (Windsor et al., 2004, p. 93)

request for proposals (**RFPs**) a call made by funding agencies to alert individuals and organizations that it will receive and review grant proposals

resources the "human, fiscal, and technical assets available" (Johnson & Breckon, 2007, p. 296) to plan, implement, and evaluate a program

Role Delineation Project a comprehensive process that led to the creation of the responsibilities and competencies of the entry-level health educator

sample a part of the whole

sampling the process of selecting a sample

sampling frame a list or quasi-list of all sampling units

sampling unit an element or set of elements considered for selection as part of the sample (Babbie, 1992), for example, individual, organization, or geographical area

scope the breadth and depth of the material covered in a curriculum

secondary building blocks assets located in the neighborhood but largely controlled by people outside

secondary data those that have been collected by someone else and available for use by the planners

seed dollars funds designated to start up a new program or project

segmentation process of identifying groups of consumers that share similar characteristics and will respond in a like way to a marketing strategy

self-assessments a process wherein an individual assesses him/herself

self-control gaining control over one's own behavior through monitoring and adjusting it

self-efficacy people's confidence in their ability to perform a certain behavior or task

self-regulation see *self-control*

self-reinforcement person reinforcing self for a behavior performed in an appropriate manner

self-report when individuals or groups answer questions about themselves

sensitivity the ability of a test to identify correctly those with a disease or condition (Mausner & Kramer, 1985)

sequence defines the order in which the content of a curriculum is presented

significant other one who has an important relationship (e.g., friend, family member, partner, spouse) with another

simple random sample (SRS) most basic process for selecting a random sample

single-step survey a means of gathering data in which collectors obtain the data from individuals or groups with a single contact

skill development/acquisition objective type of impact objective that describes the skill those in the priority population will be able to perform

sliding-scale fee a fee structure based upon one's ability to pay

SMART Social Marketing Assessment and Response Tool—a seven-phase social marketing planning model developed in 1998

SMART objectives objectives that are specific, measurable, achievable, realistic, and time-phased (CDC, 2003)

social action a form of community organizing that "is both task and process oriented" (Minkler & Wallerstein, 2005, p. 30) and deals with organizing a disadvantaged segment of the population

social assessment the first phase of PRECEDE-PROCEED wherein planners seek to subjectively define the quality of life (problems and priorities) of those in the priority population

social capital "relationships and structures within a community that promote cooperation for mutual benefit" (Minkler & Wallerstein, 2005, p. 35)

social marketing "the application of commercial marketing technologies to the analysis, planning, execution, and evaluation of programs designed to influence the voluntary behavior of target audiences in order to improve their personal welfare and that of their society" (Andreasen, 1995, p. 7)

social planning a form of community organizing that is "heavily task oriented, stressing rational-empirical problem solving" (Minkler & Wallerstein, 2005, p. 30)

social support a network of individuals that provides assistance or encouragement to a person who is engaging in a new behavior

soft money a source of funding that is not an ongoing part of the operating budget

speaker's bureau a service offered by various groups in which the organizations have experts who are willing to present information to others

specificity the ability of a test to identify correctly those who do not have a disease or condition (Mausner & Kramer, 1985)

stage a step in the change process

stage theory a theory comprised of an ordered set of categories into which people can be classified, and for which factors could be identified that could induce movement from one category to the next (Weinstein & Sandman, 2002a)

stakeholders any person or organization with a vested interest in a health program, usually decision makers, program partners, or clients

steering committee see *planning committee*

strata as it relates to sampling, subgroups of the survey population

strategy a general plan of action for affecting a health problem; it may encompass several activities (CDC, 2003)

stratified random sample a type of probability sample that first divides the survey population into strata and then randomly selects participants from each strata

subjective norm "the perceived social pressure to engage or not to engage in a behavior" (Ajzen, 2006)

summative evaluation "any combination of measurements and judgments that permit conclusions to be drawn about impact, outcome or benefits of a program or method" (Green & Lewis, 1986, p. 366)

supporting participants those who are seldom involved but help to swell the ranks and may contribute in nonactive ways or through financial contributions

survey population as it relates to sampling, those in the universe specified by time or place, and who are accessible

SWOT Strengths, Weaknesses, Opportunities, and Threats an approach to planning that minimizes planning time and moves quickly to action steps by assessing internal strengths and weaknesses as well as external opportunities and threats, usually displayed in a 2×2 matrix

Systematic Approach to Health Promotion (*Healthy People 2010*) the planning model used to develop *Healthy People 2010*

systematic sample a type of probability sample that selects participants from a sampling frame by taking every Nth person after a random start

tailored an intervention activity that is specifically created for an individual's needs, interests, and circumstances

Task Development Time Line a program management charting method that provides a graphical illustration of the time frame for tasks to be completed

termination a stage of change in which a person who has changed a behavior has zero temptation to return to the old behavior

test-retest reliability (or stability) "used to generate evidence of—stability over time" (Torabi, 1994, p. 57)

theory "a set of interrelated concepts, definitions, and propositions that presents a *systematic* view of events or situations by specifying relations among variables in order to *explain* and *predict* the events of the situations" (Glanz et al., 2002b, p. 25)

treatment see *intervention*

triple blind study an evaluation wherein neither the participants, nor those implementing the program, nor the evaluators, know which group is experimental and which group is the control

t-test a statistical test involving interval or ratio data that assesses whether the means of two groups are statistically different from each other

Type I error rejecting the null hypothesis when it is actually true

Type II error failing to reject the null hypothesis when it is, in fact, not true

Type III error failure to implement the health education intervention properly (Basch et al., 1985)

units of study "a segment of instruction focused on a particular topic" (ASCD, 2007, ¶. 3).

univariate data analysis analysis of one variable

universe as it relates to sampling, all those unspecific by time and place

unobtrusive observation when people are not aware they are being measured, assessed, or tested

validity whether an instrument correctly measures what it is intended to measure

variable a construct, characteristic, or attribute that can be measured or observed

vendors those who sell their products to program planners

vicarious reinforcement observation of another being reinforced

walk-through a type of observation completed by walking through an area at various times on different days looking for indicators of health

windshield tour a type of observation completed by driving through an area at various times on different days looking for indicators of health

References

Ad Hoc Work Group of the American Public Health Association. (1987). Criteria for the development of health promotion and education programs. *American Journal of Public Health, 77*(1), 89–92.

Agency for Healthcare Research and Quality (AHRQ). (2006). *Treating tobacco use and dependence.* Retrieved May 16, 2007, from http://www.ahrq.gov/path/tobacco.html

Airhihenbuwa, C. O., Cottrell, R. R., Adeyanju, M., Auld, M. E., Lysoby, L., & Smith, B. J. (2005). The national health educator competencies update project: Celebrating a milestone and recommending next steps for the profession. *American Journal of Health Education, 36*(6), 361–370.

Ajzen, I. (1988). *Attitudes, personality, and behavior.* Chicago: Dorsey Press.

Ajzen, I. (2006). *Theory of planned behavior.* Retrieved May 2, 2007, from http://www.people.umass.edu/aizen/tpb.html

Albrecht, T. L., & Bryant, C. (1996). Advances in segmentation modeling for health communication and social marketing campaigns. *Journal of Health Communication, 1,* 65–80.

Aldana, S. G. (2001). Financial impact of health promotion programs: A comprehensive review of the literature. *American Journal of Health Promotion, 15*(5), 296–320.

Alexander, G. (1999). Health risk appraisal. In G. C. Hyner, K. W. Peterson, J. W. Travis, J.E. Dewey, J. J. Foerster, & E. M. Framer (Eds.), *SPM handbook of health assessment tools* (pp. 5–8). Pittsburgh, PA: The Society of Prospective Medicine.

Alinsky, S. D. (1971). *Rules for radicals: A pragmatic primer for realistic radicals.* New York: Random House.

Altschuld, J. W., & Witkin, B. R. (2000). *From needs assessment to action: Transforming needs into solution strategies.* Thousand Oaks, CA: Sage Publications, Inc.

American Association for Health Education (AAHE), National Commission for Health Education Credentialing, Inc. (NCHEC), & Society for Public Health Education (SOPHE). (1999). *A competency-based framework for graduate-level health educators.* Reston, VA: Authors.

American Cancer Society. (2007). *Cancer Facts & Figures, 2007.* Retrieved March 24, 2007, from http://www.cancer.org/downloads/STT/CAFF2007PWSecured.pdf

American College Health Association (ACHA). (2002). *Healthy Campus 2010: Making it Happen.* Baltimore, MD: Author.

American College of Sports Medicine (ACSM). (2005). *ACSM's guidelines for exercise testing and prescription* (5th ed.). Philadelphia, PA: Lippincott, Williams, & Wilkins.

American Marketing Association. (2007). *Dictionary of Marketing Terms.* Retrieved April 18, 2007, from http://www.marketingpower.com

Anderson, B., Fortson, B. W., Kleindler, S. R., & Schonthal, H. (Eds.) (2002). *The American hertitage dictionary.* New York, NY: Dell Publishing.

Anderson, P., & Fenichel, E. (1989). *Serving culturally diverse families of infants and toddlers with disabilities.* Washington, DC: National Center for Clinical Infant Programs.

Andreasen, A. (1995). *Marketing social change.* Jossey-Bass, San Francisco, CA.

Andreasen, A. (1995). *Marketing sound change: Changing behavior to promote health, social development, and the environment.* San Francisco: Jossey-Bass.

Anspaugh, D. J., Dignan, M. B., & Anspaugh, S. L. (2000). *Developing health promotion programs.* Boston, MA: McGraw-Hill.

Arkin, E. B. (1990). Opportunities for improving the nation's health through collaboration with the mass media. *Public Health Reports, 105*(3), 219–223.

Armitage, C. J., & Conner, M. (1999). Distinguishing perceptions of control from self-efficacy: Predicting consumption of a low-fat diet using the theory of planned behavior. *Journal of Applied Social Psychology, 29,* 72–90.

Association for Supervision and Curriculum Development (ASCD). (2007). *A lexicon of learning.* Retrieved from http://www.ascd.org/portal/site/ascd/menuitem.4247f922ca8c9ecc8c2a9410d3108a0c/

Association for the Advancement of Health Education (AAHE). (1994). *Cultural Awareness and Sensitivity: Guidelines for Health Educators.* Reston, VA: Author.

Auld, E. (1997). Practical tips for influencing public policy. *Health Education & Behavior, 24*(3), 272–274.

Babbie, E. (1992). *The practice of social research* (6th ed.). Belmont, CA: Wadsworth Publishing Company.

Backer, T. E., & Rogers, E. M. (1998). Diffusion of innovations theory and worksite AIDS programs. *Journal of Health Communication, 1,* 17–28.

Bakker, A. B. (1999). Persuasive communication about AIDS prevention: Need for cognition determines the impact of message format. *AIDS Education and Prevention, 11,* 150–162.

Bandura, A. (1977a). Self-efficacy: Toward a unifying theory of behavioral change. *Psychological Review, 84*(2), 191–215.

Bandura, A. (1977b). *Social learning theory.* Englewood Cliffs, NJ: Prentice-Hall.

Bandura, A. (1986). *Social foundations of thought and action.* Englewood Cliffs, NJ: Prentice-Hall.

Bandura, A. (2001). Social cognitive theory: An agentic perspective. *Annual review of psychology, 52,* 1–26.

Baranowski, T., (1985). Methodologic issues in self-report of health behavior. *Journal of School Health, 55*(5), 179–182.

Baranowski, T., Perry, C. L., & Parcel, G. S. (2002). How individuals, environments, and health behavior interact. In K. Glanz, B. K. Rimer, & F. M. Lewis (Eds.), *Health behavior and health education: Theory, research, and practice* (3rd ed., pp. 165–184). San Francisco, CA: Jossey-Bass.

Barnes, M. D., Neiger, B. L., & Thackeray, R. (2003). Health communication. In R. J. Bensley & J. Brookins-Fisher (Eds.), *Community health education methods* (2nd ed., pp. 51–82). Boston, MA: Jones and Bartlett Publishers.

Bartholomew, L. K., Parcel, G. S., Kok, G., & Gottlieb, N. H. (2006). *Planning health promotion programs: An intervention mapping approach* (2nd ed.). Jossey-Bass, San Francisco, CA.

Bartlett, E. E., Windsor, R. A., Lowe, J. B., & Nelson, G. (1986). Guidelines for conducting smoking cessation programs. *Health Education, 17*(1), 31–37.

Bartol, K. M., & Martin, D. C. (1991). *Management.* New York, NY: McGraw-Hill Inc.

Basch, C. E., Sliepcevich, E. M., Gold, R. S., Duncan, D. F., & Kolbe, L. J. (1985). Avoiding type III errors in health education program evaluations: A case study. *Health Education Quarterly, 12*(3), 315–331.

Bates, I. J., & Winder, A. E. (1984). *Introduction to health education.* Palo Alto, CA: Mayfield.

Becker, M. H. (Ed.). (1974). The health belief model and personal health behavior. *Health Education Monographs, 2* (entire issue).

Becker, M. H., Drachman, R. H., & Kirscht, J. P. (1974). A new approach to explaining sick-role behavior in low income populations. *American Journal of Public Health, 64*(March), 205–216.

Becker, M. H., & Green, L. W. (1975). A family approach to compliance with medical treatment, a selective review of the literature. *International Journal of Health Education, 18*(3), 2–11.

Beckwith, H. (1997). *Selling the invisible: A field guide to modern marketing* (p. 31). New York: Warner Books.

Behrens, R. (1983). *Work-site health promotion: Some questions and answers to help you get started.* Washington, DC: Office of Disease Prevention and Health Promotion.

Belch, G. E., & Belch, M. A. (2007). *Advertising and promotion. An integrated marketing communications perspective.* New York: McGraw-Hill Irwin.

Bellicha, T., & McGrath, J. (1990). Mass media approaches to reducing cardiovascular disease risk. *Public Health Reports, 105*(3), 245–252.

Bensley, L. B. (1989). A review of the use of mass media and marketing in health education: A look at theory and practice. *Eta Sigma Gamman, 21*(1), 18–23.

Bensley, L. B. (1991). Schoolsite health promotion: Ways of sustaining interest. *Journal of Health Education, 22*(2), 86–89.

Bensley, L. B. (2003). Using theory and ethics to guide method selection and application. In R. J. Bensley & J. Brookins-Fisher (Eds.). *Community health education methods: A practical guide* (2nd ed., pp. 3–30). Sudbury, MA: Jones and Bartlett Publishers.

Berkman, L. F., & Syme, S. L. (1979). Social networks, host resistance and mortality: A nine-year follow-up of Alameda County residents. *American Journal of Epidemiology, 109*(2), 186–204.

Bertrand, J. T. (2004). Diffusion of Innovations and HIV/AIDS. *Journal of Health Communication, 9*(S1), 113–121.

Berwick, D. M. (2003). Disseminating innovations in health care. *Journal of the American Medical Association, 15,* 1969–1975.

Bhatt, S. (2006, December 13). Taxi stand provides place for tipsy to get cabs. *Seattle Times.*

Bloom, B. S. (Ed.) (1956). *Taxonomy of educational objectives. The classification of educational goals. Handbook I: Cognitive domain.* New York, NY: David McKay.

Bloomquist, K. (1981). Physical fitness programs in industry: Applications of social learning theory. *Occupational Health Nursing, 29*(7), 30–33.

Borg, W. R., & Gall, M. D. (1989). *Educational research: An introduction* (5th ed.). New York: Longman.

Borras, J. M., Fernandez, E., Schiaffino, A., Borrell, C., & LaVecchia, C. (2000). Pattern of smoking initiation in Catalonia, Spain, from 1948 to 1992. *American Journal of Public Health, 9,* 1459–1462.

Boslaugh, S. E., Kreuter, M. W., Nicholson, R. A., & Naleid, K. (2005). Comparing demographic, health status and psychosocial strategies of audience segmentation to promote physical activity. *Health Education Research 20*(4), 430–438.

Bowling, A. (2002). *Research methods in health: Investigating health and health services* (2nd ed.). Buckingham, UK: Open University Press.

Bowling, A. (2005). *Measuring health: A review of quality of life measurement scales* (3rd ed.). New York, NY: Open University Press.

Brager, G., Specht, H., & Torczyner, J. L. (1987). *Community organizing.* New York: Columbia University Press.

Braithwaite, R. L., Murphy, F., Lythcott, N., & Blumenthal, D. S. (1989). Community organization and development for health promotion within an urban black community: A conceptual model. *Health Education, 20*(5), 56–60.

Breckon, D. J. (1997). *Managing health promotion programs: Leadership skills for the 21st century.* Gaithersburg, MD: Aspen.

Breckon, D. J., Harvey, J. R., & Lancaster, R. B. (1998). *Community health education: Settings, roles, and skills for the 21st century* (4th ed.). Gaithersburg, MD: Aspen.

Breen, M. (1999). Researching grants on the Internet. *Community Health Center Management,* March/April, p. 29.

Breslow, L. (1999). From disease prevention to health promotion. *Journal of the American Medical Association, 281*(11), 1030–1033.

Brownson, R. C., Koffman, D. M., Novotny, T. E., Hughes, R. G., & Eriksen, M. P. (1995). Environmental and policy interventions to control tobacco use and prevent cardiovascular disease. *Health Education Quarterly, 22*(4), 478–498.

Bryant, C. (1998, June). *Social marketing: A tool for excellence.* Eighth annual conference on social marketing in public health, Clearwater Beach, FL.

Bryant, C., Lindenberger, J., Brown, C., Kent, E., Schreiber, J. M., Bustillo, M., & Canright, M. W. (2001). A social marketing approach to increasing enrollment in a public health program: A case study of the Texas WIC program. *Human Organization, 60*(3) 234–246.

Burdine, J. N., & McLeroy, K. R. (1992). Practitioners' use of theory: Examples from a workgroup. *Health Education Quarterly*, 19(3), 331–340.

Burns, D. M., & Warner, K. E. (2003). Smokers who have not quit: Is cessation more difficult and should we change our strategies? National Cancer Institute, Monograph 15: *Those who continue to smoke.* Retrieved April 19, 2007 from http://cancercontrol.cancer.gov/tcrb/monographs/

Butterfoss, F. D., & Whitt, M. D. (2003). Building and sustaining coalitions. In R. J. Bensley & J. Brookins-Fisher (Eds.), *Community health education methods* (2nd ed., pp. 325–356). Boston, MA: Jones and Bartlett Publishers.

Campbell, M. K., Devellis, B. M., Strecher, V. J., Ammerman, A. S., Devillis, R. F., & Sandler, R. S. (1994). Improving dietary behavior: The effectiveness of tailored messages in primary care settings. *American Journal of Public Health*, 84(5), 783–787.

Campinha-Bacote, J. (1994). Cultural competence in psychiatric mental health nursing: A conceptual model. *Nursing Clinics of North America*, 29, 1–8.

Capwell, E. M., Butterfoss, F., & Francisco, V. T. (2000). Why evaluate? *Health Promotion Practice*, 1(1), 15–20.

Centers for Disease Control and Prevention. U.S. Department of Health and Human Services. (no date). *Planned approach to community health: Guide for local coordinator*. Atlanta, GA: Author.

Centers for Disease Control and Prevention. U.S. Department of Health and Human Services. (1999a). *An ounce of prevention. . . What are the returns?* (2nd ed.). Atlanta, GA: Author.

Centers for Disease Control and Prevention. U.S. Department of Health and Human Services. (1999b). *Best practices for comprehensive tobacco control programs*. Atlanta, GA: Author.

Centers for Disease Control and Prevention. (1999c). Framework for program evaluation in public health. *Morbidity and Mortality Weekly Report*, 48 (RR-11), 1–40.

Centers for Disease Control and Prevention. (1999d). Ten great public health achievements—United States, 1900–1999. *Morbidity and Mortality Weekly Report*, 48(12), 241–243.

Centers for Disease Control and Prevention (2000). *Healthy plan-it: A tool for planning and managing public health programs. Sustainable Management Development Program*. Atlanta, GA: Author.

Centers for Disease Control and Prevention. U.S. Department of Health and Human Services. (2003). *CDCynergy 3.0: Your Guide to Effective Health Communication* (CD-ROM Version 3.0). Atlanta, GA: Author.

Centers for Disease Control and Prevention. (2003a). *The power of prevention: Reducing the health and economic burden of chronic disease*. Retrieved March 2, 2007, from http://www.cdc.gov/nccdphp/publications/PowerOfPrevention.

Centers for Disease Control and Prevention. (2006). *CDC injury fact book*. Atlanta, GA: National Center for Injury Prevention and Control.

Centers for Disease Control and Prevention. (2007). *Chronic disease prevention*. Retrieved March 2, 2007, from http://www.cdc.gov/nccdphp/index.htm

Centers for Disease Control and Prevention. (2007a). *The community guide*. Retrieved March 30, 2007, from http://www.thecommunityguide.org/index.html

Centers for Disease Control and Prevention. (2007b). *5-a-Day website*. retrieved April 24, 2007, from http://www.cdc.gov/nccdphp/dnpa/5aday/index.htm

Chaplin, J. P., & Krawiec, T. S. (1979). *Systems and theories of psychology* (4th ed.). New York: Holt, Rinehart & Winston.

Chapman, L. S. (1997). Securing support from top management. *The Art of Health Promotion, 1*(2), 1–7.

Chapman, L. S. (2003). Meta-evaluation of worksite health promotion economic return studies. *The Art of Health Promotion, 6*(6), 1–14.

Chapman, L. S. (2003a). Biometric screening in health promotion: Is it really as important as we think? *The Art of Health Promotion, 7*(2), 1–12.

Chapman, L. S. (2005). Incentives: An introduction and a story—Part I. *Absolute Advantage, 4*(7), 1–46. Retrieved May 17, 2007, from http://www.welcoa.org/freeresources/pdf/aa_vol4_no7_jul05.pdf

Chapman, L. S. (2006). Planning wellness: Getting off to a good start—Part I. *Absolute Advantage, 5*(4), 1–87. Retrieved March 24, 2007, from http://www.welcoa.org/freeresources/pdf/aa_v5.4.pdf

Checkoway, B. (1989). Community participation for health promotion: Prescription for public policy. *Wellness Perspectives: Research, Theory and Practice, 6*(1), 18–26.

Chenoweth, D. H. (1987). *Planning health promotion at the worksite*. Indianapolis: Benchmark Press.

Cho, M. K., Arruda, M., & Holtzman, N. A. (2006). *Promoting safe and effective genetic testing in the United States*. National Institutes of Health, National Human Genome Research Institute. Retrieved April 21, 2007, from http://www.genome.gov/10002407

Cinelli, B., Rose-Colley, M., & Hayes, D. M. (1988). Health promotion efforts in Pennsylvania schools. *American Journal of Health Promotion, 2*(4), 36–44.

Clark, N. M., Friedman, A. R., & Lachance, L. L. (2006). *Summing it up: Collective lessons from the experience of seven coalitions, 7*(2), 149S–152S.

Clark, N. M., Janz, N. K., Dodge, J. A., & Sharpe, P. A. (1992). Self-regulation of health behavior: The "take PRIDE" program. *Health Education Quarterly, 19*(3), 341–354.

Cleary, M. J., & Neiger, B. L. (1998). *The certified health education specialist: A self-study guide for professional competency* (3rd ed.). Allentown, PA: The National Commission for Health Education Credentialing.

Clow, K. E., & Baack, D. (2007). *Integrated advertising, promotion and marketing communications* (3rd ed.). Upper Saddle River, NJ: Pearson Prentice Hall.

Coalition of National Health Education Organizations (CNHEO). (1999). *Code of ethics.* Retrieved June 9, 2007, from. http://www.cnheo.org/

Coalition of National Health Education Organizations (CNHEO). (2007). *Health education advocate.* Retrieved June 9, 2007, from: http://www.healtheducationadvocate.org/

Cohen, J. (1960). A coefficient of agreement for nominal scales. *Educational and Psychological Measurement, 20*(1), 37–46.

Cohen, S., & Lichtenstein, E. (1990). Partner behaviors that support quitting smoking. *Journal of Consulting and Clinical Psychology, 58*, 304–309.

Colletti, G., & Brownell, K. (1982). *The physical and emotional benefits of social support: Application to obesity, smoking and alcoholism.* In M. Eisler et al. (Eds.), *Progress in behavior modification* (vol. 13). New York: Academic Press.

Conner, R. F. (1980). Ethical issues in the use of control groups. In R. Perloff & E. Perloff (Eds.), *New Directions for Program Evaluation* (pp. 63–75). San Francisco: Jossey-Bass.

Connor, D. M. (1968). *Strategies for development.* Ottawa: Development Press.

Cook, T. D., & Campbell, D. T. (1979). *Quasi-experimentation: Design and analysis issues for field settings.* Boston: Houghton Mifflin.

Coreil, J., Bryant, C. A., & Henderson, J. N. (2001). *Social and behavioral foundations of public health.* Thousand Oaks, CA: Sage.

Cottrell, R. R., Girvan, J. T., & McKenzie, J. F. (2006). *Principles and foundations of health promotion and foundations* (3rd ed.). San Francisco, CA: Benjamin Cummings.

Cottrell, R. R., Girvan, J. T., & McKenzie, J. F. (2009). *Principles and foundations of health promotion and education* (4th ed.). San Francisco, CA: Benjamin Cummings.

Cottrell, R. R., & McKenzie, J. F. (2005). *Health promotion & education research methods: Using the five chapter thesis/dissertation model.* Boston, MA: Jones & Bartlett.

Courtney, A. (2004). Using community-based prevention marketing to promote physical activity among teens. *Social Marketing Quarterly, 10*, 3–4, 58–61.

Cowdery, J. E., Wang, M. Q., Eddy, J. M., & Trucks, J. K. (1995). A theory driven health promotion program in a university setting. *Journal of Health Education, 26*(4), 248–250.

Croker, K. S., Ryan, A., Morzenti, T., Cave, L., Maze-Gallman, T., & Ford, L. (2004). Delivering prostate cancer prevention messages to the public: How the National Cancer Institute (NCI) effectively spread the word about the Prostate Cancer Prevention Trial (PCPT) results. *Urologic Oncology, 22*, 369–376.

Crosby, R. A., Kegler, M. C., & DiClemente, R. J. (2002). Understanding and applying theory in health promotion practice and research. In R. J. DiClemente, R. A. Crosby, & M. C. Kegler (Eds.), *Emerging theories in health promotion practice and research: Strategies for improving public health.* (pp. 1–15). San Francisco, CA: Jossey-Bass.

Cummings, C., Gordon, J. R., & Marlatt, G. A. (1980). Relapse: Prevention and prediction. In W. R. Miller (Ed.), *Addictive behaviors* (pp. 291–322). Oxford, U.K.: Pergamon Press.

Cummings, K., Becker, M. H., & Maile, M. (1980). Bringing the models together in an empirical approach to combining variables used to explain health actions. *Journal of Behavioral Medicine, 3*(2), 123–145.

D'Onofrio, C. N. (1992). Theory and the empowerment of health education practitioners. *Health Education Quarterly, 19*(3), 385–403.

Dane, F. C. (1990). *Research Methods.* Pacific Grove, CA: Brooks/Cole Publishing Company.

Davis, M. J., & Addis, M .E. (1999). Predictors of attrition from behavioral medicine treatments. *Annals of Behavioral Medicine, 21*, 339–349.

Davis, N. A., Lewis, M. J., Rimer, B. K., Harvey, C.M., & Koplan, J. P. (1997). Evaluation of a phone intervention to promote mammography in a managed care plan. *American Journal of Health Promotion, 11*(4), 247–249.

Davis, P. C., & Rankin, L. L. (2006). Guidelines for making existing health education programs more culturally appropriate. *American Journal of Health Education, 37*(4), 250–252.

Debus, M. (1988). *Handbook of excellence on focus group research.* Washington, DC: Academy for Educational Development.

Deeds, S. G. (1992). *The health education specialist: Self-study for professional competence.* Los Alamitos, CA: Loose Canon.

Dennis, D. L., & Rainey, J. (2007, Winter). Percentage of questions from each area of responsibility on the revised CHES examination. *The CHES Bulletin, 18*(1), 5.

DiBlase, D. (1985). Small businesses lead into wellness. *Business Insurance,* (December 2), 16.

DiClemente, R. J., Crosby, R. A., & Kegler, M. C. (Eds.). (2002). *Emerging theories in health promotion practice and research: Strategies for improving public health.* San Francisco, CA: Jossey-Bass.

Dignan, M. B. (1995). *Measurement and evaluation of health education* (3rd ed.). Springfield, IL: Charles C. Thomas.

DiIorio, C. K. (2005). *Measurement in health behavior.* San Francisco, CA: Jossey-Bass.

Dishman, R. K. (1988). *Exercise Adherence,* Champaign, IL: Human Kinetics.

Dishman, R. K., Sallis, J. F., & Orenstein, D. R. (1985). The determinants of physical activity and exercise. *Public Health Reports, 100*(2), 158–171.

Doak, C. C., Doak, L. G., & Root, J. H. (1996). *Teaching patients with low literacy skills* (2nd ed.). Philadelphia, PA: J. B. Lippincott Company.

Dunbar, J. M., Marshall, G. D., & Howell, M. F. (1979). Behavioral strategies for improving compliance. In R. B. Haynes, D. W. Taylor, & D. L. Sackett (Eds.), *Compliance in health care* (pp. 174–190). Baltimore: Johns Hopkins University Press.

Edington, D. W. (2001). Emerging research: A view from one research center. *American Journal of Health Promotion, 15*(5), 341–349.

Educational Resource Information [ERIC]. (2007). *Eric.* Retrieved April 6, 2007, from http://www.eric.ed.gov/

Edwards, R. W., Jumper-Thurman, P., Plested, B. A., Oetting, E. R., & Swanson, L. (2000). Community readiness: Research to practice. *Journal of Community Psychology, 28*(3), 291–307.

El-Askari, G., & Walton, S. (2005). Local government and resident collaboration to improve health: A case study in capacity building and cultural humility. In M. Minkler (Ed.). *Community organizing and community building for health* (2nd ed., pp. 254–271). New Brunswick, NJ: Rutgers University Press.

Emont, S. L., & Cummings, K. M. (1989). Adoption of smoking policies by automobile dealerships. *Public Health Reports, 104*(5), 509–514.

Eng, E., & Blanchard, L. (1990-91). Action-oriented community diagnosis: A health education tool. *International Quarterly of Community Health Education, 11*(2), 96–97.

Erfurt, J. C., Foote, A., Heirich, M. A., & Gregg, W. (1990). Improving participation in worksite wellness: Comparing health education classes, a menu approach, and follow-up counseling. *American Journal of Health Promotion, 4*(4), 270–278.

Erickson, A. C., McKenna, J. W., & Romano, R. M. (1990). Past lessons and new uses of the mass media in reducing tobacco consumption. *Public Health Reports, 105*(3), 239–244.

Feldman, R. H. L. (1983). Strategies for improving compliance with health promotion programs in industry. *Health Education, 14*(4), 21–25.

Ferrence, R. (1996). Using diffusion theory in health promotion: The case of tobacco. *Canadian Journal of Public Health, Supp2,* 24–27.

Fink, A., & Kosecoff, J. (1978). *An evaluation primer.* Washington, DC: Capitol Publications.

Finkler, S. A. (1992). *Budgeting concepts for nurse managers* (2nd ed.). Philadelphia: W. B. Saunders.

Fishbein, M. (Ed.) (1967). *Readings in attitudes theory measurement.* New York, NY: Wiley.

Fishbein, M., & Ajzen, I. (1975). *Belief, attitude, intention and behavior: An introduction to theory and research*. Reading, MA: Addison-Wesley.

Fitzpatrick, J. L., Sanders, J. R., & Worthen, B.R. (2004). *Program evaluation: Alternative approaches and practical guidelines* (3rd ed.). Boston, MA: Pearson, Allyn & Bacon.

Forster, J., Jeffery, R., Sullivan, S., & Snell, M. (1985). A worksite weight control program using financial incentives collected through payroll deduction. *Journal of Occupational Medicine, 27*(11), 804–808.

Forthofer, M. S., & Bryant, C. A. (2000). Using audience-segmentation techniques to tailor health behavior change strategies. *American Journal of Health Behavior, 24*(1), 36–43.

Frankish, C. J., Lovato, C. Y., & Shannon, W. J. (1998). Models, theories, and principles of health promotion with multicultural populations. In R. M. Huff & M. V. Kline (Eds.), *Promoting health in multicultural populations* (pp. 41–72). Thousand Oaks, CA: Sage.

Frederiksen, L. (1984). Using incentives in worksite wellness. *Corporate Commentary, 1*(2), 51–57.

Freimuth, V. S., & Mettger, W. (1990). Is there a hard-to-reach audience? *Public Health Reports, 105*(3), 232–238.

Freire, P. (1973). *Education: The practice of freedom*. London: Writer's and Reader's Publishing.

Freire, P. (1974). *Pedagogy of the oppressed*. New York: Seabury Press.

French, S. A., Jeffery, R. W., & Oliphant, J. A. (1994). Facility access and self-reward as methods to promote physical activity among healthy sedentary adults. *American Journal of Health Promotion, 8*(4), 257–259, 262.

French, S. A., Jeffery, R. W., Story, M., Hannan, P., & Snyder, M. P. (1997). A pricing strategy to promote low-fat snack choices through vending machines. *American Journal of Public Health, 87*(5), 849–851.

Gagne, R. (1985). *The conditions of learning* (4th ed.). New York, NY: Holt, Rinehart, Winston.

Galer-Unti, R. A., Tappe, M. K., & Lachenmayr, S. (2004). Advocacy 101: Getting started in health education advocacy. *Health Promotion Practice, 5*(3), 280–288.

General Services Administration (GSA), Office of Chief Acquisition Officer, Regulatory and Federal Assistance Division. (2007). *The Catalog of Federal Domestic Assistance*. Retrieved June 8, 2007, from http://12.46.245.173/cfda/cfda.html

Gilbert, G., & Sawyer, R. (2000). *Health education: Creating strategies for school and community health* (2nd ed.). Boston: Jones and Bartlett Publishers.

Gilmore, G. D., & Campbell, M. D., (2005). *Needs and capacity assessment strategies for health education and health promotion* (3rd ed.). Sudbury, MA: Jones & Bartlett Publishers.

Gilmore, G. D., Olsen, L. K., Taub, A., & Connell, D. (2005). Overview of the national health educator competencies update project, 1998–2004. *Health Education & Behavior, 32*(6), 725–737.

Gittelsohn, J., Dyckman, W., Tan, M. L., Boggs, M. K., Frick, K. D., Alfred, J., Winch, P. J., Haberle, H., & Palafox, N. A. (2006). Development and implementation of a food store-based intervention to improve diet in the Republic of the Marshall Islands. *Health Promotion Practice, 7*(4), 396–405.

Glanz, K., Lewis, F. M., & Rimer, B. K. (Eds.). (1996). *Health behavior and health education: Theory, research, and practice* (2nd ed.). San Francisco, CA: Jossey-Bass.

Glanz, K., Lewis, F. M., & Rimer, B. K. (Eds.). (2002a). *Health behavior and health education: Theory, research, and practice*. San Francisco, CA: Jossey-Bass.

Glanz, K., Lewis, F. M., & Rimer, B. K., (2002b). Theory, research, and practice in health behavior and health education. In K. Glanz, B. K. Rimer, & F. M. Lewis (Eds.), *Health behavior and health education: Theory, research, and practice.* (3rd ed, pp. 22–39.) San Francisco, CA: Jossey-Bass.

Glanz, K., & Rimer, B. K. (1995). *Theory at a glance: A guide for health promotion practice* [NIH Pub. No. 95–3896]. Washington, DC: National Cancer Institute.

Glasgow, R. E. (2002). Evaluation of theory-based interventions: The RE-AIM model. In K. Glanz, B. K. Rimer, & F. M. Lewis (Eds.), *Health behavior and health education: Theory research, and practice* (3rd. ed, pp. 530–544). San Francisco, CA: Jossey-Bass.

Glasgow, R. E., Vogt, T. M., & Boles, S. M. (1999). Evaluating the public health impact of health promotion interventions: The RE-AIM framework. *American Journal of Public Health, 89*(9), 1322–1327.

Godin, G., & Kok, G. (1996). The theory of planned behavior: A review of its applications to health-related behaviors. *American Journal of Health Promotion, 11*(2), 87–98.

Goetzel, R. Z., Anderson, D. R., Whitmer, R. W., Ozminkowski, R. J., Dunn, R. L., & Wasserman, J., The Health Enhancement Research Organization (HERO) Research Committee. (1998). The relationships between modifiable health risks and health care expenditures. *Journal of Occupational and Environmental Medicine, 40*(10), 843–854.

Golaszewski, T. (2001). Shining lights: Studies that have most influenced the understanding of health promotion's financial impact. *American Journal of Health Promotion, 15*(5), 332–340.

Goldman, K. D. (1998). Promoting new ideas on the job: Practical theory-based strategies. *The Health Educator, 30*(1), 49–52.

Goldman, K. D., & Schmalz, K. J. (2006). Logic models: The picture worth ten thousand words. *Health Promotion Practice, 7*(1), 8–12.

Goldsmith, M. (2006). Ethics in health education: Issues, concerns, and future directions. *The Health Education Monograph Series, 23*(1), 33–37.

Goldstein, M. G., DePue, J., Kazura, A., & Niaura, R. (1998). Models for provider-patient interaction: Applications to health behavior change. In S. A. Shumaker, E. B. Schron, J. K. Ockene, & W. L. McBee (Eds.), *The handbook of health behavior change* (2nd ed., pp. 85–113). New York: Springer.

Goodlad, J. I., & Su, Z. (1992). Organization and the curriculum. In P. W. Jackson (Ed.). *Handbook of research in the curriculum* (pp. 327–344). New York, NY: Macmillan Publishing Company.

Goodman, R. M., McLeroy, K. R., Steckler, A.B., & Hoyle, R. H. (1993). Development of level of institutionalization scales for health promotion programs. *Health Education Quarterly, 20*(2), 161–178.

Goodman, R.M., Speers, M. A., McLeroy, K., Fawcett, S., Kegler, M., Parker, E., Smith, S. R., Sterling, T. D., & Wallerstein, N. (1999). Identifying and Defining the Dimensions of Community Capacity to Provide a Basis for Measurement. *Health Education and Behavior, 25*(3), 258–278.

Goodman, R. M., & Steckler, A. (1989). A model for the institutionalization of health promotion programs. *Family and Community Health, 11*(4), 63–78.

Granat, J. P. (1994). *Persuasive advertising for entrepreneurs and small business owners: How to create more effective sales messages.* Binghamton, NY: Haworth Press.

Green, L. W. (1974). Toward cost-benefit evaluations of health education: Some concepts, methods, and examples. *Health Education Monographs, 2* (Suppl. 1), 34–64.

Green, L. W. (1975). Evaluation of patient education programs. Criteria and measurement techniques. In *Rx: Education for the patient: Proceedings of the Continuing Education Institution, Southern Illinois University* (pp. 89–98). Carbondale, IL: Southern Illinois University Press.

Green, L. W. (1976). Methods available to evaluate the health education components of preventive health programs. In *Preventive Medicine*, USA (pp. 162–171). New York: Prodist.

Green, L. W. (1979). National policy on the promotion of health. *International Journal of Health Education, 22,* 161–168.

Green, L. W. (1980). Healthy People: The Surgeon General's report and the prospects. In W. J. McNervey (Ed.), *Working for a healthier America* (pp. 95–110). Cambridge, MA: Ballinger.

Green, L. W. (1981a). Emerging federal perspectives on health promotion. In J. P. Allegrante (Ed.), *Health Promotion Monographs* (28 pp.). New York: Teachers College, Columbia University.

Green, L. W. (1981b). The objectives for the nation in disease prevention and health promotion: A challenge to health education training. *Proceedings of the National Conference for Institutions Preparing Health Educators,* (DHHS Publication No. 81-50171) (pp. 61–73). Washington, DC: U.S. Office of Health Information and Health Promotion.

Green, L. W. (1982). Reconciling policy in health education and primary care. *International Journal of Health Education, 24* (Suppl. 3), 1–11.

Green, L. W. (1983a). New policies in education for health. *World Health* (April–May), 13–17.

Green, L. W. (1983b). *New policies for health education in primary health care* (Background document for the technical discussions of the 36th World Health Assembly, May 1983). Geneva: World Health Organization.

Green, L. W. (1984a). A triage and stepped approach to self-care education. *Medical Times, 111,* 75–80.

Green, L. W. (1984b). Health education models. In J. D. Matarazzo, S. M. Weiss, & J. A. Herd (Eds.), *Behavioral health: A handbook of health enhancement and disease prevention* (pp. 181–198). New York: Wiley.

Green, L. W. (1984c). La educacion para la salud en el medio urbano. In *Conferencia InterAmericana de Educacion Para La Salud* (pp. 80–82). Mexico City: Sector Salud, SEP, and International Union for Health Education and World Health Organization.

Green, L. W. (1984d). Modifying and developing health behavior. *Annual Review of Public Health, 5,* 215–236.

Green, L. W. (1986a, October). *Applications and trials of the PRECEDE framework for planning and evaluation of health programs.* Paper presented at the meeting of the American Public Health Association, Las Vegas, NV.

Green, L. W. (1986b). Evaluation model: A framework for the design of rigorous evaluation of efforts in health promotion. *American Journal of Health Promotion, 1*(1), 77–79.

Green, L. W. (1986c). *New policies for health education in primary health care.* Geneva: World Health Organization.

Green, L. W. (1986d). Research agenda: Building a consensus on research questions. *American Journal of Health Promotion, 1*(2), 70–72.

Green, L. W. (1986e). The theory of participation: A qualitative analysis of its expression in national and international health policies. In W. B. Ward (Ed.), *Advances in Health Education and Promotion* (pp. 211–236). Greenwich, CT: JAI Press.

Green, L. W. (1987a). How physicians can improve patients' participation and maintenance in self-care. *Western Journal of Medicine, 147,* 346–349.

Green, L. W. (1987b). *Program planning and evaluation guide for Lung Associations.* New York: American Lung Association.

Green, L. W. (1989, March). *The health promotion program of the Henry J. Kaiser Family Foundation.* Paper presented at a public lecture at Mankato State University, Mankato, MN.

Green, L. W. (1990). The revival of community and the public obligation of academic health centers. In R. E. Bulger and S. J. Reiser (Eds.), *Integrity in institutions: Humane environments for teaching* (pp. 163–178). Iowa City: University of Iowa Press.

Green, L. W. (1999). Health education's contributions to public health in the twentieth century: A glimpse through health promotion's rear-view mirror. In J. E. Fielding, L.B. Lave, & B. Starfield (Eds.), *Annual review of public health* (pp. 67–88). Palo Alto, CA: Annual Reviews.

Green, L. W., & Allen, J. (1980). *Toward a healthy community: Organizing events for community health promotion* (PHS Publication No. 80–50113). Washington, DC: USDHHS, Office of Disease Prevention and Health Promotion.

Green, L. W., Glanz, K., Hochbaum, G. M., Kok, G., Kreuter, M. W., Lewis, F. M., Lorig, K., Morisky, D., Rimer, B. K., & Rosenstock, I.M. (1994). Can we build on, or must we replace, the theories and models of health education? *Health Education Research, 9*(3), 397–404.

Green, L. W., & Kreuter, M. W. (1991). *Health promotion planning: An educational and environmental approach* (2nd ed.). Mountain View, CA: Mayfield.

Green, L. W., & Kreuter, M. W. (1992). CDC's planned approach to community health as an application of PRECEDE and an inspiration for PROCEED. *Journal of Health Education, 23*(3), 140–147.

Green, L. W., & Kreuter, M. W. (1999). *Health promotion planning: An educational and ecological approach* (3rd ed.). Mountain View, CA: Mayfield.

Green, L. W., & Kreuter, M. W. (2005). *Health program planning: An educational and ecological approach* (4th ed.). Boston, MA: McGraw-Hill.

Green, L. W., Kreuter, M. W., Deeds, S. G., & Partridge, K. B. (1980). *Health education planning: A diagnostic approach.* Palo Alto, CA: Mayfield.

Green, L. W., Levine, D. M., & Deeds, S. G. (1975). Clinical trials of health education for hypertensive outpatients: Design and baseline data. *Preventive Medicine, 4*, 417–425.

Green, L. W., & Lewis, F. M. (1986). *Measurement and evaluation in health education and health promotion.* Palo Alto, CA: Mayfield.

Green, L. W., & McAlister, A. L. (1984). Macro-intervention to support health behavior: Some theoretical perspectives and practical reflections. *Health Education Quarterly, 11*, 323–339.

Green, L. W., Mullen, P. D., & Friedman, R. (1986). An epidemiological approach to targeting drug information. *Patient Education and Counseling, 8*, 255–268.

Green, L. W., Wang, V. L., Deeds, S. G., Fisher, A. A., Windsor, R., & Rogers, C. (1978). Guidelines for health education in maternal and child health programs. *International Journal of Health Education, 21* (suppl.), 1–33.

Green, L. W., Wilson, A. L., & Lovato, C. Y. (1986). What changes can health promotion achieve and how long do these changes last? The tradeoffs between expediency and durability. *Preventive Medicine, 15*, 508–521.

Green, L. W., Wilson, R. W., & Bauer, K. G. (1983). Data required to measure progress on the objectives for the nation in disease prevention and health promotion. *American Journal of Public Health, 73*, 18–24.

Greenberg, J. (1978). Health education as freeing. *Health Education, 9*(2), 20–21.

Gurley, L. (2007, April). *Assessing progress on the nation's health promotion agenda: Healthy People 2010.* Presentation at a public lecture at Ball State University, Muncie, IN.

Guyer, M. (1999). Grants: Finding a funding source. *Grant Source* (pp. 1–3). Columbus, OH: Office of the Auditor, State of Ohio.

Haider, M., & Kreps, G. L. (2004). Forty years of diffusion of innovations: Utility and value in public health. *Journal of Health Communication, 9*, 3–11

Hall, C. L. (1943). *Principles of behavior.* New York: Appleton-Century-Crofts.

Hallfors, D., & Godette, D. (2002). Will the principles of effectiveness improve prevention practice? Early findings from a diffusion study. *Health Education Research, 4*, 461–470.

Hancock, T., & Minkler, M. (2005). Community health assessment or healthy community assessment: Whose Community? Whose health? Whose assessment? In M. Minkler (Ed.). *Community organizing and community building for health* (2nd ed., pp. 138–157). New Brunswick, NJ: Rutgers University Press.

Hanlon, J. J. (1974). *Administration of public health.* St. Louis: C. V. Mosby.

Harris, J. H. (2001). Selecting the right vendor for your health promotion program. *Absolute Advantage, 1*(4), 4–5.

Harris, J. H. (2003). Increasing participation: An expert interview. Retrieved May 17, 2007, from http://www.welcoa.org/freeresources/pdf/harris_interview_incentives.pdf

Harris, J. H., & McKenzie, J. F (2004). *Checklist for selecting health promotion vendors.* Retrieved May 28, 2007 from http://www.welcoa.org/freeresources/pdf/vendor_checklist.pdf

Harris, J. H., McKenzie, J. F., & Zuti, W. B. (1986). How to select the right vendor for your company's health promotion program. *Fitness in Business, 1* (October), pp. 53–56.

Hayden, J. (2000). *The health education specialist: A study guide for professional competence* (4th ed.). Allentown, PA: The National Commission for Health Education Credentialing, Inc.

Health Insurance Association of America. (1983). *Your guide to wellness at the worksite.* Pamphlet issued by the Public Relations Division of the Health Insurance Association of America, Washington, DC.

Healthy people: The Surgeon General's report on health promotion and disease prevention. (1979). (Publication No. 79–55071). Washington, DC: Department of Health, Education, and Welfare (Public Health Service).

Hellerstedt, W. L., & Jeffery, R. W. (1997). The effects of a telephone-based intervention on weight loss. *American Journal of Health Promotion, 11*(3), 177–182.

Hertoz, J. K., Finnegan, J. R., Rooney, B., Viswanath, K., & Potter, J. (1993). *Health Communication, 5*(1), 21–40.

Hinkle, D. E., Oliver, J. D., & Hinkle, C. A. (1985). How large should the sample be? Part II—the one-sample case for survey research. *Educational and Psychological Measurement 45*(2), 271–280.

Hochbaum, G. M., Sorenson, J. R., & Lorig, K. (1992). Theory in health education practice. *Health Education Quarterly, 19*(3), 295–313.

Hopkins, K. D., Stanley, J. C., & Hopkins, B. R. (1990). *Educational and psychological measurement and evaluation* (7th ed.). Englewood Cliffs, NJ: Prentice-Hall.

Horman, S. (1989). The role of social support on health throughout the lifestyle. *Health Education, 20*(4), 18–21.

Horne, W. M. (1975). Effects of a physical activity program on middle-aged, sedentary corporation executives. *American Industrial Hygiene Journal,* (March), 241–245.

Hosokawa, M. C. (1984). Insurance incentives for health promotion. *Health Education, 15*(6), 9–12.

Huff, R. M., & Kline, M. V. (1999). Health promotion in the context of culture. In R. M. Huff & M. V. Kline (Eds.), *Promoting health in multicultural populations* (pp. 3–22). Thousand Oaks, CA: Sage.

Hunnicutt, D. (2001). *A dynamic incentive campaign. . . Step-by-step: Walking your way to wellness.* Retrieved May 17, 2007, from http://www.welcoa.org/freeresources/pdf/stepbystep_ic.pdf

Hunnicutt, D. (2007). The 10 secrets of a successful worksite wellness teams. *Absolute Advantage, 6*(3), 6–13. Retrieved March 30, 2007, from http://www.welcoa.org/freeresources/pdf/10_secrets.pdf

Hunt, W. A., Barnett, L. W., & Branch, L. G. (1971). Relapse rates in addiction programs. *Journal of Clinical Psychology, 27*(4), 455–456.

Hurlburt, R. T. (2003). *Comprehending behavioral statistics* (3rd ed.). Belmont, CA: Wadsworth/Thomson Learning.

Hyner, G. C., Peterson, K. W., Travis, J. W., Dewey, J. E., Foerster, J. J., & Framer, E.M. (Eds.). (1999). *SPM handbook of health assessment tools.* Pittsburgh, PA: The Society of Prospective Medicine.

Institute of Medicine (IOM). (1988). *The future of public health.* Washington, DC: National Academy Press.

Institute of Medicine (IOM). (2001). *Health and behavior: The interplay of biological, behavioral, and societal influences.* Washington, DC: National Academy Press.

Israel, B. A., Checkoway, B., Schulz, A., & Zimmerman, M. (1994). Health education and community empowerment: Conceptualizing and measuring perceptions of individual, organizational, and community control. *Health Education Quarterly, 21*(2), 149–170.

Jacobsen, D., Eggen, P., & Kauchak, D. (1989). *Methods for teaching: A skills approach* (3rd ed.). Columbus, OH: Merrill, an imprint of Macmillan Publishing Company.

Jadad, A. R., & Gagliardi, A. (1998). Rating health information on the Internet. *Journal of the American Medical Association, 279,* 611–614.

Janz, N. K., & Becker, M. H. (1984). The health belief model: A decade later. *Health Education Quarterly, 11*(1), 1–47.

Janz, N. K., Champion, V. L., & Strecher, V. J. (2002). The health belief model. In K. Glanz, B. K. Rimer, & F. M. Lewis (Eds.), *Health behavior and health education: Theory, research, and practice* (3rd. ed., pp. 45–66). San Francisco, CA: Jossey-Bass.

Jason, L. A., Jayaraj, S., Blitz, C. C., Michaels, M. H., & Klett, L. E. (1990). Incentives and competition in a worksite smoking cessation intervention. *American Journal of Public Health, 80*(2), 205–206.

Jeffery, R. W., Epstein, L. H., Wilson, G. T., Drewnowski, A., Stunkard, A. J., & Wing, R. R. (2000). Long-term maintenance of weight loss: current status. *Health Psychology, 19* (Suppl.1), 5–16.

Jeffery, R. W., Forster, J. L., Baxter, J. E., French, S. A., & Kelder, S. H. (1993). An empirical evaluation of the effectiveness of tangible incentives in increasing participation and behavior change in a worksite health promotion program. *American Journal of Health Promotion, 8*(2), 98–100.

Jessor, R., & Jessor, S. L. (1977). *Problem behavior and psychosocial development: A longitudinal study of youth.* New York: Academic Press.

John, R., Kerby, D. S., & Landers, P. S. (2004). A market segmentation approach to nutrition education among low-income individuals. *Social Marketing Quarterly, 10,* 3–4, 24–38.

Johnson, G., Scholes, K., & Sexty, R. W. (1989). *Exploring strategic management.* Scarborough, Ontario: Prentice Hall.

Johnson, J. A., & Breckon, D. J. (2007). *Managing health education and health promotion programs:*

Leadership skills for the 21st century (2nd ed.). Sudbury, MA: Jones and Bartlett Publishers.

Joint Committee on Terminology. (2001). Report of the 2000 Joint Committee on Health Education and Promotion Terminology. *American Journal of Health Education, 32*(2), 89–103.

Kaplan, B., & Cassel, J. (1977). Social support and health. *Medical Care, 15*(5), 47–58.

Kendall, R. (1984). Rewarding safety excellence. *Occupational Hazards,* (March), 45–50.

Kerlinger, F. N. (1986). *Foundations of behavioral research.* (3rd ed.). Austin, TX: Holt, Rinehart, & Winston.

Keyser, B. B., Morrow, M. J., Doyle, K., Ogletree, R., & Parsons, N. P. (1997). *Practicing the application of health education skills and competencies.* Boston, MA: Jones and Bartlett Publishers.

Kinzie, M. B. (2005). Instructional design strategies for health behavior change. *Patient Education and Counseling, 56,* 3–15.

Kirschenbaum, J., & Russ, L. (2005). Community mapping and geographic information systems. In M. Minkler (Ed.). *Community organizing and community building for health* (2nd ed., pp. 450–454). New Brunswick, NJ: Rutgers University Press.

Kittleson, M. J. (1995). Comparison of the response rate between e-mail and postcards. *Health Values, 19*(2), 27–29.

Kittleson, M. J. (1997). Determining effective follow-up of e-mail surveys. *American Journal of Health Behavior, 21*(3), 193–196.

Kittleson, M. J. (2003). Suggestions for using the web to collect data. *American Journal of Health Behavior, 27*(2), 170–172.

Kline, M. V., & Huff, R. M. (1999). Tips for the practitioner. In R. M. Huff & M. V. Kline (Eds.), *Promoting health in multicultural populations* (pp. 103–111). Thousand Oaks, CA: Sage.

Koffman, D. M., Lee, J. W., Hopp, J. W., & Emont, S. L. (1998). The impact of including incentives and competition in a workplace smoking cessation program on quit rates. *American Journal of Health Promotion, 13*(2), 105–111.

Kotecki, J. E., & Chamness, B. E. (1999). A valid tool for evaluating health-related WWW sites. *Journal of Health Education, 30*(1), 56–59.

Kotler, P., & Clarke, R. N. (1987). *Marketing for health care organizations.* Englewood Cliffs, NJ: Prentice-Hall.

Kotler, P., & Keller, K. L. (2007). *A framework for marketing management.* (3rd Ed.) Upper Saddle River, NJ: Pearson/Prentice Hall.

Kotler, P., & Lee, N. (2006). *Marketing in the public sector.* Upper Saddle River, NJ: Wharton School Publishing.

Kotler, P., Robert, N., & Lee, N. (2002). *Social marketing: Improving the quality of life* (2nd ed.). Thousand Oaks: Sage.

Kretzmann, J. P., & McKnight, J. L. (1993a). *Building communities from the inside out: A path toward finding and mobilizing a community's assets.* Evanston, IL: Institute for Policy Research, Northwestern University.

Kretzmann, J. P., & McKnight, J. L. (1993b). Introduction from *Building communities from the inside out: A path toward finding and mobilizing a community's assets.* Retrieved May 25, 2007, from http://northwestern.edu/ipr/publications/community/introd-building.html

Kreuter, M. W. (1992). PATCH: Its origin, basic concepts, and links to contemporary public health policy. *Journal of Health Education, 23*(3), 135–139.

Kreuter, M. W., Bull, F. C., Clark, E. M., & Oswald, D. L. (1999). Understanding how people process health information: A comparison of tailored and nontailored weight-loss materials. *Health Psychology, 18,* 487–494.

Kreuter, M. W., Farrell, D., Olevitch, L., & Brennan, L. (2000). *Tailoring health messages: Customizing communication with computer technology.* Hillsdale, NJ: Erlbaum.

Kreuter, M. W., Nelson, C. F., Stoddard, R. P., & Watkins, N. B. (1985). *Planned approach to community health.* Atlanta, GA: Centers for Disease Control.

Kreuter, M. W., Vehige, E., & McGuire, A. G. (1996). Using computer-tailored calendars to promote childhood immunization. *Public Health Reports, III* (March/April), 176–178.

Krosnick, J. A., & Petty, R. E. (1995). Attitude strength: An overview. In R. E. Petty & J.A. Krosnick (Eds.), *Attitude strength: Antecedents and consequences* (pp.1–24). Hillsdale, NJ: Erlbaum.

Kviz, F. J., Crittenden, K. S., Madura, K. J., & Warnecke, R. B. (1994). Use and effectiveness of buddy support in a self-help smoking cessation program. *American Journal of Health Promotion, 8*(3), 191–201.

Lalonde, M. (1974). *A new perspective on the health of Canadians: A working document.* Ottawa, Canada: Minister of Health.

Landers, J., Mitchell, P., Smith, B., Lehman, T., & Conner, C. (2006). "Save the crabs, then eat 'em": A culinary approach to saving the Chesapeake Bay. *Social Marketing Quarterly, 12*(1), 15–28.

Lando, J., Williams, S. M., Sturgis, S., & Williams, B. (2006). A logic model for the integration of mental health into chronic disease prevention and health promotion. *Preventing Chronic Disease, 3*(2), 1–5. [serial online]. Retrieved February 24, 2007, from http://www.cdc.gov/ped/issues/2006/apr/05_0215.html

Last, J. M. (Ed.). (2007). *A Dictionary of Public Health* (4th ed.). New York, NY: Oxford University Press.

Lefebvre, R. C. (2006). Partnerships for social marketing programs: an example from the National Bone Health Campaign. *Social Marketing Quarterly, 12*(1) 41–54.

Lefebvre, R. C., & Flora, J. A. (1988). Social marketing and public health intervention. *Health Education Quarterly, 15*(3), 299–315.

LeMaster, P. L., & Connell, C. M. (1994). Health education interventions among native Americans: A review and analysis. *Health Education Quarterly, 21*(4), 521–538.

Leventhal, H., & Cleary, P. D. (1980). The smoking problem: A review of the research and theory in behavioral risk modification. *Psychological Bulletin, 88*(2), 370–405.

Levin, H. M., & McEwan, P. J. (2001). *Cost-effectiveness analysis: Methods and applications.* Thousand Oaks, CA: Sage.

Levine, R. J. (1988). *Ethics and regulations of clinical research.* New Haven, CT: Yale University Press.

Lewin, K. (1935). *A dynamic theory of personality.* New York: McGraw-Hill.

Lewin, K. (1936). *Principles of topological psychology.* New York: McGraw-Hill.

Lewin, K., Dembo, T., Festinger, L., & Sears, P. S. (1944). Level of aspiration. In J. Hunt (Ed.), *Personality and the behavior disorders* (pp. 333–378). New York: Ronald Press.

Lindsey, L. L. M., Carter, H. K., Prue, C. E., Flores, A. L., Kopfman, J. E., Correa-Sierra, E. & Valencia, D. (in press). Understanding optimal nutrition among women of childbearing age in the United States and Puerto Rico: Employing formative research to lay the foundation for national birth defects prevention campaigns. *Journal of Health Communication.*

Linkins, R. W., Dini, E. F., Watson, G., & Patriarca, P. A. (1994). A randomized trail of the effectiveness of computer-generated telephone messages in increasing immunization visits among preschool children. *Archives of Pediatric and Adolescent Medicine, 148*(9), 908–914.

Ludman, E. J., Curry, S. J., Meyer, D., & Taplin, S. H. (1999). Implementation of outreach telephone counseling to promote mammography participation. *Health Education* & Behavior, 26*(5), 689–702.

Luquis, R. R., & Pérez, M. A. (2003). Achieving cultural competence: The challenges for health educators. *American Journal of Health Education, 34*(3), 131–138.

Luquis, R., Pérez, M., Young, K. (2006). Cultural competence development in health education professional preparation programs. *American Journal of Health Education, 37*(4), 233–241.

Luszczynska, A., & Sutton, S. (2005). Attitudes and expectations. In J. Kerr, R. Weitkunat, & M. Moretti (Eds.), *ABC of behavior change: A guide to successful disease prevention and health promotion,* (pp. 71–84). Edinburgh: Elsevier.

MacAskill, S., Stead, M., MacKintosh, A. M., & Hastings, G. (2002). "You cannae just take cigarettes away from somebody and no' gie them something back"; Can social marketing help solve the problem of low-income smoking? *Social Marketing Quarterly, 8*(1), 19–34.

Maibach, E., Shenker, A., & Singer, S. (1997). Results of the Delphi survey. *Journal of Health Communication, 2,* 304–307.

Marcarin, S. (Ed.). (1995). *Cumulative index to nursing & allied health literature: CINAHL.* Volume 40, Part A. Glendale, CA.

Marcus, B. H., Emmons, K. M., Simkin-Silverman, L., Linnan, L. A., Taylor, E. R., Bock, B. C., Roberts, M. B., Rossi, J. S., & Abrams, D. B. (1998). Evaluation of motivationally-tailored versus standard self-help physical activity interventions at the workplace. *American Journal of Health Promotion, 12*(4), 246–253.

Marlatt, G. A. (1982). Relapse prevention: A self-control program for treatment of addictive behaviors. In R. B. Sturat (Ed.), *Adherence, compliance, and generalization in behavioral medicine* (pp. 329–377). New York: Brunner/Mazel.

Marlatt, G. A. (1985). Relapse prevention: Theoretical rationale and overview of the model. In G. A. Marlatt & J. R. Gordon (Eds.), *Relapse prevention* (pp. 3–70). New York: Guilford Press.

Marlatt, G. A., & George, W. H. (1998). Relapse prevention and the maintenance of optimal health. In S. A. Shumaker, E. B. Schron, J.K. Ockene, & W. L. McBee (Eds.), *The handbook of health behavior change* (2nd ed., pp. 33–58). New York: Springer.

Mason, J. O., & McGinnis, J. M. (1990). "Healthy people 2000": An overview of the national health promotion and disease prevention objectives. *Public Health Reports, 105*(5), 441–446.

Matson, D. M., Lee, J. W., & Hopp, J. W. (1993). The impact of incentives and competitions on participation and quit rates in worksite smoking cessation programs. *American Journal of Health Promotion, 7*(4), 270–280, 295.

Mausner, J. S., & Kramer, S. (1985). *Epidemiology— An introductory text* (2nd ed.). Philadelphia, PA: W. B. Saunders Company.

McCaul, K. D., Bakdash, M. B., Geoboy, M. J., Gerbert, B., et al. (1990). Promoting self-protective health behaviors in dentistry. *Annals of Behavioral Medicine, 12*, 156–160.

McDade-Montez, E., Cvengros, J., Christensen, A. (2005). Personality and individual differences. In J. Kerr, R. Weitkunat, & M. Moretti (eds.), *ABC of behavior change: A guide to successful disease prevention and health promotion*, (pp. 57–70). Edinburgh: Elsevier.

McDermott, R. J., & Sarvela, P. D. (1999). *Health education evaluation and measurement: A practitioner's perspective* (2nd ed.). New York: WCB/McGraw-Hill.

McDowell, I., Newell, C., & Rosser, W. (1989a). Computerized reminders for blood pressure screening in primary care. *Medical Care, 27*(3), 297–305.

McDowell, I., Newell, C., & Rosser, W. (1989b). Computerized reminders to encourage cervical screening in family practice. *Journal of Family Practice, 28*(4), 420–424.

McGinnis, J. M., & Foege, W. H. (1993). Actual causes of death in the United States. *Journal of the American Medical Association, 270*, 2207–2212.

McGinnis, J. M., Williams-Russo, P. & Knickman, J. R. (2002). The case for more active policy attention to health promotion. *Health Affairs, 21*(2), 78–93.

McGuire, W. J. (1983). A contextual theory of knowledge: Its implications for innovation and reform in psychological research. *Advances in Experimental Social Psychology, 16*, 1–47.

McKenzie, J. F. (1986). Cost-benefit and cost-effectiveness as a part of the evaluation of health promotion programs. *The Eta Sigma Gamman, 18*(2), 10–16.

McKenzie, J. F. (1988). Twelve steps in developing a schoolsite health education/promotion program for faculty and staff. *The Journal of School Health, 58*(4), 149–153.

McKenzie, J. F., Wood, M. L., Kotecki, J. E., Clark, J. K., & Brey, R. A. (1999). Establishing content validity: Using qualitative and quantitative steps. *American Journal of Health Behavior, 23*(4), 311–318.

McKenzie, J. F., Pinger, R. R., & Kotecki, J. E. (2005). *Introduction to community health* (5th ed.). Sudbury, MA: Jones and Bartlett Publishers.

McKenzie, J. F., Pinger, R. R., & Kotecki, J. E. (2008). *Introduction to community health* (6th ed.). Sudbury, MA: Jones and Bartlett Publishers.

McKenzie, J. F., Luebke, J., & Romas, J. A. (1992). Incentives: A means of getting and keeping workers involved in health promotion programs. *Journal of Health Education, 23*(2), 70–73.

McKnight, J. L., & Kretzmann, J. P. (2005). Mapping community capacity. In M. Minkler (Ed.), *Community organizing and community building for health.* (pp. 158–172). New Brunswick, NJ: Rutgers University Press.

McLeroy, K. R. (1993). Theory and practice in health education: Which practice, which theory? *American Public Health Association, Public Health Education and Health Promotion Section Newsletter,* Summer, 7–8.

McLeroy, K. R., Bibeau, D., Steckler, A., & Glanz, K. (1988). An ecological perspective on health promotion programs. *Health Education Quarterly, 15*, 351–377.

McLeroy, K. R., Steckler, A., Goodman, R. & Burdine, J. N. (1992). Health education research, theory, and practice: Future directions. *Health*

Education Research, Theory, and Practice, 7(1), 1–8.

Meyer, J., & Rainey, J. (1994). Writing health education material for low-literacy populations. *Journal of Health Education, 25*(6), 372–374.

Mikanowicz, C. K., & Altman, N. H. (1995). Developing policies on smoking in the workplace. *Journal of Health Education, 26*(3), 183–185.

Miniño, A. M., Heron, M., Smith, B. L, & Kochanek, K. D. (2006). *Deaths: Final data for 2004. Health E-Stats.* Retrieved March 2, 2007, from http://www.cdc.gov/nchs/products/pubs/pubd/hestats/finaldeaths04/finaldeaths04.htm#Fig1

Minkler, M. (Ed.). (2005). *Community organizing and community building for health* (2nd ed.). New Brunswick, NJ: Rutgers University Press.

Minkler, M. (Ed.). (2005a). Introduction to community organizing and community building. In M. Minkler (Ed.). *Community organizing and community building for health* (2nd ed., pp. 1–21). New Brunswick, NJ: Rutgers University Press.

Minkler, M. (Ed.). (2005b). Community organizing with the elderly poor in San Francisco's Tenderloin district. In M. Minkler (Ed.). *Community organizing and community building for health* (2nd ed., pp. 272–287). New Brunswick, NJ: Rutgers University Press.

Minkler, M., & Wallerstein, N. (2005). Improving health through community organization and community building: A health education perspective. In M. Minkler (Ed.). *Community organizing and community building for health* (2nd ed., pp. 26–50). New Brunswick, NJ: Rutgers University Press.

Modell, M. E. (1996). *A professional's guide to system analysis* (2nd ed.). Boston, MA: McGraw-Hill.

Mokdad, A. H., Marks, J. S. Stroup, D. F., & Gerberding, J. L. (2004). Actual causes of death, in the United States, 2000. *Journal of the American Medical Association, 291*(10), 1238–1245.

Mokdad, A. H., Marks, J. S., Stroup, D. F., & Greberding, J. L. (2005). Correction: Actual causes of death in the United States, 2000. *Journal of the American Medical Association, 293*(3), 293–294.

Mondros, J. B., & Wilson, S. M. (1994). *Organizing for power and empowerment.* New York: Columbia Press.

Montano, D. E., & Kasprzyk, D. (2002). The theory of reasoned action and the theory of planned behavior. In K. Glanz, B. K. Rimer, & F. M. Lewis (Eds.), *Health behavior and health education: Theory, research, and practice* (3rd. ed., pp. 67–98). San Francisco, CA: Jossey-Bass.

Montano, D., Kasprzyk, D., von Haeften, I., & Fishbein, M. (2001). Toward an understanding of condom use behaviors: A theoretical and methodological overview of the project SAFER. *Psychology, Health, & Medicine, 6*(2), 139–150.

Montano, D., Phillips, W., & Kasprzyk, D. (2000). Explaining physician rates of providing flexible sigmoidoscopy. *Cancer Epidemiology, Biomarkers, & Prevention, 9,* 665–669.

Montano, D., Thompson, B., Taylor, V. M., & Mahloch, J. (1997). Understanding mammography intention and utilization among women in an inner city public hospital clinic. *Prevention Medicine, 26,* 817–824.

Morreale, M. (no date). Understanding public health research: A primer for youth workers. *Issue Brief.* Washington, DC: National Network for Youth.

Morris, L. L., Fitz-Gibbon, C. T., & Freeman, M. E. (1987). *How to communicate evaluation findings.* Newbury Park, CA: Sage.

Murphy, E. (2004). Diffusion of Innovations: Family Planning in Developing Countries. *Journal of Health Communication, 9* (S1), 123–129.

National Association of County Health Officials (NACHO). (1991). *APEX/PH, Assessment protocol for excellence in public health.* Washington, DC: Author.

National Association of County and City Health Officials (NACCHO). (2001). *Mobilizing for action through planning and partnerships (MAPP).* Washington, DC: Author.

National Cancer Institute (NCI). (2002). *Making health communication programs work* (NIH Publication No. 02-5145). Washington, DC: U.S. Department of Health and Human Services.

National Center for Health Statistics [NCHS]. (2006). *Health United States, 2006 With Chartbook on Trends in the Health of Americans.* Hyattsville, MD: U.S. Government Printing Office.

National Commission for Health Education Credentialing, Inc. [NCHEC], (1985). *A framework for the development of competency-based curricula for entry-level health educators.* New York, NY: Author.

National Commission for Health Education Credentialing, Inc. (NCHEC). (1996). *A competency-based framework for professional development of certified health education specialists.* New York: Author.

National Commission for Health Education Credentialing, Inc. [NCHEC], (2006). *Competencies Update Project.* Retrieved February 24, 2007, from http://www.nchec.org/aboutnchec/cup/cup.html

National Commission for Health Education Credentialing, Inc. [NCHEC], Society for Public Health Education [SOPHE], & American Association for Health Education [AAHE]. (2006). *A competency-based framework for health educators.* Whitehall, PA: Author.

The National Commission for the Protection of Human Subjects of Biomedical and Behavioral Research. (1979). *The Belmont Report: Ethical Principles and Guidelines for the Protection of Human Subject Research.* Retrieved June 9, 2007, from http://www.nihtraining.com/ohsrsite/guidelines/belmont.html

National Highway Traffic Safety Administration [NHTSA]. (2007). Traffic safety facts. Retrieved March 30, 2007, from http://www.nhtsa.dot.gov/people/injury/TSFLaws/PDFs/810725W.pdf

National Institutes for Health. (n.d.). *Informed consent and assent.* Retrieved May 25, 2003, from http://www.cc.nih.gov/ccc/protomechanics/chap_3.html# whatareinformca

National Institutes for Health (NIH). (2004). *Guidelines for the conduct of research involving human subjects at the National Institutes for Health.* (5th printing). Retrieved June 9, 2007, from http://www.nihtraining.com/ohsrsite/guidelines/GrayBooklet82404.pdf

National Library of Medicine [NLM]. (2006). *Fact sheet MEDLINE®.* Retrieved April 6, 2007, from http://www.nlm.nih.gov/pubs/factsheets/medline.html

National Task Force on the Preparation and Practice of Health Educators, Inc. (1985). *A framework for the development of competency-based curricula for entry-level health educators.* New York: Author.

Neiger, B. L., & Thackeray, R. (1998). *Social marketing: Making public health sense.* Paper presented at the annual meeting of the Utah Public Health Association, Provo, UT.

Neiger, B. L., & Thackeray, R. (2002). Application of the SMART Model in two successful social marketing campaigns. *American Journal of Health Education, 33,* 291–293.

Neiger, B. L., Thackeray, R., Merrill, R. M., Miner, K. M., Larsen, L., & Chalkley, C. M. (2001). The impact of social marketing on fruit and vegetable consumption and physical activity among public health employees at the Utah department of health. *Social Marketing Quarterly, 7,* 9–28.

Nelson, D. E., Brownson, R. C., Remington, P.L., & Parvanta, C. (Eds.). (2002). *Communicating public health information effectively: A guide for practitioners.* Washington, DC: American Public Health Association.

Net.MBA. (2002–2007). *CPM-critical path method.* Retrieved June 12, 2007, from http://www.netmba.com/operations/project/cpm/

Newcomer, K. E., & Wirtz, P. W. (2004). Using statistics in evaluation. In J. S. Wholey, H. P. Hatry, & K. E. Newcomer (Eds.). *Handbook of practical program evaluation* (2nd ed., pp. 439–478). San Francisco, CA: Jossey-Bass.

Norwood, S. L. (2000). *Research strategies for advanced practice nurses.* Upper Saddle River, NJ: Prentice-Hall, Inc.

Novelli, W. D. (1988). Marketing health and social issues: What works? In R. Dunmire (Ed.), *Social marketing: Accepting the challenge in public health.* Atlanta, GA: Centers for Disease Control.

Nutbeam, D., & Harris, E. (1999). *Theory in a nutshell: A guide to health promotion theory.* Sydney, Australia: The McGraw-Hill Companies, Inc.

Nye, R. D. (1979). *What is B. F. Skinner really saying?* Englewood Cliffs, NJ: Prentice-Hall.

Nye, R. D. (1992). *The legacy of B. F. Skinner: Concepts and perspectives, controversies, and misunderstandings.* Pacific Grove, CA: Brooks/Cole.

O'Donnell, M. P. (1996). Editor's notes. *American Journal of Health Promotion, 10*(4), 244.

Office of Minority Health (OMH). (2001). National standards on culturally and linguistically appropriate services (CLAS). Retrieved June 8, 2007, from http://www.omhrc.gov/templates/browse.aspx?lvl=2&lvlID=15

Ogbu, J. (1987). Cultural influences on plasticity in human development. In J. L. Gallagher & C. T.

Ramey (Eds.), *The malleability of children* (pp. 155–169). Baltimore, MD: Paul H. Brookes.

Ornstein, A. C., & Hunkins, F. P. (1998). *Curriculum: Foundations, principals, and issues* (3rd ed.). Boston, MA: Allyn & Bacon.

Pahnos, M. L. (1992). The continuing challenge of multicultural health education. *Journal of School Health, 62*(1), 24–26.

Parcel, G. S. (1983). Theoretical models for application in school health education research. *Health Education, 15*(4), 39–49.

Parcel, G. S. (1995). Diffusion research: The smart choices project. *Health Education Research: Theory and Practice, 10*(3), 279–281.

Parcel, G. S., & Baranowski, T. (1981). Social learning theory and health education. *Health Education, 12*(3), 14–18.

Parkinson, R. S., & Associates. (1982). *Managing health promotion in the workplace: Guidelines for implementation and evaluation.* Palo Alto, CA: Mayfield.

Pasick, R. J., D'Onofrio, C. N., & Otero-Sabogal, R. (1996). Similarities and differences across cultures: Questions to inform a third generation for health promotion research. *Health Education, 23* (Suppl.), S142–S161.

Patton, M. Q. (1988). *How to use qualitative methods in evaluation.* Newbury Park, CA: Sage.

Patton, R. P., Corry, J. M., Gettman, L. R., & Graff, J. S. (1986). *Implementing health/fitness programs.* Champaign, IL: Human Kinetics.

Pavlov, I. (1927). *Conditional reflexes.* Oxford: Oxford University Press.

Pealer, L. N., & Dorman, S. M. (1997). Evaluating health-related web sites. *Journal of School Health, 67*(1), 232–235.

Pellmar, T. C., Brandt, Jr., E. N., & Baird, M. (2002). Health and behavior: The interplay of biological, behavioral, and social influences: Summary of an Institute of Medicine Report. *American Journal of Health Promotion, 16*(4), 206–219.

Penner, M. (1989). Economic incentives to reduce employee smoking: A health insurance surcharge for tobacco using state of Kansas employees. *American Journal of Health Promotion, 4*(1), 5–11.

Perlman, J. (1978). Grassroots participation from neighborhood to nation. In S. Langton (Ed.), *Citizen participation in America* (pp. 65–79). Lexington, MA: Lexington Books.

Pescatello, L. S., Murphy, D., Vollono, J., Lynch, E., Bernene, J., & Costanzo, D. (2001). The cardiovascular health impact of an incentive worksite health promotion program. *American Journal of Health Promotion, 16*(1), 16–20.

Petersen, D. J., & Alexander, G. R. (2001). *Needs assessment in public health: A practical guide for students and professionals.* New York, NY: Kluwer Academic/Plenum Publishers.

Petty, R. E., Barden, J., & Wheeler, S. C. (2002). The elaboration likelihood model of persuasion. In R. J. DiClemente, R. A. Crosby, & M. C. Kegler (Eds.), *Emerging theories in health promotion practice and research: Strategies for improving public health.* (pp.71–99). San Francisco, CA: Jossey-Bass.

Petty, R. E., Wheeler, S. C., & Bizer, G. Y. (1999). Is there one persuasion process or more? Lumping versus splitting in attitude change theories. *Psychology Inquiry, 10,* 156–163.

Pickett, G. E., & Hanlon, J. J. (1990). *Public health: Administration and practice.* St. Louis: Mosby-Year Book, Inc.

Piniat, A. J. (1984). How to put spirit in an incentive program. *National Safety News,* (January), 46–49.

Pollock, M. L., Foster, C., Salisburg, R., & Smith, R. (1982). Effects of a YMCA starter fitness program. *The Physician and Sportsmedicine, 10*(1), 89–91, 95–99, 120.

Poole, K., Kumpfer, K., & Pett, M. (2001). The impact of an incentive-based worksite health promotion program on modifiable health risk factors. *American Journal of Health Promotion, 16*(1), 21–26.

Powell, D. R., & Frank, E. (2002).The future of workplace health promotion. In M. P. O'Donnell (Ed.). *Health promotion in the workplace* (3rd ed., pp. 590–603). Albany, NY: Delmar.

Price, J. H., Telljohann, S. K., Roberts, S. M., & Smit, D. (1992). Effects of incentives in an inner city junior high school smoking prevention program. *Journal of Health Education, 23*(7), 388–396.

Prochaska, J. (2005). Stages of change, readiness, and motivation. In J. Kerr, R. Weitkunat, & M. Moretti (Eds.), *ABC of behavior change: A guide to successful disease prevention and health promotion,* pp. 111–123. Edinburgh: Elsevier.

Prochaska, J. O. (1979). *Systems of psychotherapy: A transtheoretical analysis*. Homewood, IL: Dorsey Press.

Prochaska, J. O., DiClemente, C. C., & Norcross, J. C. (1992). In search of how people change: Applications to addictive behaviors. *American Psychologist, 47*(9), 1102–1114.

Prochaska, J. O., Johnson, S., & Lee, P. (1998). The transtheoretical model of behavior change. In S. A. Shumaker, E. B. Schron, J.K. Ockene, & W. L. McBee (Eds.), *The handbook of health behavior change* (2nd ed., pp. 59–84). New York: Springer.

Prochaska, J. O., Norcross, J. C., Fowler, & J. L., Follick, M. J., & Abrams, D. B. (1992). Attendance and outcome in a worksite weight control program: Processes and stages of change as process and predictor variables. *Addictive Behaviors, 17*, 35–45.

Prochaska, J. O., Redding, C. A., Harlow, L. L., Rossi, J. S., & Velicer, W. F. (1994). The transtheoretical model of change and HIV prevention: A review. *Health Education Quarterly, 21*(4), 471–486.

Prochaska, J. O., Reeding, C. A., & Evers, K. E. (2002). The transtheoretical model and stages of change. In K. Glanz, B. K. Rimer, & R. M. Lewis (Eds.), *Health behavior and health education: Theory, research, and practice* (3rd. ed, pp. 99–120). San Francisco, CA: Jossey-Bass.

Rakich, J. S., Longest, B. B., & O'Donovan, T. R. (1977). *Managing health care organizations*. Philadelphia: W. B. Saunders.

Ramaprasad, J. (2005). Warning signals, wind speeds and what next: a pilot project for disaster preparedness among residents of central Vietnam's lagoons. *Social Marketing Quarterly, 11*(2), 41–53.

Redding, C. A., Rossi, J. S., Rossi, S. R., Velicer, W. F., & Prochaska, J. O. (1999). Health behavior models. In G. C. Hyner, K. W. Peterson, J. W. Travis, J. E. Dewey, J. J. Foerster, & E. M. Framer (Eds.), *SPM handbook of health assessment tools* (pp. 83–93). Pittsburgh, PA: The Society of Prospective Medicine.

Rice, R. E., & Atkin, C. K. (1989). Trends in communication campaign research. In R.E. Rice & C. K. Atkin (Eds.), *Public communication campaigns* (2nd ed.). Newbury Park, CA: Sage.

Rich, R. F., & Sugrue, N. M. (1989). Health promotion, disease prevention, and public policy.

Wellness Perspectives: Research, Theory and Practice, 6(1), 27–35.

Riedel, J. E. (1999). The cost-effectiveness of health promotion. In G. C. Hyner, K. W. Peterson, J. W. Travis, J. E. Dewey, J. J. Foerster, & E. M. Framer (Eds.), *SPM handbook of health assessment tools* (pp. 111–118). Pittsburgh, PA: The Society of Prospective Medicine.

Rimer, B. K., & Glanz, K. (2005). *Theory at a glance: A guide for health promotion practice* (2nd ed.). [NIH Pub. No. 05–3896]. Washington, DC: National Cancer Institute.

Riner, M. E., Cunningham, C. & Johnson, A. (2004). Public health education and practice using geographic information system technology. *Public Health Nursing, 21*(1), 57–65.

Robbins, L. C., & Hall, J. H. (1970). *How to practice prospective medicine*. Indianapolis, IN: Methodist Hospital of Indiana.

Robison, J. (1998). To reward?. . . or not to reward?: Questioning the wisdom of using external reinforcement on health promotion programs. *American Journal of Health Promotion, 13*(1), 1–3.

Rogers, E. M. (1962). *Diffusion of innovations*. New York: Free Press of Glencoe.

Rogers, E. M. (1983). *Diffusion of innovations* (3rd ed.). New York: Free Press.

Rogers, E. M. (2002). Diffusion of prevention innovations. *Addictive Behaviors, 6*, 989–993.

Rogers, E. M. (2003). *Diffusion of innovations* (5th ed.). New York, NY: Free Press.

Romer, D., & Kim, S. (1995). Health interventions for African American and Latino youth: The potential role of mass media. *Health Education Quarterly, 22*(2), 172–189.

Rosenstock, I. M. (1966). Why people use health services. *Milbank Memorial Fund Quarterly, 44*, 94–124.

Rosenstock, I. M., Strecher, V. J., & Becker, M.H. (1988). Social learning theory and the health belief model. *Health Education Quarterly, 15*(2), 175–183.

Ross, H. S., & Mico, P. R. (1980). *Theory and practice in health education*. Palo Alto, CA: Mayfield.

Ross, M. G. (1967). *Community organization: Theory, principles, and practice*. New York: Harper & Row.

Rothman, J., & Tropman, J. E. (1987). Models of community organization and macro practice perspectives: Their mixing and phasing. In F. M. Cox, J. L. Erlich, J. Rothman, & J. E. Tropman (Eds.), *Strategies of community organization: Macro practice* (pp. 3–26). Itasca, IL: F. E. Peacock.

Rotter, J. B. (1954). *Social learning and clinical psychology.* New York: Prentice-Hall.

Rubin, H. J., & Rubin, I. S. (1992). *Community organizing and development* (2nd ed.). New York: Macmillan.

Ruof, J., Mittendorf, T., Pirk, O., & von der Schulenberg, J. M. (2002). Diffusion of innovations: Treatment of Alzheimer's disease in Germany. *Health Policy, 1,* 59–66.

Saunders, R. P., Evans, M. H., & Joshi, P. (2005). Developing a process-evaluation plan for assessing health promotion program implementation: A how-to guide. *Health Promotion Practice, 6*(2), 134–147.

Schechter, C., Vanchieri, C., & Crofton, C. (1990). Evaluating women's attitudes and perceptions in developing mammography promotion messages. *Public Health Reports, 105*(3), 253–257.

Schmid, T. L., Pratt, M., & Howze, E. (1995). Policy as intervention: Environmental and policy approaches to the prevention of cardiovascular disease. *American Journal of Public Health, 85,* 1207–1211.

Schwarzer, R. (2001). Social-cognitive factors in changing health-related behaviors. *Current Directions in Psychological Science, 10,* 47–51.

Selig, S., Tropiano, E., & Greene-Moton, E. (2006). Teaching cultural competence to reduce health disparities. *Health Promotion Practice, 7*(3), 247S–255S.

Shea, S., & Basch, C. E. (1990). A review of five major community-based cardiovascular disease prevention programs: Part I, rationale, design and theoretical framework. *American Journal of Health Promotion, 4*(3), 203–213.

Shepard, M. (1985). Motivation: The key to fitness compliance. *The Physician and Sportsmedicine, 13*(7), 88–101.

Sherrill, W. W., Crew, L., Mayo, R. M., Mayo, W. F., Rogers, B. L., & Haynes, D. F. (2005). Educational and health services innovation to - improve care for rural Hispanic communities in the US. *Education for Health, 18*(3), 356–367.

Shim, J. K., & Siegel, J. G. (1994). *Complete budgeting workbook and guide.* New York: New York Institute of Finance.

Silberg, W. M., Lundberg, G. D., & Musacchio, R. A. (1997). Assessing, controlling, and assuring the quality of medical information on the Internet. *Journal of the American Medical Association, 277,* 1244–1245.

Simkin, L. R., & Gross, A. M. (1994). Assessment of coping with high-risk situations for exercise relapse among healthy women. *Health Psychology, 13,* 274–277.

Simmons, R. (1998). Quitting by phone. *Health Education & Behavior, 25*(6), 686–687.

Simons-Morton, B. G., Greene, W. H., & Gottlieb, N. H. (1995). *Introduction to health education and health promotion* (2nd ed.). Prospect Heights, IL: Waveland Press.

Simons-Morton, D. G., Simons-Morton, B. G., Parcel, G. S., & Bunker, J. F. (1988). Influencing personal and environmental conditions for community health: A multilevel intervention model. *Family and Community Health, 11*(2), 25–35.

Skinner, B. F. (1953). *Science and human behavior.* New York: Free Press.

Skinner, C. S., Strecher, V. J., & Hospers, H. (1994). Physicians' recommendations for mammography; Do tailored messages make a difference? *American Journal of Public Health, 84*(1), 43–49.

Slater, M. D., Kelly, K. J., & Thackeray, R. (2006). Segmentation on a Shoestring: Health Audience Segmentation in Limited-Budget and Local Social Marketing Interventions. *Health Promotion Practice, 7,* 170–173

Snow, L. (2001). *The organization of hope: A workbook for rural asset-based community development.* Evanston, IL: Institute for Policy Research, Northwestern University.

Soet, J. E., & Basch, C. E. (1997). The telephone as a communication medium for health education. *Health Education & Behavior, 24*(6), 759–772.

Solomon, D. D. (1987). Evaluating community programs. In F. M. Cox, J. L. Erlich, J. Rolhman, & J. E. Tropman (Eds.), *Strategies of community organization: Macro practices* (pp. 366–368). Itasca, IL: F. E. Peacock.

Sorensen, G., Rigotti, N., Rosen, A., Pinney, J., & Prible, R. (1991). Effects of a worksite nonsmoking policy: Evidence for increased cessation. *American Journal of Public Health, 81*(2), 202–204.

Speers, M. (1992). Preface. *Journal of Health Education, 23*(3), 132–133.

Spencer, L., Adams, T. B., Malone, S., Roy, L., & Yost, E. (2006). Applying the transtheoretical model to exercise: A systematic and comprehensive review of the literature. *Health Promotion Practice, 7*(4), 428–443.

SPM Board of Directors (SPMBoD). (1999). Ethics guidelines for the development and use of health assessments. In G. C. Hyner, K. W. Peterson, J. W. Travis, J. E. Dewey, J.J. Foerster, & E. M. Framer (Eds.), *SPM handbook of health assessment tools* (p. xxiii). Pittsburgh, PA: The Society of Prospective Medicine.

Springett, J. (2003). Issues in participatory evaluation. In M. Minkler & N. Wallerstein (Eds.), *Community-based participatory research for health* (pp. 263–288). San Francisco, CA: Jossey-Bass.

Stacy, R. D. (1987). Instrument evaluation guides for survey research in health education and health promotion. *Health Education, 18*(5), 65–67.

Staten, L. K., Birnbaum, A. S., Jobe, J. B., & Elder, J. P. (2006). A Typology of Middle School Girls: Audience Segmentation Related to Physical Activity. *Health Education Behavior, 33*(1), 66–80.

Steckler, A., Goodman, R. M., McLeroy, K. R., Davis, S., & Koch, G. (1992). Measuring the diffusion of innovative health promotion programs. *American Journal of Health Promotion, 6*(3), 214–224.

Steckler, A., & Linnan, L. (Eds.). (2002). *Process evaluation for public health interventions and research*. San Francisco, CA: Jossey-Bass.

Steckler, A., McLeroy, K. R., Goodman, R. M., Bird, S. T., & McCormick, L. (1992). Toward integrating qualitative and quantitative methods: An introduction. *Health Education Quarterly, 19*(1), 1–8.

Strecher, V. J., DeVellis, B. M., Becker, M. H., & Rosenstock, I. M. (1986). The role of self-efficacy in achieving health behavior change. *Health Education Quarterly, 13*(1), 73–91.

Strecher, V. J., Kreuter, M. W., Den Boer, D. J., Kobrin, S., Hospers, H. J., & Skinner, C. S. (1994). The effects of computer-tailored smoking cessation messages in family practice. *Journal of Family Practice, 39*(3), 262–270.

Strecher, V. J., & Rosenstock, I. M. (1997). The health belief model. In K. Glanz, F. M. Lewis, & B. K. Rimer (Eds.), *Health behavior and health education: Theory, research, and practice* (pp. 41–59). San Francisco: Jossey-Bass.

Strycker, L. A., Foster, L. S., Pettigrew, L., Donnelly-Perry, J., Jordan, S., & Glasgow, R. E. (1997). Steering committee enhancements on health promotion program delivery. *American Journal of Health Promotion, 11*(6), 437–440.

Stunkard, A. J., & Braunwell, K. D. (1980). Worksite treatment for obesity. *American Journal of Psychiatry, 137,* 252–253.

Suggs, L. S. (2006). A 10–year retrospective on research in new technologies for health communication. *Journal of Health Communication, 11*(1), 61–74.

Sullivan, D. (1973). Model for comprehensive, systematic program development in health education. *Health Education Report, 1*(1) (November-December), 4–5.

Svenkerud, P. J., & Singhal, A. (1998). Enhancing the effectiveness of HIV/AIDS prevention programs targeted to unique population groups in Thailand: Lessons learned from applying concepts of diffusion of innovation and social marketing. *Journal of Health Communication, 3,* 193–216.

Syre, T. R., & Wilson, R. W. (1990). Health care marketing: Role evolution of the community health educator. *Health Education, 21*(1), 6–8.

Taylor, S. M., Elliott, S., & Riley, B. (1998). Heart health promotion: predisposition, capacity and implementation in Ontario public health units, 1994–1996. *Canadian Journal of Public Health, 6,* 410–414.

TechTarget. (2007). *Gantt chart*. Retrieved June 9, 2007, from http://searchsoftwarequality.techtarget.com/sDefinition/0,,sid92_gci331397,00.html

TechTarget. (2007a). *PERT chart*. Retrieved June 9, 2007, from http://searchsoftwarequality.techtarget.com/sDefinition/0,,sid92_gci331391,00.html

Thorndike, E. L. (1898). Animal intelligence: An experimental study of the associative processes in animals. *Psychological Monographs, 2*(8).

Tillman, H. N. (1997). Evaluating quality on the web [Online]. Available: http://tiac.net/users/hope/findqual.html

Timmreck, T. C. (1997). *Health services cyclopedic dictionary* (3rd. ed.). Boston, MA: Jones and Bartlett Publishers.

Timmreck, T. C. (2003). *Planning, program development, and evaluation* (2nd ed.). Boston, MA: Jones and Bartlett Publishers.

Torabi, M. R. (1994). Reliability methods and numbers of items in development of health instruments. *Health Values, 18*(6), 56–59.

Toufexis, A. (1985). Giving goodies to the good. *Time* (November 18), 98.

Truman, B. I., Smith-Akin, C. K., Hinman A. R., Gebbie, K. M., Brownson, R., Novick, L. F., Lawrence, R. S., Pappaioanou, M., Fielding, J., Evans, C. A., Guerra, F. A., Vogel-Taylor, M., Mahan, C. S., Fullilove, M., & Zaza, S. (2000). Developing the Guide to Community Preventive Services—overview and rationale. The Task Force on Community Preventive Services. *American Journal of Preventive Medicine, 18*(1 Suppl) 18–60.

Turnock, B. J. (2004). *Public health: What is it and how it works* (3rd ed.). Sudbury, MA: Jones and Bartlett Publishers.

U.S. Census Bureau (USCB). (2006). *Americans marrying older, living alone more, see households shrinking, Census Bureau reports.* Retrieved May 25, 2007 from http://www.census.gov/Press-Release/www/releases/archives/families_households/

U.S. Department of Health and Human Services, Centers for Disease Control and Prevention. (no date). *Planned approach to community health: Guide for local coordinator.* Atlanta, GA: Author.

U.S. Department of Health and Human Services, Office of Disease Prevention and Health Promotion. (1997). *Developing objectives for healthy People 2010.* Washington, DC: U.S. Government Printing Office.

U.S. Department of Health and Human Services, Office of Substance Abuse Prevention. (1991). *The fact is. . . you can prepare easy-to-read materials.* Rockville, MD: Author.

U.S. Department of Health and Human Services. (1980). *Promoting health/preventing disease: Objectives for the nation.* Washington, DC: U.S. Government Printing Office.

U.S. Department of Health and Human Services. (1986b). *The 1990 health objectives for the nation: A midcourse review.* Washington, DC: U.S. Government Printing Office.

U.S. Department of Health and Human Services. (1989). *Making health communication programs work: A planner's guide* (NIH Publication No. 89–1493). Washington, DC: U.S. Government Printing Office.

U.S. Department of Health and Human Services. (1990a). *Healthy People 2000: National health promotion disease prevention objectives* (DHHS Publication No. [PHS] 90–50212). Washington, DC: U.S. Government Printing Office.

U.S. Department of Health and Human Services. (1994). *Healthy People 2000 Review, 1993* (DHHS Publication No. [PHS] 94–1232–1). Washington, DC: U.S. Government Printing Office.

U.S. Department of Health and Human Services. (1995). *Healthy People 2000: Midourse review and 1995 revisions.* Washington, DC: U.S. Government Printing Office.

U.S. Department of Health and Human Services. (2001a). *Healthy people in healthy communities: A community planning guide using healthy people 2010.* Washington, DC: Author.

U.S. Department of Health and Human Services. (2001b). *Healthy workforce 2010: An essential health promotion sourcebook for employees, large and small.* Retrieved April 21, 2007, from http://www.prevent.org/images/stories/Files/publications/Healthy_Workforce_2010.pdf

U.S. Department of Health and Human Services. (2007b). *HP 2010 Midcourse Review: Appendix C: Technical Appendix.* Retrieved April 21, 2007, from http://www.healthypeople.gov/data/midcourse/default.html

U.S. Department of Health and Human Services. (2007d). *Office of Civil Rights—HIPAA.* Retrieved June 11, 2007, from: http://www.hhs.gov/ocr/hipaa/

U.S. Department of Health and Human Services. (2003). *Prevention Makes Common "Cents."* Retrieved March 24, 2007, from http://aspe.hhs.gov/health/prevention/

U.S. Department of Health and Human Services. (2000a). *Reducing Tobacco Use: A Report of the Surgeon General—Executive Summary.* Atlanta, GA: U.S. Department of Health and Human Services, Centers for Disease Control and Prevention, National Center for Chronic Disease Prevention and Health Promotion, Office on Smoking and Health.

U.S. Department of Health and Human Services. (2001c). *Youth violence: A report of the surgeon general.* Retrieved June 10, 2007, from http://www.surgeongeneral.gov/library/youthviolence/default.html

U.S. Department of Health and Human Services, Office of Civil Rights. (2006). *Medical privacy—National standards to protect the privacy of personal health information.* Retrieved April 6, 2007, from http://www.hhs.gov/ocr/hipaa/

U.S. Department of Health and Human Services. (2006). *Healthy People 2010: Midcourse Review Executive Summary.* Retrieved April 21, 2007, from http://www.healthypeople. gov/data/midcourse/html/introduction.html

U.S. Department of Health and Human Services. (2007a). *Healthy People.* Retrieved April 21, 2007, from http://www.healthypeople.gov/default.htm

U.S. Department of Health and Human Services. (2007c). *About GRANTS.GOV.* Retrieved June 8, 2007 from http://www.grants. gov/about-grants/about_grants_gov.jsp

U.S. Department of Labor. (2007). *Employment characteristics of families in 2006.* Retrieved May 25, 2007, from http://www.bls.gov/news.release/pdf/famee.pdf

U.S. Government Printing Office. (2004). *Federal Register: About.* Retrieved June 8, 2007, from http://www. gpoaccess.gov/fr/about.html

United Nations. (1955). *Social progress through community development.* New York, NY: Author.

University of Kansas. (2007). *Community Toolbox.* Retrieved March 20, 2007, from http://ctb.ku.edu/about/en

University of Wisconsin–Extension. (2002a). *Enhancing Program Performance with Logic models.* Retrieved February 25, 2006, from http://www.uwex.edu/ces/lmcourse)

University of Wisconsin–Extension. (2002b). *Logic Model.* Retrieved February 25, 2007, from www.uwex.edu/ces/pdande/evaluation/evallogicmodel.html

Valente, T. W. (2002). *Evaluating health promotion programs.* New York, NY: Oxford University Press.

van Ryn, M., & Heaney, C. A. (1992). What's the use of theory? *Health Education Quarterly, 19*(3), 315–330.

Venditto, G. (1997, January). Critic's choice: Six sites that rate the Web. *Internet World,* pp. 82–96.

Vogele, C. (2005). Education. In J. Kerr, R. Weikunat, & M. Moretti (Eds.), *ABC of behavior change: A guide to successful disease prevention and health promotion* (pp. 271–287). Edinburgh: Elsevier Churchill Livingstone.

Wagner, E. H., & Guild, P. A. (1989). Choosing an evaluation strategy. *American Journal of Health Promotion, 4*(2), 134–139.

Walker, R. A., & Bibeau, D. (1985/1986). Health education as freeing—Part II. *Health Education, 16*(6), (December/January), 4–8.

Wallerstein, N. (1994). Empowerment education applied to youth. In A. C. Matiella (Ed.), *The multicultural challenge in health education* (pp. 153–176). Santa Cruz, CA: ETR Associates.

Wallerstein, N., & Bernstein, E. (1988). Empowerment education: Freier's ideas adapted to health education. *Health Education Quarterly, 15*(4), 379–394.

Wallston, K. A. (1992). Hocus-pocus, the focus isn't strictly on locus: Rotter's social learning theory modified for health. *Cognitive Therapy and Research, 16,* 183–199.

Wallston, K. A. (1994). Theoretically based strategies for health behavior change. In M. P. O'Donnell, & J. S. Harris (Eds.), *Health promotion in the workplace* (2nd ed., pp. 185–203). Albany, NY: Delmar.

Wallston, K. A., Wallston, B. S., & DeVellis, R. (1978). Development of the multidimensional health locus of control (MHLC) scales. *Health Education Monographs, 6,* 160–170.

Walsh, D. C., Rudd, R. E., Moeykens, B. A., & Moloney, T. W. (1993). Social marketing for public health. *Health Affairs, 12,* 104–119.

Walter, C. L. (1997). Community building practice: A conceptual framework. In M. Minkler (Ed.), *Community organizing and community building for health* (pp. 68–83). New Brunswick, NJ: Rutgers University Press.

Wanderman, A., Goodman, R. M., & Butterfoss, F. D. (2005). Understanding coalitions and how they operate as organizations. In M. Minkler (Ed.). *Community organizing and community building for health* (2nd ed., pp. 292–313). New Brunswick, NJ: Rutgers University Press.

Wang, C. C. (2005). *Photovoice.* Retrieved April 1, 2007, from http://www.photovoice.com/index.html

Wang, C. C., & Burris, M. A. (1994). Empowerment through photovoice: Portraits of participation. *Health Education Quarterly, 21*(2), 171–186.

Wang, C. C., & Burris, M. A. (1997). Photovoice: Concept, methodology, and use for participatory needs assessment. *Health Education and Behavior, 24*(3), 369–387.

Warren, M. R. (1963). *The community in America.* Chicago, IL: Rand McNally.

Watson, J. B. (1925). *Behaviorism.* New York: W.W. Norton.

Watts, G. F., Donahue, R. E., Eddy J. M. & Wallace, E. V. (2001). Use of an ecological approach to worksite health promotion. *American Journal of Health Studies, 17*(3), 144–147.

Weinreich, N. K. (1999). *Hands-on social marketing: A step by step guide.* Thousand Oaks, CA: Sage Publications.

Weinstein, N. D. (1988). The precaution adoption process. *Health Psychology, 7,* 355–386.

Weinstein, N. D., & Rothman, A. J., & Sutton, S.R. (1998). Stage theories of health behavior: Conceptual and methodological issues. *Health Psychology, 17,* 290–299.

Weinstein, N. D., & Sandman, P. M. (1992). A model of the precaution adoption process: Evidence from home radon testing. *Health Psychology, 11,* 170–180.

Weinstein, N. D., & Sandman, P. M. (2002a). The precaution adoption process model. In K.Glanz, B. K. Rimer, & F. M. Lewis (Eds.), *Health behavior and health education: Theory, research, and practice* (3rd. ed., pp. 121–143). San Francisco, CA: Jossey-Bass.

Weinstein, N. D., & Sandman, P. M. (2002b). The precaution adoption process model and its application. In R. J. DiClemente, R.A. Crosby, & M. C. Kegler (Eds.), *Emerging theories in health promotion practice and research: Strategies for improving public health.* (pp. 16–39). San Francisco, CA: Jossey-Bass.

Weiss, C. H. (1984). Increasing the likelihood of influencing decisions. In L. Rutman (Ed.), *Evaluation research methods: A basic guide* (2nd ed., pp. 159–190). Beverly Hills, CA: Sage.

Weiss, C. H. (1998). *Evaluation* (2nd ed.). Upper Saddle River, NJ: Prentice-Hall.

Wilbur, C. (1983). Live for life—The Johnson & Johnson program. *Preventive Medicine, 12*(5), 672–681.

Wilcox, C. (2006). *Impact of a recognized diabetes education program with telephonic and letter follow-up on the glycosylated hemoglobin (HbA1c) levels and quality of life of patients with type II diabetes.* Unpublished master's thesis. Ball State University, Muncie, IN.

Williams, B., & Suen, H. (1998). Formal vs. informal assessment methods. *American Journal of Health Behavior, 22*(4), 308–313.

Williams, J. E., & Flora, J. A. (1995). Health behavior segmentation and campaign planning to reduce cardiovascular disease risk among Hispanics. *Health Education Quarterly, 22*(1), 36–38.

Wilson, M. G. (1990). Factors associated with, issues related to, and suggestions for increasing participation in workplace health promotion programs. *Health Values, 14*(4), 29–36.

Windsor, R., Clark, N., Boyd, N., & Goodman, R. M. (2004). *Evaluation of health promotion, health education, and disease prevention programs* (3rd ed.). Boston, MA: McGraw-Hill.

W. K. Kellogg Foundation. (2004). *Logic Model Development Guide.* Battle Creek, MI: Author.

Wolfe, R., Slack, T., & Rose-Hearn, T. (1993). Factors influencing the adoption and maintenance of Canadian, facility-based worksite health promotion programs. *American Journal of Health Promotion, 7*(3), 189–198.

Wong, F., Huhman, M., Heitzler, C., Asbury, L., Bretthauer-Mueller, R., McCarthy, S., & Londe, P. (2004). VERB™—A Social Marketing Campaign to Increase Physical Activity Among Youth. *Preventing Chronic Disease, 1*(3) 1–7.

Wright, P. A. (Ed.). (1994). *Technical assistance bulletin: A key step in developing prevention materials is to obtain expert and gatekeepers' reviews.* Bethesda, MD: Center for Substance Abuse Prevention (CASP) Communications Team.

Wurzbach, M. E. (Ed.). (2002). *Community health education and promotion: A guide to program design and evaluation* (2nd ed.). Gaithersburg, MD: Aspen Publishers, Inc.

Yamane, T. (1973). *Statistics: An introductory analysis* (3rd ed.). New York, NY: Harper & Row, Publishers.

Zara, S., Briss, P. A., & Harris, K. W. (Eds.). (2005). *Guide to community preventive services: What works to promote health.* New York, NY: Oxford University Press.

Name Index

AARP, 284

Academy for Educational Development, 313

Ad Hoc Work Group, American Public Health Association (APHA), 226, 232

Agency for Healthcare Research and Quality (AHRQ), 226

Airhihenbuwa, C. O., 7

Ajzen, I., 168, 169, 199

Albrecht, T. L., 41

Aldana, S. G., 63

Alexander, G., 91

Alinsky, S. D., 240

All About Marketing website, 313

Altschuld, J. W., 81

American Association of Health Education (AAHE), 6, 80, 120, 163

American Cancer Society (ACS), 158, 283
  Cancer Facts and Figures, 62
  smoking cessation program, 276

American College Health Association (ACHA), 155, 158

American College of Obstetricians and Gynecologists, 226

American College of Sports Medicine (ACSM), 226

American Evaluation Association (AEA),

American Heart Association (AHA), 158, 284
  Health advocacy page, 234

American Lung Association (ALA), 284

American Marketing Association, 287, 307, 313

American Public Health Association (APHA), 226

American Society for Quality (ASQ), 333

Anderson, B., 201

Andreason, A., 32, 293

Anspaugh, D. J., 81, 317, 319, 320

Arkin, E. B., 205

Assessment Protocol for Excellence in Public Health (APEX-PH), 46

Asset-Based Community Development (ABCD) Institute, 258

Asian Development Bank (ADB), 389

Association for Community Health Improvement, 57

Association of State and Territorial Health Officials (ASTHO), 77, 389

Association for Supervision and Curriculum Development (ASCD), 270

Auld, E., 217

Babbie, E., 128, 129, 131

Backer, T. E., 296

Bakker, A. B., 231

Bandura, A., 180, 184–186

Baranowski, T., 83, 185–186

Barnes, M. D., 215

Bartholemew, L. K., 50–51, 81, 203, 317

Bartlett, E. E., 226

Bartol, K. M., 47

Basch, C. E., 330

Bates, I. J., 10, 54

Becker, M. H., 171, 172, 224

Behrens, R., 60

Belch, G. E. and M. A., 301, 305

Bellicha, T., 203

Belmont Report: Ethical Principles and Guidelines for the Protection of Human Subjects in Research, 327, 333

Bensley, L. B., 221, 222, 309, 327, 327

Berkman, L. E., 224

Bertrand, J. T., 296

Berwick, D. M., 296

Bhatt, S., 304

Bioethicsline database, 97

Bloom, B. S., 116

Bloomquist, K., 222

Borg, W. R., 134

Borras, J. M., 296

Boslaugh, S. E., 290

Bowling, A., 83, 119, 122, 128

Brager, G., 245, 246, 254

Braithwaite, R. L., 244

Breckon, D. J., 11, 58, 319

Breslow, L., 2, 4

Brownson, R. C., 210

Bryant, C., 41

Burdine, J. N., 192–194

Burns, D. M., 308

Butterfoss, F. D., 247, 248

Campbell, M. K., 231

Canadian Evaluation Society (CES), 349

Cancer Prevention Resource Center (CPRC), University of Rhode Island, 198

Capwell, E. M., 341

Catalog of Federal Domestic Assistance (CFDA), 278, 285

Centers for Disease Control and Prevention (CDC), 2
  5 a Day website, 355
  CDCynergy, 141

Subject Index